# PRIMAL PANACEA

# PRIMAL
# PANACEA

by Thomas E. Levy, MD, JD

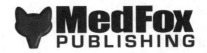

To order additional copies of this book, contact:
MedFox Publishing, LLC
1-866-359-5589
www.MedFoxPub.com
Orders@MedFoxPub.com
2505 Anthem Village Drive, Suite E-582
Henderson, NV 89052

# Foreword

## By Garry Gordon, MD

For years I have highly prized Dr. Tom Levy's significant scientific contributions regarding the miraculous healing powers of vitamin C. I have heavily relied upon and referenced his previous book, *Curing the Incurable: Vitamin C, Infectious Diseases and Toxins*, for many years in treating patients and teaching practitioners all over the world.

Through the extensive published literature compiled by Dr. Levy (with over 1,200 scientific references), many now know which forms and in what dosages vitamin C is most beneficial — proving that the accepted daily requirements of vitamin C are far too low for maintaining healthy cellular function and fighting off infections. Vitamin C in what appears to be mega doses of 5,000 to 20,000 milligrams or more orally – and 20 to 200 grams intravenously – can and has saved lives even after all else has failed.

This book comes at a time when our healthcare system is failing. We are losing our personal rights to choose the type of medical care we want. We are losing availability to quality hospitals and services, and we are losing doctors as they close down their practices because of oppressive governmental restrictions and legislation.

"Corruption is authority plus monopoly minus transparency." This anonymous quote describes the current functioning of our corporate controlled government today. We must not sit idly by thinking that the Obama healthcare bill, unconstitutionally forced into law against the people's will, is going to make things better. If it is not repealed, we will only experience more of the same and worse.

Currently we spend more on healthcare in this country than any other country in the world, yet we are getting fatter and sicker while taking more and more pharmaceutical drugs. Deadly drugs are mass marketed by corporations making trillions of dollars off sickness and suffering. Prescriptions are pushed and peddled through slick, happy commercials targeting every demographic, from infants to the elderly — and even the unborn.

How can one deny the legitimacy of a drug commercial showing a smiling and relaxed person – strolling along a beautiful beach at sunset, or enjoying a family gathering with loved ones — now happy and healthy because their "diagnosis" of depression, or heart disease, or cancer, or high cholesterol, or erectile dysfunction, has finally been cured with the newest wonder drug? These commercials also urge you to "ask your doctor" about said drug if you suspect you might have any of the symptoms or conditions described... and don't pay any attention to the dozens of ill effects listed quickly and quietly as a disclaimer at the end. If your trusted physician believes in it, and if it is approved by the FDA, then it must be the safest and the best course of treatment, right?

Wrong! It's all about money — and control. Most drugs only mask symptoms, ignoring the real underlying causes of disease, all the while generating new illnesses and conditions that will require another drug. The drug companies know this, and knowingly hide it from you.

Sadly, the *Wall Street Journal* reports that more than a quarter of U.S. kids and teens today are taking a prescription medication on a chronic basis, with nearly 7% of those on two or more drugs. Flu vaccines and antidepressants are being prescribed to pregnant women, with known adverse effects upon the fetus, resulting in long-term chronic conditions for the child later in life. And according to the CDC, half of all Americans take prescription drugs on a consistent basis; approximately one-third use two or more pharmaceutical drugs daily, and more than 10% of all Americans are frequently on five or more drugs at a time. In light of those statistics it should come as no surprise that the *Journal of The American Medical Association* (JAMA) has reported that fatal adverse drug reactions (FADR's) are now the leading cause of death in the U.S. today.

The unsavory relationship between government control, mainstream medicine, and the pharmaceutical industry has been uncovered by none other than Harvard Medical School's Dr. Marcia Angell, who is also the former Editor-in-Chief at the *New England Journal of Medicine*, one of the most respected medical journals on earth. An outspoken critic of the current U.S. healthcare system and the pharmaceutical industry, Dr. Angell is the author of the book, *The Truth About the Drug Companies: How They Deceive Us and What to Do About It*, and an excellent article in the *New York Review of Books* called "Drug Companies & Doctors: A Story of Corruption." Revealing the financially-driven corrupt ties between current healthcare practices in the U.S. and industry-backed clinical research, she wrote:

> "No one knows the total amount provided by drug companies to physicians, but I estimate from the annual reports of the top 9 U.S.-based drug companies that it comes to tens of billions of dollars a year in North America alone. By such means, the pharmaceutical industry has gained enormous control over how doctors evaluate and use its own products. Its extensive ties to physicians, particularly senior faculty at prestigious medical schools, affect the results of research, the way medicine is practiced, and even the definition of what constitutes a disease."

Mainstream medicine and the media, under the control of the FDA and their pharmaceutical company "clients," have done everything in their power to keep things like vitamin C and other natural, affordable forms of self-treatment from being routinely used as the first line of response to any health issue we encounter.

Why do they do this?

Because nutritional supplements are not patentable and so they aren't able to make trillions of dollars through proprietary ownership like they do with pharmaceutical drugs. That does not mean they aren't continually trying to find a way to control our healthcare options, pursuing control through propaganda, misinformation, and furtive legislation, all in the name of "public safety". In July of 2011 the FDA and Illinois Senator Dick Durbin (D) introduced yet another bill —the Dietary Supplement Labeling Act of 2011 (S.1310) — specifically designed to suffocate the nutritional supplement industry through ridiculous labeling and redundant notification requirements.

They do not want the public to know the unbelievable power that high doses of oral and intravenous vitamin C (taken orally in daily dosages of 4 to 20 or more grams a day and when needed, intravenously in doses of 30 to 200 or more grams a day) provide to help mankind deal with some of our most challenging chronic and acute health problems.

We must all learn what we can do to help ourselves deal with the myriad of healthcare problems we encounter, from minor accidents to the antibiotic resistant infections that kill over 100,000 each year. We must become fully informed of all options and fight the system for our inalienable right to choose natural remedies over conventional practices.

Dr. Levy shows us how to save lives. We need more champions like him, and champions like Ralph Fucetola, JD, known as "The Vitamin Lawyer," who has received numerous awards for his role in the 1995 DHEA Cases on behalf of the Life Extension Foundation, and brilliant Constitutional

Attorney Jonathan Emord, who has defeated the FDA in federal court a total of eight times so far on behalf of First Amendment rights and the rights of citizens' access to alternative and experimental therapies. Many "alternative" modalities can be incorporated into mainstream medicine by consumer demand – that will follow when the public becomes more informed about the numerous other life-saving modalities available.

For this latest and most welcome book, Dr. Tom Levy has accurately and rightfully chosen the powerful name "Primal Panacea." We are experiencing very challenging times on a toxic planet that is going through substantial magnetic and atmospheric earth changes — which are contributing to the epidemic of chronic degenerative diseases we are seeing today from heart disease, cancer, obesity, diabetes, et cetera. It takes an expert and driven proponent like him and others to inform the general public about all these amazingly effective, virtually non-toxic therapies that are all too frequently utilized in America only after all "standard" medical approaches have failed.

There is no question in my mind that vitamin C is truly as close to a cure-all that we have today. Every health problem will respond to treatment and recover better when patients are receiving adequate levels of vitamin C.

We need a revolution in medicine and Dr. Thomas E. Levy is undeniably one of the most important voices helping to guide us all towards true health and longevity.

# Preface

I was awestruck as I witnessed an event that forever changed the direction of my life and the way in which I would practice medicine. That day I watched a very ill patient with multiple sclerosis rapidly display a striking clinical improvement that just was not supposed to happen. Certainly, if I hadn't seen it with my own eyes, I would have said, "Impossible!" Although this event had been surrounded by many other similar, but not quite as dramatic observations, the patient's change was so striking and occurred so rapidly that it radically altered my understanding of physiology, disease, and medicine.

It happened in the summer of 1993 in Colorado Springs, Colorado. Up to that time, my private medical practice kept me totally occupied. Cardiology had been my specialty field of choice since my first year in medical school — with a sense of direction and determination not shared by most of my classmates. Even as a young lad I wanted to be a doctor. Throughout the rest of my medical training and for nearly all of the years of my private practice, I was completely happy with what I was doing. I felt I was making a very positive difference in the lives of my patients.

In about 1992 a slight twinge of dissatisfaction began to gnaw at me. Somehow, the practice of cardiology just seemed to fall short. Although I had no doubts that I had helped many patients achieve greater degrees of health, I still felt that something was missing. To the relatively few people in whom I confided, I expressed my disquieting sense that there was something more important that I should be doing, even though I had absolutely no idea what this new something was supposed to be.

About a year later I met Dr. Hal Huggins, a true medical pioneer who fully realized that many illnesses begin in the dental chair. Revered by many and perhaps reviled by even more, Dr. Huggins challenged many of the foundational, yet flawed practices of modern dentistry. He had concrete evidence that many standard dental procedures profoundly and negatively impact the general health of the body.

Dr. Huggins was truly one of the first healthcare practitioners I'd met who treated the entire patient. As a dentist, he did not practice medicine, but he did address much more than the dental problems of his patients. He and his team of assistants addressed issues of nutrition, diet, supplementation, and general lifestyle. When medical problems were encountered during examination and treatment, he made sure that his patients sought the care of qualified physicians.

At that time, Dr. Huggins had a large practice that specialized in the removal of dental toxins, including mercury fillings and chronically infected teeth. Although the idea of dental toxins was not a completely new idea to me, it was never much of a consideration when I evaluated and treated my cardiac patients. I never considered the possibility that previous dental treatments — especially endodontic treatments ("root canals") — were responsible for so much of the chest pain, blocked arteries, and heart attacks suffered by many of my patients.

Shortly after I met him, Dr. Huggins invited me to come by his clinic to see what he was doing. I went with an open mind, but I wasn't even remotely prepared for what I was about to see and experience.

I subsequently visited Dr. Huggins' clinic on several more occasions. Curiosity and amazement grew as I watched one patient after another respond in ways that radically challenged what my medical training had taught me to expect. A majority of his patients were extremely ill. Advanced cases of multiple sclerosis, amyotrophic lateral sclerosis (Lou Gehrig's disease), Parkinson's disease, and Alzheimer's disease were common. Many patients were already confined to wheelchairs. Certainly, I had never seen, or even heard of such patients showing significant clinical improvement — regardless of the protocol or intervention. Yet, in this clinic, substantial improvements were the rule. Only rarely did a patient fail to demonstrate any clear benefit after the typical two weeks of care.

All patients were tracked extensively with pre- and post-treatment laboratory testing. Abnormal blood and urine tests would routinely normalize or show near-normalization by the end of the two weeks in the clinic. Gout-like levels of uric acid would plummet, and abnormal liver and muscle enzymes would rapidly respond. The more I visited the clinic, the more the basic pillars of my medical education were shaken. Dr. Huggins consistently demonstrated a vastly greater knowledge of physiology and chemistry than any physician I had ever known, and the clinical responses of his patients consistently validated his methodology.

When all of this information finally sank in, I realized that a host of chronic degenerative diseases were not, in fact, irreversible sentences of suffering and premature death. I was an eyewitness to clear and consistent ways to treat nearly all such diseases and to expect positive results.

Although much of my medical understanding had already been challenged during my early visits to Dr. Huggins' clinic, it was soon to be changed to the core.

On that life-changing day, a very sick, listless patient was wheeled into the dental suite by her caregiver. This woman was just one of the many wheelchair-bound, advanced cases of multiple sclerosis that found their way into the clinic. She had a mouth X-ray that revealed a great deal of dental pathology, even to my relatively untrained eye. Many teeth were missing, a few dental implants and root canal-treated teeth were present, and the overall bone mass in the jaw appeared to be decreased. Despite her general state of poor health, she was subjected to several hours of dental surgery that day. There were extractions, cavitation revisions (the cleaning of infected holes in the jawbone), and the replacement of a few mercury amalgam fillings with bio-compatible composite materials.

At the time, I quietly thought this was far too much dental work for an initial visit to the dental chair by this very ill and obviously delicate patient. After all, I knew young, healthy friends who had several wisdom teeth removed by their dentists in one visit. Most often they became effectively bedridden for several days while their strength gradually returned and good healing kicked in.

But that was not the case with this patient. Almost immediately after the end of her dental surgery, she began smiling, joking a bit, proclaiming her energy was greatly improved, and even declaring she wanted to go "out on the town" that night with her caregiver and try to eat a steak with the few remaining good teeth she had on the left side of her mouth. I was flabbergasted, to say the least. Intuitively, I knew that getting toxins out of the body was a good thing, but this good and this quickly?

I confessed my confusion and disbelief to Dr. Huggins. He smiled and just pointed to the IV bag that was still infusing into the patient. This didn't seem like much of an answer, as I had administered thousands of IVs in my life and never witnessed such an impressive patient response. He then said that it was a vitamin C infusion.

Vitamin C? I was even more confused. Like everyone else on the planet, I knew that vitamin C was something good, but that it only got into the body from good food or supplements, and usually in amounts of no more than 50 to 250 milligrams at a time. However, this IV had 50 grams (50,000 milligrams) in it, and it had been infused for the entire duration of the dental work.

Although I had no idea why the vitamin C was helping this patient, I immediately knew that I had found a new weapon for my arsenal of treatment options. Even then, I had no real clue as to how powerful that new weapon was. But it marked the beginning of my second, and certainly most important, medical education. As I look back now, I realize my earlier training was little more than a reasonably good foundation for what I would learn after meeting Dr. Huggins. Ironically, a dentist taught me more about clinical medicine and physiology than all the medical doctors in my life combined.

As I continued to research the literature about vitamin C, I only became increasingly amazed. I found that vitamin C was vastly more than a vitamin required in tiny daily amounts to prevent the development of the deficiency disease scurvy. It is arguably the most important nutrient that we can ingest.

Contrary to the blindly repeated mantra of the mainstream medical community that "there are no studies," I discovered a wealth of information, much of it in the most accepted and respected medical journals. Study after study demonstrated vitamin C's ability to singularly eradicate, neutralize, or otherwise cure an incredibly large and diverse array of infectious diseases, especially viral diseases. Furthermore, there appeared to be no type of poisoning or toxin exposure that a high enough amount of properly administered vitamin C could not remedy.

In the 1940s Frederick Klenner, MD, pioneered the use of mega-gram intravenous doses of vitamin C to effectively treat and often cure many different infections. These included ones even now considered to be incurable, such as polio, tetanus, and encephalitis. He also led the way in demonstrating the ability of vitamin C to act as the ultimate antidote in reversing the toxicity of otherwise fatal doses of agents such as carbon monoxide, pesticides, barbiturates, and even heavy metals.

Other medical practitioners have followed since then, and those using the dosing regimens suggested by Dr. Klenner have seen similar results. My own direct experiences with vitamin C have been just as stunning from any reasonable clinical perspective. As a cardiologist, I have never had the opportunity to treat the many infections and toxin exposures that Dr. Klenner encountered. Nevertheless, I have successfully treated a number of conditions that modern medicine still approaches only with bed rest, supportive care, and the guarded optimism that the immune system may eventually prevail.

In two of only two cases of West Nile viral infection that I was asked to treat, both patients were completely well after only three days of vitamin C infusion therapy. Both of these individuals had been ill for months, and one had such extensive infection that his laboratory results showed he had developed hepatitis as well. Nevertheless, this resolved promptly and completely along with all of the other associated signs and symptoms. Similarly, two of two patients who presented with infectious mononucleosis responded just as dramatically after three days of intravenous vitamin C. Both were young, and one of the individuals had been so ill for months that he had already dropped out of college.

While visiting friends in Colombia, South America, I treated a 15 year-old girl with hemorrhagic Dengue fever. Intravenous vitamin C was not available so I used 10 grams of oral vitamin C in a special liposome-encapsulated form. This simple protocol completely cured her within three days.

Even Lyme disease has shown great response to vitamin C therapy. However, unlike many other infections treated with vitamin C, it is only acute Lyme disease that I have seen definitively cured after several days of intravenous vitamin C. Chronic Lyme disease, present for months to years, has consistently responded well to high doses of vitamin C, but without a definitive eradication or cure. Nevertheless, I have had numerous Lyme disease patients return to a sense of clinical normalcy on vitamin C therapy, even though the associated microbes might not be totally cleared from the body. With Lyme and other chronic infections such as AIDS and chronic hepatitis C, vitamin C can often restore the patient to a symptomless or near-symptomless state. This state can allow them to "coexist" indefinitely with their infections and even enjoy a normal lifespan.

Vitamin C is also the best way to maintain good health. Infections rarely have the opportunity to take hold when vitamin C levels are normal in the body. Similarly, most cancers begin when there are areas of increased oxidative stress in certain tissues, which is another way of saying that not enough vitamin C is present in those areas. As will be discussed in this book, it is also a deficiency of vitamin C in the inner lining of the coronary arteries ("focal scurvy") that provokes and allows the development of blockages leading to a heart attack.

Any doctor who has routinely administered 50- to 100-gram doses of vitamin C intravenously has had the opportunity to witness clinical responses that the bulk of the medical profession still regards as coincidental or just plain impossible.

In 2009 intravenous vitamin C cured a comatose swine flu patient who was literally at the point of being removed from life support. He had also been diagnosed with white-out pneumonia and "hairy cell" leukemia. This incredible story, entitled "Living Proof?" was documented and aired by New Zealand's version of *60 Minutes* in August 2010. The attending doctors had wanted to "pull the plug" that had been sustaining this patient's life for the prior month, but the family insisted that Klenner-sized doses of vitamin C be tried first. The clinical response was quick and stunning. Almost immediately, the patient's lungs began to clear and he recovered enough to be taken off life support. Within a few weeks, he walked out of the hospital. Furthermore, his leukemia appeared to have resolved along with the swine flu. Even with this miraculous turnaround and no other explanation, nearly all of the doctors reviewing the case concluded that his recovery was a coincidence — that his healing had nothing to do with the infusions of vitamin C.

After over 15 years of research and personal observation, I can categorically say that high-dose vitamin C is a clinical miracle when compared to all of our modern drugs. Furthermore, volumes of studies exist that say it works. It's one of the safest substances known to man — we have yet to discover a toxic dose for vitamin C, a bit of a miracle itself. Even when hundreds of grams have been administered within a few days, the only side effect is good health. Its cost is microscopic compared to the cost of most prescription drugs and therapies. Many of the diseases and conditions that vitamin C has been shown to cure remain "incurable" with conventional medications.

So why is there an almost universal refusal to consider the merits of high-dose vitamin C, or even to look at the evidence for it? I'll leave it to the reader to answer that question. But regardless of motive, this is inexcusable! Unless and until the public forces the medical profession to be the noble profession it pretends to be, nothing will change.

As you read this book and consider all the compelling scientific data that has been accummulated on vitamin C, ask yourself why such a therapy is not better known and more extensively used. The evidence unequivocally shows that mega-gram doses of vitamin C can prevent and cure a vast list of conditions that plague mankind. It is both inexpensive and completely safe. My conclusion: vitamin C is the "Primal Panacea." I trust you will agree.

Thomas E. Levy, MD, JD

# Table of Contents

Chapter Eight — High-Dose Vitamin C: Revolution Required

# Are profits more important than people?          110

Chapter Nine — High-Dose Vitamin C: How to Benefit

# Where do we go from here?          126

Special Resources

# FOR THOSE WHO WANT MORE SUBSTANTIATION

# RESOURCE A: How Vitamin C Works          139

# RESOURCE H: Published studies supporting the use of vitamin C in the treatment of infectious diseases and toxin exposures

## Chapter One

High-Dose Vitamin C: The Universal Antimicrobial

# Don't you dare say "CURE"

We "put cancer in remission," get heart disease, diabetes, and arthritis "under control"... but we don't really "cure" anything! Considering the trillions of dollars and decades of time already spent on pharmaceutical research, shouldn't there be a "cure" for man's most dreaded conditions?

Medical people **do not** use the word "cure" and those who are selling supplements **dare not** use it. Advertising language for supplements cannot use the word "cure" even when referring to a nutrient deficiency disease like scurvy (*a vitamin C deficiency*) or beriberi (*a vitamin B deficiency*). Even with overwhelming scientific evidence to show that a food or supplement can "cure," "prevent," or even help "treat" a disease, the FDA considers a reference to that evidence as a "drug claim." A food or supplement seller making such claims can be subject to the following:

- Search and/or seizure of bank accounts
- Search and/or seizure of all records
- Seizure of product
- Substantial fines
- Time in prison

On the other hand, drug companies don't ever promise a cure. One has to wonder whether they are even looking for one.

Consult the medical reference book found in the office of most MDs and you'll find there is "no effective treatment" for the majority, if not all, of viral infections. In layman's terms, the standard protocol for a viral infectious disease victim is: "make patient comfortable... hope (pray) patient's immune system prevails."

*How criminal... when one of the*
- Most studied
- Safest
- Least expensive
- Wildly effective

*antimicrobials has been available for decades!*

High-dose vitamin C has been proven to be a successful treatment — and in many cases it's a complete cure — for most viral and many bacterial infections. So why does it continue to be ignored?...ridiculed?...shunned?...penalized?

## Four Apparently "Untreatable" Deadly Conditions

Unfortunately, there are four deadly conditions that seem to be unaffected by high-dose vitamin C:
- Ignorance
- Cynicism
- Fear of being proven wrong
- Greed

Lest I be accused of overstating my point, I offer a recent example that was brought to light in two powerful New Zealand *60 Minutes* health documentaries that aired in 2010.

The first, called "Living Proof?", told the story of a New Zealand farmer who contracted an extremely severe case of H1N1. Medical tests confirmed the diagnosis of swine flu, white-out pneumonia, and hairy cell leukemia. His lungs were so filled with infection that he had to be hooked to a device — called ECMO — that bypasses and functions for the lungs outside the body. After nearly four weeks in an induced coma with aggressive medical intervention his condition was no better. The intensive care specialists met to consider Allan Smith's prognosis. Their conclusion was that "with his lung failure, Mr. Smith cannot survive." After a second meeting the same specialists wrote, "The group is in unanimous agreement that Mr. Smith should be removed from ECMO and be allowed to die. Continuing is only pro-longing his inevitable death."[1]

The family protested that the doctors hadn't tried everything. They vehemently lobbied for the administration of high-dose, intravenous vitamin C. Two days before Allan's scheduled removal from life support, the doctors consented to allow the vitamin C therapy even while stating, "We are all in agreement that vitamin C will be of no benefit."[1]

After only two 25-gram infusions of vitamin C, x-rays revealed a significant clearing of the lungs. The vitamin C therapy was continued at a rate of 100 grams per day. Within a few days, Allan had rapidly improved to the point where he could breathe on his own and he was removed from ECMO.

Then Allan's condition started to deteriorate. When questioned, the hospital admitted that the vitamin C had been discontinued. His family pushed for a resumption of the therapy. The doctors capitulated, but only continued at a meager two grams per day. The patient did start to improve again, but at a very slow rate. Why the doctors resumed vitamin C at a dose that was only two percent of the earlier beneficial dose defies logic if Mr. Smith's welfare was the only significant concern.

When Mr. Smith improved to the point he could be moved to a hospital closer to home, the new set of doctors again discontinued the C therapy. Predictably, Allan started to worsen. This time, the family had to hire an attorney to force a resumption of the C therapy. But, the new hospital would only administer two grams per day. Even so, the patient started to recover. As soon as Allan was able to swallow, his family fed him large doses of an oral liposome-encapsulated vitamin C. To the doctors' amazement, Allan walked out of the hospital several weeks before they thought it possible. Furthermore, there was no longer evidence of hairy cell leukemia.

Perhaps the most amazing part of this story is that those in the medical community with bedside seats to this amazing drama were unconvinced that vitamin C *had any part* in Allan Smith's return to health! One reviewing physician who refused to believe vitamin C had any positive effect in Allan Smith's recovery theorized that his turn-around could just as reasonably be attributed to the passing of a bus outside Allan's hospital room.[2]

In another H1N1 case covered by *60 Minutes*, a 25 year-old Australian woman was also put on an ECMO machine. Her brother, Mark, had seen the earlier segment, "Living Proof?" and decided to track down the Smith family to get more information about high-dose vitamin C. Convinced that the therapy might help his sister, Mark pushed the hospital to administer intravenous vitamin C. They finally relented. As in the Allan Smith case, her heavily-infected lungs started to clear with a couple of treatments. Finally, the patient improved to the point that the ECMO was discontinued. At the same time, after convincing the patient's mother that its continued administration could somehow be dangerous, the doctors discontinued the vitamin C. Her health rapidly deteriorated and within a few days she passed away.[2]

A majority of physicians blindly accept the false notion that there is "no evidence" and there are "no studies" showing the effectiveness of high-dose vitamin C in the treatment of anything but scurvy. The fact is, there are thousands of studies and much evidence! Yet, even when the proof mag-nificently displays itself — right before their eyes — most in the medical community refuse to see it.

The obvious reality did not escape the attention of the general population, however. These documentaries have created such a groundswell of outrage in New Zealand that the people are forcing a radical change in the way medicine is practiced there. Once the *60 Minutes* documentaries were put on the internet, people all over the world began to hear the truth. Coincidentally (or not), shortly after all this attention, the U.S. Food and Drug Administration (FDA) prevented the company in America that supplied the intra-venous vitamin C shown in both programs from producing any more. This draconian action transcends ignorance and cynicism. And more malicious restriction of high-dose vitamin C appears to be on the way *(see Chapter Eight)*.

Dr. Ian Brighthope, a nutritional and environmental medicine specialist familiar with the power of high-dose vitamin C, summarized it best in the *60 Minutes* docu-mentary: "People are dying because of the attitude of the medical profession."[2]

## *Some Medical "Treatments" are Downright Barbaric*

Since the discovery of penicillin many antibiotics have been added to the arsenal of chemical agents doctors deploy against bacterial infections. But, for a number of reasons, many strains of bacteria are totally unaffected by them. Even now, pharmaceutical companies are losing the race to develop antibiotics that are effective against increasingly drug-resistant bacteria.

In 2008, Dr. Kenneth Todar, bacteriologist, helped identify the enormity of this growing problem:

> "Nowadays, about 70 percent of the bac-
> teria that cause infections in hospitals
> are resistant to at least one of the drugs
> most commonly used for treatment. Some
> organisms are resistant to all approved
> antibiotics and can only be treated with
> experimental and potentially toxic drugs."[3]

So what happens in a traditional medical environment when a patient develops a raging, antibiotic-resistant infection? The answer depends on where the infection is. If it's in an organ — barring a miracle — the patient dies. But if the uncontrollable infection is isolated in a limb, there's a more effective therapy: AMPUTATION!

In most, if not all cases, this is unnecessary. The late Maureen Kennedy Salaman, President of the National Health Federation, tells of a frightening experience with her husband, Frank. During an attempt to bathe Sam, their pet cat, the feline became more than excited at the sound and feel of a hair dryer. Sam bit into the bone of her husband's right index finger. An emergency room doctor checked the bite, administered a tetanus shot, and prescribed an antibiotic.

During the next four days Frank's right hand swelled to twice its normal size, became discolored, and caused him intolerable pain that medication could not quell. Doctors at the emergency hospital were unanimous in their diagnosis: osteomyelitis (infection of the bone). In Maureen Salaman's words:

> "The bacteria had eaten away the bone,
> the joint, and the knuckle, and continued
> to travel down the hand. The laboratories
> were unable to identify the bacteria. Grim-
> faced doctors told me it would most proba-
> bly cost Frank his hand — and possibly his
> life. He was put on intravenous antibiotics

> around the clock. His hand was slashed open across the palm and down both sides of the finger to the bone and washed every two hours in an attempt to stop the raging infection."

> "I went before the hospital board to try to get vitamin C administered to him intra-venously. I was told that they were sure it was a good treatment, but they knew noth-ing about it, and they did not allow treat-ments of which they had no knowledge."[4]

After five weeks of this ineffective therapy, the Sal-amans were told there was only one way to save Frank's life: AMPUTATION! Through consultation with Robert Cathcart, MD, a vitamin C expert, they decided to leave the hospital and treat the infection with high-dose vitamin C. Doctors inside and outside the hospital counseled them that their decision would probably cost Frank his life. Nevertheless, in anticipation of things continuing to worsen, the surgical appointment for amputation was allowed to stand.

The Salamans drove from the hospital directly to a local clinic that routinely administered high-dose vitamin C. Immediately the doctors started an intravenous infusion of vitamin C, giving Frank 60 to 75 grams per day via this route. Frank was also taking 30 grams of oral vitamin C per day and packing a poultice of garlic and red clay on his hand each night.

Within *two* treatments the pain, which had been requiring two codeine tablets every four hours, stopped! After nine days of treatment, the infection and the swelling were totally gone. The deep open wounds from the surgery had healed with only hairline scars left as a reminder. Again, in Maureen Salaman's words:

"Frank kept his appointment for the planned amputation. With a broad smile, he held out a no longer misshapen or discolored right hand to shake the hand of a very shaken surgeon. "They had 'never seen this happen before'. 'One in a million,' they said."

"As I watched their shocked faces, a scripture verse came to mind: 'God has chosen the simple things of the world to confound the wise.'"[4]

Perhaps more alarming than the case just recounted is the pandemic of a related problem: sepsis. Commonly called "blood poisoning," sepsis occurs as a result of the body's inability to cope with a microbial infection as well as the toxins generated by the infection. Even though seven in ten adults have never heard of sepsis, it claims the lives of one American every 2.5 minutes. Other victims of sepsis are "saved" through amputation. Thousands of studies support the fact that high-dose vitamin C is a broad-spectrum antimicrobial *(Resource H)* and that it neutralizes all toxins *(Chapter Two and Resource H)*.

Every day high-dose vitamin C could be saving the lives of sepsis victims. Every day countless fingers, toes, hands, feet, arms, and legs could remain attached and healthy if the medical community would simply hear and respond to the facts with scientific integrity.

## *Vitamin C Can Cure Viral Infections*

Vitamin C has been shown to prevent, put into remission, and even cure many viral infections (*see Resource H for details*). Here's a partial listing:

- AIDS/HIV
- Ebola

- Encephalitis
- Hepatitis
- Herpes
- Pneumonia
- Polio
- Shingles
- Swine Flu

On the other hand, drug companies have yet to develop any drugs that will reliably kill viruses. Instead, vaccination is modern medicine's answer to viral infections. Without delving into the controversies surrounding vaccination, this strategy is not without significant health risks. In addition, many viruses, such as those causing influenza, can evolve into new strains that are unaffected by the antibodies that were developed in response to a previous vaccination. For example, this year's flu vaccination — which was created from last year's virus — may have little or no effect against the flu virus currently making the rounds.

Given the fact that modern medicine has no effective therapy for all viral and many bacterial infectious diseases, why aren't doctors turning to high-dose vitamin C to save the lives of their patients? For decades, men in places of influence have tried to keep the knowledge of high-dose vitamin C locked away. When that has not worked, they have tried to discredit it. Here's where it all started...

## Modern Medicine's Scorn for High-Dose Vitamin C: The Beginning

Most Americans under the age of 30 know little, if anything, about polio. Thankfully, it rarely occurs any longer in the United States. During the late 1940s and early 1950s, however, it rose to epidemic proportions. Many of the polio victims "fortunate" enough to survive the acute infection spent the remainder of their lives crippled. Polio devastated the lives of many patients and families.

Polio was one of the first viral diseases treated with high-dose vitamin C. The clinical results were awe-inspiring and the response of the medical community was totally dumbfounding!

On June 10, 1949, in Atlantic City, New Jersey, Frederick Klenner, MD, presented a summarization of his polio work at the Annual Session of the American Medical Association (AMA).[5,6] At that time he had cured **60** out of **60** cases of polio with high-dose injectable vitamin C. He made the following remarks:

> "It might be interesting to learn how poliomyelitis was treated in Reidsville, N.C., during the 1948 epidemic. In the past seven years, virus infections have been treated and cured in a period of 72 hours by the employment of massive frequent injections of ascorbic acid, or vitamin C. I believe that if vitamin C in these massive doses — **6,000** to **20,000mg** in a twenty-four hour period — is given to these patients with poliomyelitis none will be paralyzed and there will be no further maiming or epidemics of poliomyelitis."[6]
> [*Note: These doses were used on infants and small children, equating into doses well in excess of 100 grams daily for an adult.*]

Polio cured! 72 hours or less! Simple injections of vitamin C! No further maiming! No more epidemics! Shockingly, there were no questions, no challenges, no suggestions to investigate the protocol... not even a question from those doctors in attendance! It is noteworthy to mention that a Dr. Jonas Salk and a Dr. Albert Sabin were well into their work to develop polio vaccines at this time. Eight years later, in 1957, when the polio epidemic was already over, Salk announced his injectable vaccine to the world. Thirteen years after Dr. Klenner reported his polio cure, Sabin licensed his oral polio vaccine (the sugar cube).

I can hardly describe the flood of emotions that came over me when I first came across Dr. Frederick Klenner's work with polio patients. The fact that the polio virus was so easily eradicated by vitamin C was not surprising. My own successful experiences in using high-dose vitamin C with a number of different medical conditions had already convinced me of its potent virus-killing abilities. What over-whelmed me now was the new realization that vitamin C had been shown to cure this disease BEFORE countless people had been killed or crippled by it. Even now my heart aches when I see the pictures of polio victims in iron lungs, wheelchairs, and leg braces... and then I get angry! If just a few in the medical community would have opened their eyes, it could have been much different.

This criminal negligence should cause the researchers, politicians, drug company executives, government officials, and physicians who have fought to keep vitamin C out of the mainstream to hang their heads in shame. Yet, in the words of the obnoxious TV infomercial announcer, "But wait, there's more!"

## Herpes Infections and High-Dose Vitamin C

In 1936 scientists published results of groundbreaking research establishing vitamin C as a potential treatment for herpes virus infections. Their research clearly proved that vitamin C is a powerful virus-killing agent — it kills every known herpes virus for which it has been tested upon contact, including the kind that causes shingles.[7] Additional testing confirmed their findings the following year.[8] Still other studies have further validated the findings.[9,10]

Shingles, a type of herpes infection, develops from a reactivation of the chickenpox virus — often many years after the initial experience with chickenpox. The lesions that result from shingles are very painful and can persist for weeks. Over 50 years ago, a medical doctor was able to resolve shingles outbreaks with a daily combination of two to three grams of vitamin C via injection with another gram given orally.

Perhaps the most impressive study of high-dose vitamin C and shingles was published in 1950. The researcher reported a complete resolution in *327 out of 327* shingles patients treated with intravenous vitamin C — all within 72 hours from the start of treatment.[11]

What are the chances your doctor will recommend high-dose vitamin C if you were to walk into his office with a full-blown case of shingles? If your doctor is a traditionally trained MD, I can safely say there's no chance! Why? Because the use of high-dose vitamin C was conspicuously absent from his medical textbooks and continues to be absent to this day. In other words, he doesn't know!

### AIDS and High-Dose Vitamin C

Although at present there is insufficient evidence to make a strong curative claim for high-dose vitamin C in the treatment of AIDS, many vitamin C studies show positive results in treating this disease.

In 1990, Robert Cathcart, MD, reported his experience in the vitamin C treatment of over 250 HIV-positive patients, including ones with full-blown AIDS. In this article he noted that clinical improvement for any given patient seemed to be dependent on two major factors:

1) the amount of vitamin C given and

2) the level of illness at the beginning of treatment.

He asserted that any AIDS patient could be put into remission if enough vitamin C were taken to neutralize the toxicity produced by the virus and adequately treat any secondary infections.[12]

Basically, Dr. Cathcart routinely contained the HIV infection, allowing most of his patients to live out a normal lifespan in an asymptomatic state. Although not technically a cure, his patients peacefully coexisted with their infections.

## Vitamin C Can Also Prevent and Cure Non-Viral Infections

A considerable list of bacterial, parasitic, and other non-viral infections continues to plague mankind. Many respond poorly to antibiotics or do not respond at all.

Even here, vitamin C has been shown to prevent, speed recovery, and even cure many of these infections (*see Resource H for details*). Here's a partial listing:

- Diphtheria
- Dysentery
- Leprosy
- Malaria
- Pertussis
- Pneumonia
- Pseudomonas Infections
- Rheumatic Fever
- Staph Infections
- Strep Infections
- Tetanus
- Trichinosis
- Tuberculosis
- Typhoid Fever

Researchers report that all of these diseases create a deficiency of vitamin C in the host. This happens because all pathogens produce excessive oxidative stress, depleting available blood and tissue levels of vitamin C in the process. As has been reported for viral diseases like polio and encephalitis, when extremely large doses of vitamin C are used to combat the infection, immediate and curative results almost always ensue. And, even when small doses are employed, vitamin C will often noticeably improve the patient's condition. Remember Allan Smith's case, where his rate of improvement dramatically slowed when his doctors inexplicably dropped his daily vitamin C from 50-100 grams to two grams. However, this will not always be the case. Often a complete clinical relapse will occur when vitamin C dosage is reduced too early and too drastically, allowing viral or microbe titers to rebound.

Furthermore, it is clear that a certain blood concentration or tissue saturation of vitamin C is always needed before a positive clinical response can be observed. So, when tiny doses have been tested against many different infections, researchers often report that vitamin C had no positive clinical effect. Many seemingly unethical studies appear to have employed this fact to discredit vitamin C's efficacy by purposely testing with very small amounts. The researchers then conclude that vitamin C was of no value at all, rather than just ineffective at a tiny dose.

## Conclusion

### Consider the facts:

- Traditional methods of preventing and treating many infectious diseases are woefully inadequate
- Pathogens always deplete vitamin C levels in the body *(see Resource H)*

- Even when insufficient doses of vitamin C are used, the outcomes of many infectious diseases have been greatly improved
- When high-dose vitamin C is employed, "incurable" infectious diseases are routinely cured (e.g. polio and viral encephalitis)
- Vitamin C fuels and empowers the immune system in many different ways *(see Resource B)*
- Unlike antibiotics and vaccinations, vitamin C has no unhealthy side effects *(see Chapter Seven)*
- Vitamin C has no known toxicity *(see Chapter Seven)*

The argument for employing high-dose vitamin C in the treatment of infectious disease is overwhelming when the evidence is actually reviewed rather than arbitrarily dismissed as simplistic or unbelievable. A thorough review of Resource H will make an even more compelling case. And yet the traditional medical community flat-out refuses to use vitamin C. Some researchers and clinicians claim there is a purposeful "stonewalling"[13] against this natural substance. Why? I must leave that to the reader to determine. But, unless the public collectively demands the incorporation of high-dose vitamin C into the routine practice of medicine, we will all be saddled with vastly more expensive, less efficacious, and decidedly toxic drugs and therapies.

As Dr. Klenner said, "Ascorbic acid [vitamin C] is the safest and the most valuable substance available to the physician. Many headaches and many heartaches will be avoided with its proper use."[14]

Finally, if high-dose vitamin C were only efficacious for the prevention and treatment of infectious disease, that alone should be sufficient to recommend its universal use in the practice of medicine and as an essential supplement for the population at large. But vitamin C's value extends far beyond its unequalled antimicrobial properties, as you'll soon see...

## Chapter Two

# "9-1-1, HELP! My 10 month-old just swallowed some..."

In 2009, unintentional poisoning sent over 700,000 people to the hospital. Any emergency is stressful, but few are as terrifying as finding a child lying listless beside a cabinet filled with open, overturned containers. The poison must be identified, the amount swallowed needs to be determined, and quite possibly the CDC's Poison Control number needs to be called. Poison-specific directions need to be closely followed, even though you might not be sure what was ingested, how much was ingested, or how long it's been since the poisoning occurred.

What if there was a safe, proven, inexpensive, and exceptionally potent antidote that could immediately begin to neutralize and reverse the damage regardless of the type of poison? And, what if the paramedics could administer this antitoxin — even while the CDC was called and the specifics of the poisoning reported?

***There is!***

A quick scan of Resource H will provide a sampling of studies that show high-dose vitamin C can quickly neutralize a vast array of toxins and venoms like:

- Drug overdoses *(examples: alcohol, barbiturates, amphetamines)*
- Dangerous chemicals *(examples: aromatic hydrocarbons, cyanides, arsenic, mercury, lead)*
- Lethal gases *(examples: carbon monoxide, fluorine)*
- Pesticides and herbicides
- Poisonous mushrooms
- Deadly spider bites and snakebites
- Radiation *(examples: UV sunlight, X-rays, CAT scans, nuclear accidents)*

Shouldn't it be available to every rescue squad and in every emergency room in the country?

***Unfortunately, it's not!***

In fact, to my knowledge, it's not available to **ANY** rescue squad or in **ANY** emergency room in the U.S. Why? Because most traditionally-trained medical professionals are completely ignorant about high-dose vitamin C!

This was not always true. In at least one emergency room... the one manned by Dr. Klenner in Reidsville, North Carolina from the mid-1950s to the early 1970s, this ultimate antidote was available. Here are but a few of the many cases he reported:

## Pesticide Exposure

Three young boys were heavily exposed to the pesticide spray of a crop-dusting airplane. The youngest boy, aged seven years, received little exposure because the other two boys shielded him. The oldest boy, aged 12 years, was given **10,000 mg** of vitamin C with a 50 cc syringe every eight hours. This child was discharged to his home on the second hospital day. The third child did not receive any vitamin C but only received "supportive care." He developed a chemical burn and dermatitis, and died on the fifth day of hospitalization.[1]

## Black Widow Spider Bite

In another case, a three-and-a-half year-old girl remembered "knocking a big black bug off her stomach" while playing during the day. She suddenly fell ill, with a loss of appetite and a "severe gripping pain" in her stomach. She had nausea almost immediately and began vomiting about six hours later. The vomiting continued intermittently throughout the night, and after 12 hours she developed a fever. Her mother noted redness around the child's navel. There was "considerable swelling and rigidity." Touching the area elicited severe pain. Over the next few hours the child's condition deteriorated dramatically. Her "speech became incoherent" as she became progressively "stuporous."

When Klenner first saw the little girl about 18 hours after the onset of symptoms, he was able to identify the "obvious" fang marks of the spider bite with a magnifying glass. Klenner noted that the child was non-responsive to his questions, nearly comatose, and had developed labored breathing. Her abdomen was described as "board-like."

After multiple administrations of much vitamin C, some by injection and more by mouth over a period of four days, the swelling subsided, her appetite returned, and the girl fully recovered. Klenner reported that he had successfully treated "eight proven cases of black widow bite" during his medical practice.[2]

## Barbiturate Overdose

Excess barbiturates in the body result in depression of the central nervous system, often resulting in death. Dr. Klenner reported dramatic success in reversing a serious barbiturate overdose with vitamin C. The patient's blood pressure had fallen to 60/0 — barely alive — when he arrived in the emergency room. Immediately Dr. Klenner administered *12,000 mg* of vitamin C with a syringe as quickly as the vein would allow, followed by a slower intravenous drip. Within just 10 minutes the patient's blood pressure was up to 100/60. The patient woke up three hours later and completely recovered, having received a total of *125,000 mg* of vitamin C over a 12-hour period![3]

In another case, a patient with a barbiturate overdose awoke after *42,000 mg* of vitamin C was "given by vein as fast as a 20 gauge needle could carry the flow." Ultimately this patient received *75,000 mg* of vitamin C intravenously and *30,000 mg* more by mouth over a 24-hour period.

Klenner asserted that the success of his vitamin C protocol "in no less than 15 cases of barbiturate poisoning" indicated that "no death should occur" in this condition. In discussing the dramatic effects of vitamin C on barbiturate poisoning (and carbon monoxide poisoning), he commented that "the results are so dramatic that it borders on malpractice to deny this therapy."[4]

Dr. Klenner's assertion that it "borders" on malpractice was much too kind. The scientifically proven efficacy of vitamin C in the treatment of severe toxin/poison exposure screams "criminal negligence" when such therapy is ignored. But the herd mentality of most physicians provides great comfort and legal security in the world of medical incompetence.

## Highland Moccasin Snake Bite

A four year-old girl received a "full strike" from a mature highland moccasin. She immediately complained of severe pain in her leg and was "already vomiting within twenty minutes after the bite." Dr. Klenner first gave her 4,000 mg of vitamin C intravenously. The child stopped crying within 30 minutes, took fluids by mouth, and even had occasion to laugh. She commented while sitting on the emergency room table, "Come on daddy, I'm all right now, let's go home." Because of a slight fever and persistent tenderness in the leg, Klenner gave her another 4,000 mg of vitamin C intravenously, and finally another 4,000 mg late in the day. No antibiotics and no antivenin were ever given. In Klenner's words, "38 hours after being bitten, she was completely normal."[5,6]

In contrast, Dr. Klenner reported on a 16 year-old girl who had been bitten by a moccasin and received only "accepted" medical treatment. Judging from the appearance of the fang marks, he calculated the moccasin was roughly the same size as the one that had bitten the little girl. This older patient did not receive any vitamin C but was given three doses of antivenin. Her arm swelled to four times the size of the opposite arm, and she required morphine for pain control. Ultimately, she required three weeks of hospitalization.[5]

Dr. Klenner used high-dose vitamin C to successfully treat cases of drug overdose and miscellaneous poisonings, as well as venomous bites, for nearly two decades. His case studies were consistently published in peer-reviewed medical journals. Like his results with polio, Dr. Klenner's many successes using vitamin C as an antitoxin were met with deafening silence.

But it's not just Klenner who has been ignored. Thousands of articles about the truly remarkable properties of vitamin C have been ignored as well, without any regard to their important relevance to modern medicine. Even worse, many supporters of "traditional" medicine consistently attack vitamin C — they not only belittle its value, but they also question the intelligence of anyone who would dare to promote its virtues. Unfortunately, this unforgivable and even malicious negligence means countless men, women, and children will continue to die needless, and often horribly painful, deaths.

## Mushroom Poisoning

Fatal poisoning often results when adventurous cooks fail to distinguish poisonous mushrooms from nonpoisonous varieties. *Amanita phalloides*, also known as the "death cap," is a species of mushroom that is especially toxic. Within 24 hours the toxins from this mushroom will often cause irreversible damage to the heart, liver, and kidneys. Ingestion of as little as one-quarter mushroom cap, approximately 2/3 of an ounce, usually results in death. Short-term survivors often suffer enough liver damage that they require a liver transplant to achieve long-term survival.

In the 1950s, a French physician by the name of Bastien developed a successful vitamin C treatment protocol for mushroom poisoning. The method consisted of giving intravenous vitamin C, along with a couple of antibiotics, for three days. By 1969 he had successfully treated 15 patients for poisoning. He was so convinced of the efficacy of his protocol that he publicly consumed what would have easily been a fatal dose of mushrooms (about 2.5 ounces) and then successfully treated his own poisoning. ***And, not just once, but twice!*** It should also be noted that there are no examples in the literature of an antibiotic effectively neutralizing a deadly toxin. Therefore, it is highly unlikely the two antibiotics Bastien used played any significant role in the recovery of the patients he treated. It's much more likely that vitamin C did the job alone.

For a time, Dr. Bastien's method became the treatment of choice at a number of medical centers in France. Then the protocol fell into obscurity until it was rediscovered in 1984, resurrected, published, and added to the dusty stacks of unread medical literature.[7] We'll never know how many mushroom-poisoning victims have left this world writhing in pain because emergency physicians were (and continue to be) ignorant of vitamin C . How wonderful it would be for this ultimate antidote to be available to all who may need it in the future.

Thankfully, however, statistics show that the vast majority of people will never be victims of an acute, potentially fatal, poisoning crisis. Fortunately, most of us will never experience a venomous snakebite, a barbiturate overdose, being sprayed with pesticide, eating a poisonous mushroom...

We all face a much different challenge: a very slow, minute-by-minute, microgram-by-microgram poisoning from an array of other sources.

## The Daily Need for the Ultimate Antidote

Much is made of the toxicity of our modern world. Frequently we're told that still another substance in our surroundings has been linked to cancer, heart disease, Alzheimer's disease, or some other degenerative malady. There's mercury in your tuna, pesticides on your lettuce, hormones and antibiotics in your chicken, PCBs in your water, poisonous exhaust in the air you breathe, cancer-causing UV light from the sun, and toxic chemicals — all with names that are too long to pronounce — in your clothes, your carpet, your car, your shampoo, your deodorant...

Vitamin C has the proven ability to neutralize virtually any toxic substance and even the dangerous effects of radiation. Arguably, it's the safest substance on the planet. Therefore, it makes perfect sense that copious vitamin C supplementation should be part of everyone's defense against the daily onslaught of environmental toxins.

It's not complicated. Credible science proves a direct correlation between vitamin C blood levels and mortality rates. Data from large population studies indicate that mortality rates could be cut in half — from all causes — if people substantially increased their blood levels of vitamin C.[8]

But, rather than follow the science, our government, with the backing of the medical establishment, pushes a totally unfounded mantra: "The average dietary intake provides 100% of our requirement for vitamin C… and much more just creates expensive urine."

Think about it. The amount of water needed to put out a fire depends on the size of the blaze. In a house fire, the firemen furiously pump water on the inferno until the flames subside, and then a lot more for good measure to quench the remaining heat. To simply toss one bucket on a fire, regardless of size, and then to suggest that using any more will just create expensive steam is maliciously reckless.

Just as firemen use as much water as is necessary to extinguish a fire, vitamin C-pioneer Dr. Klenner continued to administer vitamin C until he obtained the desired clinical response. And then, he typically continued high-dose vitamin C for several more days to assure there was no relapse. As his legacy demonstrates, it's a safe, reasonable, and life-saving strategy, as long as you give enough of it for a long enough time.

## Conclusion

### Consider the facts:

- Determining the type or quantity of an offending poison or venom is not always possible
- Locating a traditionally-approved antivenin or antidote for a specific toxin can exhaust invaluable treatment time
- Many antivenins and antidotes have their own significant toxicity
- All humans are subjected to a daily barrage of toxic substances linked to the development of cancer, organ diseases, and aging diseases of the brain

- Vitamin C has clearly neutralized a host of otherwise fatal toxins and venoms *(see Resource H)*
- High blood levels of vitamin C lowers mortality from all causes
- Vitamin C has no unhealthy side effects *(see Chapter Seven)*
- Vitamin C has no known toxicity *(see Chapter Seven)*
- There is no downside in giving vitamin C before even evaluating the patient, as Dr. Klenner often did

A change in the way healthcare institutions treat patients is long overdue. The needed change will NOT be initiated by drug companies, politicians, government bureaucrats, medical schools, insurance companies, hospital administrators, or mainstream medical practitioners. So don't look for a wide acceptance of vitamin C therapies in traditional emergency treatment centers in the near future *(more about this is discussed in Chapters Seven and Eight)*.

Until then, personal vitamin C supplementation is more than an option; it's an opportunity that will pay huge dividends. Even if you never fall prey to an infectious disease or are never accidentally exposed to a life-threatening toxin or venom, there are many compelling reasons to add several grams of vitamin C to your daily intake. In fact, the most compelling facts, benefits, and reasons are ahead...

## Chapter Three

High-Dose Vitamin C: Nature's Perfect Panacea

# "Once upon a time..." primal past provides powerful insight

Nearly all animals — birds, fish, reptiles, amphibians, and mammals — typically enjoy a full and healthy life, eventually dying of old age. They rarely have strokes, heart attacks, cancer, or contract infectious diseases. And they do not spend a large percentage of their lives in a chronically ill state.

Unfortunately, man does not share this wealth of health.

## *Why Are Humans So Much More Susceptible to Disease?*

It's ALARMING to consider that:

- 50% of American men will develop cancer
- 34% of American women will develop cancer
- 50% of all Americans over age 50 will develop Coronary Heart Disease.
- The incidence of diabetes will jump by 200% in the next 20 years
- The incidence of Alzheimer's disease will jump by 400% in the next 50 years

- Millions will die from lung, kidney, or liver disease in the next 12 months

It's a pretty safe bet to assume that all of us would prefer to die in our old age... in our sleep... of natural causes. It's a much safer bet that most of us will not! Any random scan through the obituaries reveals that it is very, very rare for humans to die from "natural causes."

Why?

Man is one of the sickliest of all the earth's occupants; a few scientists have known this for a long time, although the fact still remains as unappreciated as the value of vitamin C itself. Over 70 years ago researchers discovered that:

> **The mammals most susceptible to infectious disease — man, monkey, and the guinea pig — were those that were unable to synthesize vitamin C.**[1]

Yes, the vast majority of other mammals produce their own vitamin C, as do most birds, fish, reptiles, and amphibians. For all of these animals, vitamin C plays an essential role in protecting them from pathogens and toxins.

Humans, on the other hand, must satisfy their need for vitamin C through diet or supplementation. The fact that guinea pigs share this inability to synthesize their own vitamin C is the primary reason these animals are used for research. Guinea pigs can be made sick or toxic much more easily than a vitamin C-producing animal, allowing many experiments to be performed more quickly and efficiently.

The impact of this inability to synthesize vitamin C is huge! A large population study at Cambridge University supports the conclusion that much of the illness seen in our sickly populations is related to low vitamin C levels in the blood.

The Cambridge study showed that individuals with the highest blood levels of vitamin C had nearly half the death rate of those with the lowest levels — from all causes.[2] In other words, high vitamin C levels slashed the number of deaths from cancer, deaths from heart disease, deaths from infectious disease, deaths from kidney or liver failure, deaths from brain disease... deaths from all causes... by nearly 50%!

The study doesn't reveal how the people with the highest levels obtained them or if still higher levels might even produce better results, but it does clearly establish that higher levels of vitamin C translate into significantly lower mortality.

## A Little-Known Genetic Secret...

If just one little enzyme — L-gulonolactone oxidase (GLO) — were present in the liver of man, he would be able to make loads of vitamin C from the sugar (glucose) in his blood. The abundant presence of this enzyme would eliminate man's need to ingest vitamin C, substantially reduce the incidence of infectious disease, better equip him to meet toxic challenges, protect him from a host of degenerative diseases, and virtually eliminate diabetes.

### It gets even more interesting...

Researchers have now identified the gene that would give man the ability to make the missing enzyme. And we also know this gene already exists in the DNA code of all humans. In other words, the complete instructions that would allow us to produce GLO are passed to each one of us from our parents.[3] But the ability of liver cells to follow these instructions is deficient or completely missing. The logical, scientific conclusion is that:

*It is almost certain humans once synthesized their own vitamin C, as most other animals still do today.*

Unfortunately, researchers have yet to determine why the GLO code present in our DNA remains "untranslated" — that is, why the recipe for GLO is present but not carried out. It seems likely that a genetic mutation resulting in an inborn error of metabolism occurred in the past.

Scientists almost universally assume that all humans share a complete absence of GLO, although it doesn't appear that any serious study has ever been conducted to verify that assumption. It is possible that this defect may not be as universal as is assumed. There are certain groups of people with a reputation for living well into their hundreds (like the Hunzas[4]) who may owe their longevity to an ability to produce at least some GLO and some vitamin C synthesis. Further evidence comes from the fact that some individuals enrolled in vitamin C depletion studies were dropped from those studies when no symptoms of scurvy developed or when vitamin C levels did not drop significantly over an extended period of time.[5-7]

## Nature's Recommended Daily Allowance (RDA) for Goats

Although they can produce some vitamin C, domestic dogs and cats make much less than wild animals. This may explain why our favorite domestic pets eventually suffer with the same diseases as humans.

But in the wild, and even on the farm, healthy mammals produce much more. When not facing significant health stresses, goats produce roughly 13 times more vitamin C than cats or dogs. An adult goat, with a body size roughly that of an adult human, makes about 13,000 mg daily.[9] And the U.S. government still advises a recommended daily allowance (RDA) of only 75 to 90 mg!

Furthermore, when under a significant challenge, C-making animals can dramatically increase production. They can push output to 10 times (or more) beyond baseline levels.[10] When faced with life-threatening diseases or severe toxic challenges, goats can produce as much as 100,000 mg of vitamin C a day!

This natural increase in vitamin C output, in the face of disease and toxin overload, explains why so many wild animals tend to remain vibrantly healthy until they succumb to old age. It also highlights the human need to supplement vitamin C with variable daily amounts based on current health status — low challenges and minimal stress call for lower daily intake while progressively greater levels of illness and stress require increasingly more.

In spite of all the scientific evidence that has accumulated on vitamin C over the last 75 years, the U.S. government has never recommended a daily intake of more than 90 mg. When adjusting for the difference in body mass we find that cats synthesize up to 15 times more vitamin C per day than the government's RDA for humans. The same type of comparison reveals that a normal goat produces nearly 130 times more than the RDA. And the same goat under severe health challenges may produce an incredible 1,000 times more!

Is it possible that nature knows something the U.S. government does not?

## Conclusion

### Consider the facts:

- Most animals synthesize their own vitamin C
- Although defective, humans carry the gene that would provide the ability to synthesize vitamin C
- C-synthesizing animals produce vastly more vitamin C than the 90 mg government RDA

- C-producing animals radically increase production when faced with severe health challenges
- Non-C-producing humans are much more susceptible to disease than animals in the wild
- Individuals with the highest blood levels of vitamin C have a much lower risk of mortality

It is reasonable to conclude that primal man synthesized large and variable amounts of vitamin C. For some unknown reason, he lost that capacity and with the loss came a greater susceptibility to infectious and degenerative diseases. But, even if man never made substantial amounts of vitamin C internally, he clearly benefits from regular large doses of it. Studies support this conclusion by drawing a direct link between higher blood levels of vitamin C and a lower susceptibility to these diseases.

In comparison to the daily quantities of vitamin C synthesized by C-producing animals, the U.S. government's RDA is pathetically small and inadequate. Although governments are attempting to limit access to vitamin C above the RDA *(see Chapter Eight)*, there is no good medical reason for such limits. In fact, there are many reasons to abandon the RDA altogether and supplement our need for vitamin C with amounts that our current health status, toxic environmental exposures, and risk of infection would dictate.

### *A final thought: Could it be that vitamin C is...*

- *Unparalleled* as a universal antimicrobial...
- *Unequalled* as the ultimate antidote...
- *Uniquely effective* in protecting against degenerative diseases...
- *Completely safe* and nontoxic to humans...
- *"At home"* in the human body...

- In other words, *the perfect panacea...*

### because it was intended to be so from the primal past?

We live in an age of unparalleled access to information. No longer do we need to blindly trust our doctors to give us the best guidance for our health. Instead, our relationship with all health providers needs to change. We must become active participants in our health care. Doctors who refuse to consider anything beyond the "traditional" knowledge passed to them through outdated textbooks and biased training — or through aggressive marketing by pharmaceutical companies — do not deserve our unqualified trust. Blind faith in such physicians will only compromise your health care. The history of vitamin C therapy is glaring proof of this fact. Many doctors will not even believe their own eyes when it threatens what their textbooks dictate. So, trust your doctor if you must, but verify...

## Chapter Four

# Coming unglued: The heart of the problem

Coronary heart disease (atherosclerosis) is a malady that sends millions of Americans to an early grave every year... millions more to emergency rooms... and thousands of patients to a cardiac surgery suite every day (at an average cost of over $100,000).[1] Although these facts are alarming, they're not news.

*Here's some real news...*

## ALL coronary arterial blockages have a solitary root cause!

What is this root cause? Is it excessively high triglycerides or fats in the blood? No. These are only indicators of disease risk since they play an important role in the worsening of arterial narrowings — but only after the disease has taken hold. What about high serum cholesterol or high blood pressure? No. These too, are only factors that worsen rather than initiate blockages. Currently there are over 20 commonly accepted risk factors for this major killer... but none of them, individually, or in combination, *initiate* coronary heart disease.[2]

Coronary heart disease starts when the innermost protective lining (the intima) of the coronary arteries begins to come unglued. This lining is comprised of a single layer of cells that functions like ceramic tiles on a shower wall. And just like the cement and grout that hold the tiles in place, there is a gel-like substance (called ground substance) in between and under the protective cells that holds them on the arterial wall. As long as the ground substance remains firm and healthy, these cells stay in place and the artery is protected from disease.[3-7] When the ground substance becomes watery, however, open spaces between these lining cells appear, allowing plaque-building substances in the

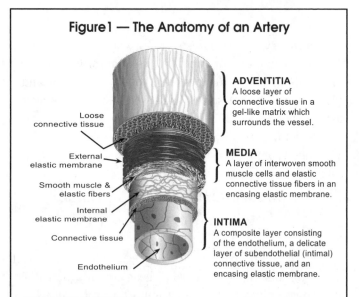

**Figure 1 — The Anatomy of an Artery**

Loose connective tissue

External elastic membrane

Smooth muscle & elastic fibers

Internal elastic membrane

Connective tissue

Endothelium

**ADVENTITIA**
A loose layer of connective tissue in a gel-like matrix which surrounds the vessel.

**MEDIA**
A layer of interwoven smooth muscle cells and elastic connective tissue fibers in an encasing elastic membrane.

**INTIMA**
A composite layer consisting of the endothelium, a delicate layer of subendothelial (intimal) connective tissue, and an encasing elastic membrane.

**THE GROUND SUBSTANCE**
The gel-like material that acts as the glue that holds cells together in bodily structures like arteries, ligaments, tendons, muscles, and others. Ample supplies of vitamin C are required to make and maintain the ground substance. It is the structural "mortar" that holds the endothelial cells found in the intima and it requires sufficient supplies of vitamin C to remain in its normal gel-like state.

**CONNECTIVE TISSUE**
Fibrous material that is used to pack, fill, and connect dissimilar structures together. The primary protein substance in connective tissue is collagen. Collagen requires sufficient supplies of vitamin C for its creation and maintenance.

blood to enter more easily.[8-10] The process of plaque formation, and the subsequent clogging of the artery, requires this initial change in the consistency of ground substance from gel-like to watery.

**Question:** What causes the deterioration of the ground substance?

*Answer:* A localized deficiency of vitamin C in the coronary arteries — called a focal scurvy — results in a breakdown of the ground substance. In contrast, a continuous and generous supply of vitamin C to the arterial linings keeps the ground substance in its healthy, gel-like state.[11-17]

*That means...*

## the solitary root cause of all coronary arterial blockages is a vitamin C deficiency in the coronary arteries!

Furthermore, vitamin C is required for the formation and maintenance of strong and resilient collagen. Since collagen is one of the main structural components of the arterial wall, a continuing deficiency of vitamin C is responsible for more than initiating arterial disease. The C-deficient environment also results in an unrestrained build-up of plaque as the body attempts to fortify arteries continually weakened by a declining quality and quantity of collagen.

For decades, "traditional" medicine has addressed coronary heart disease by treating symptoms and attempting to limit risk factors without addressing, or even acknowledging, its root cause: a focal scurvy of the coronary arteries.

As a consequence, Americans spend billions of dollars every year on expensive drugs and even more expensive procedures that only retard the progression of this lethal disease. All the while, effective vitamin C supplementation would prevent the disease in many who do not already have it. A thorough review of the scientific evidence indicates that coronary arteries with uninterrupted, abundant access to vitamin C would **NEVER** develop artery-plugging plaques. If all of us maintained a C-rich environment in our coronary arteries, the massively lucrative heart disease industry would dry up overnight.

And for those who already have coronary heart disease, there are effective vitamin C protocols that would halt the progression — and in many cases even dissolve — the proliferating, life-endangering plaque that clogs their arteries. In a published case study, for example, an angiogram revealed a 75% blockage in the right coronary artery and 50% blockages in other arteries of a 62 year-old female. A treatment combination featuring vitamin C, lysine, and proline was used to treat her for approximately 19 months. At the end of the treatment period a repeat angiogram revealed that the 75% blockage was reduced to 40% and the 50% blockages had disappeared altogether.[18]

This level of blockage reversal is considered impossible by "traditional" cardiac medicine! But the case above, as well as studies published *over 50 years ago*, show that the "arterial-plaque-buildup-is-irreversible" mantra is simply not true.[19,20] It also shows that the reversal of significant blockages can be a very realistic goal for many heart patients.

## *Understanding the Heart Disease Process*

This may seem a bit simplistic, but for the vast majority of coronary heart disease victims, the process starts and progresses as follows:

1) A localized vitamin C deficiency develops in the coronary arteries.

2) Injury to the artery results from a breakdown in the protective lining of the

artery as the ground substance becomes watery. The artery then loses its ability to securely affix and seal the interior, protective cells on the arterial wall.

3) Plaque begins to form as calcium, cholesterol, fats, and other substances floating in the blood penetrate the arterial wall through the gaps left by the deteriorating ground substance. Sensing an evolving weakness in the artery, the body compensates by trying to patch, seal, and fortify it. The body will even synthesize wads of collagen fibers over the arterial lining in an attempt to strengthen the failing vessel.

4) As all this compensatory activity continues, the arterial walls harden, thicken, and begin to block the flow of blood through the vessel.

5) If the C-deficiency is quickly and adequately addressed, the artery will heal and the blockages will shrink. If not, the blockages will continue to grow and eventually endanger the life of the victim.

An all out C-deficiency (general scurvy) can certainly produce this disease-causing focal scurvy in the arteries. However, such patients die long before arterial blockages become a problem. Multiple factors that contribute to a vitamin C deficiency include the following:

- Normal, everyday toxic exposures
- Ever-present pathogens *(even when no infection exists)*
- Free radicals from normal metabolism

## Figure 2 — Early Progression of Arterial Scurvy

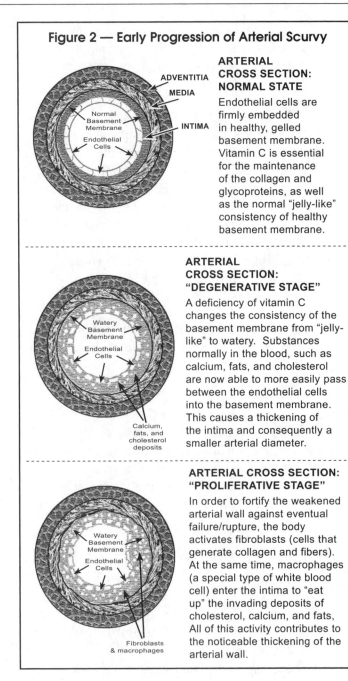

**ARTERIAL CROSS SECTION: NORMAL STATE**

Endothelial cells are firmly embedded in healthy, gelled basement membrane. Vitamin C is essential for the maintenance of the collagen and glycoproteins, as well as the normal "jelly-like" consistency of healthy basement membrane.

**ARTERIAL CROSS SECTION: "DEGENERATIVE STAGE"**

A deficiency of vitamin C changes the consistency of the basement membrane from "jelly-like" to watery. Substances normally in the blood, such as calcium, fats, and cholesterol are now able to more easily pass between the endothelial cells into the basement membrane. This causes a thickening of the intima and consequently a smaller arterial diameter.

**ARTERIAL CROSS SECTION: "PROLIFERATIVE STAGE"**

In order to fortify the weakened arterial wall against eventual failure/rupture, the body activates fibroblasts (cells that generate collagen and fibers). At the same time, macrophages (a special type of white blood cell) enter the intima to "eat up" the invading deposits of cholesterol, calcium, and fats, All of this activity contributes to the noticeable thickening of the arterial wall.

- The many bodily processes that require vitamin C
- Acute or chronic infections
- Humans no longer synthesize their own vitamin C

Additionally, all of the accepted risk factors for coronary heart disease contribute to a vitamin C deficiency and/or are made worse by it.[21] The link between vitamin C and all these risk factors will not be covered here but a list of them, with supporting studies, can be reviewed in Resource D. Because cholesterol, high blood pressure, and diabetes are especially high-profile risk factors, they will be given special attention later in this chapter.

## Specific Causes of Arterial C-Deficiency

In addition to the universal C-depleting mechanisms listed above, there are certain factors that especially deplete vitamin C in and around the heart. Disease-causing microbes and toxins from the mouth are the biggest drains on vitamin C stores in the body for most people. Generally poor dental health, mercury-containing amalgam fillings, gum disease, and root canal-treated teeth dump a continual flood of C-destroying toxins and pathogens into the blood, with the coronary arteries being the first arteries reached.[22-26]

A thorough discussion of dental infections and their associated toxins requires a book of its own *(for any who would like more detail, such a book already exists: The Roots of Disease, by Robert Kulacz, DDS and myself)*. But suffice it to say, the mouth is often the primary source for the toxins and malicious microbes that initiate and fuel degenerative diseases such as cancer, heart disease, and others.[27]

Here's a primary example of a disease-spreading dental procedure: the root canal. First, it is important to note that all root canal-treated teeth are infected by the time the procedure is completed, if not earlier. The procedure is not performed on a healthy tooth, but only on one that is diseased. In an attempt to "save" the tooth, the nerves and their supporting blood vessels in the tooth are removed. This provides freedom from future discomfort, but it also eliminates the body's only route by which the immune system can fight the infection.

Aggressive canal drilling removes some of the infection, but never enough to reach sterility, which is essential for a healthy tooth. It is a "fatally-flawed" procedure that assures a chronically infected tooth every time it is done. Prior to capping off the tooth, in a noble attempt to "disinfect" any remaining infection in the tooth, a sterilizing agent is pushed into the freshly drilled canals. Unfortunately, there are an average of three miles of capillary-sized tubes in each tooth where the disinfectant is unable to go, so the infection and resultant toxins remain and multiply.

Weston Price, DDS found that it was nearly impossible to sterilize extracted root canal-treated teeth — even **outside** the body, using measures too extreme for a tooth still in the mouth! In one of many studies, Dr. Price extracted a root canal-treated tooth from a patient suffering from a severe disease involving the central nervous system. This single extracted tooth was consecutively placed under the skins of 31 rabbits. All the rabbits rapidly developed a similar central nervous system disease. Worst yet, all died![27]

This same type of experiment was tried with many different root canal-treated teeth extracted from patients with a wide variety of ailments. In nearly every case, the lab animals developed the same disease as the one displayed by the patient from whom the tooth had been extracted. This proves to me that any theory claiming root canals are safe is simply wrong.

Over 5,000 successive extracted root canals were tested for very potent toxins, and 100% of them were found to have these toxins. The presence of these toxins, along with the infections that produce them, make root canals the most significant depleters of vitamin C in the body. Because of this:

## Root canals cause more heart disease and more cancer than any other single factor.

The ramifications of this information for heart health are terrifying because infected root canal-treated teeth literally squirt C-depleting, disease-causing pathogens and toxins into the surrounding network of blood vessels with every chew. The freshly-contaminated blood is then pumped back toward the heart through the veins and eventually into the first of the arteries encountered: the coronaries. As a result, vitamin C in the coronary arteries that should be keeping the ground substance and arterial collagen firm and healthy becomes completely spent as it tries to neutralize the incoming onslaught of infectious microbes and harmful toxins. This localized deficiency of vitamin C opens the door to the first stage of atherosclerosis and the resultant build-up of plaque from the many well-known risk factors.

Of course, dentists who perform root canals believe the procedure is completely safe. At least, that is what they say. They have been taught to discredit any challenges as being silly, radical, uninformed, and even ridiculous. And the well-funded American Dental Association (ADA) — an organization established to protect dentists and promote modern dentistry, not patient health — provides promotional and legal help in squelching all opposing voices.

## The Admitted "Temporary Fix" of Current Therapies

When asked, most cardiologists will admit that bypass surgeries, angioplasties, and stent placements rarely result in a permanent solution. They know that arterial blockages will continue to progress. This is often the case for three reasons:

1) The source of vitamin C depletion is not treated.

2) The amount of vitamin C ingested by the patient usually remains at the original, insufficient levels.

3) The vitamin C does not adequately penetrate into the most deficient areas of the arteries.

Several years ago, a close friend had a "Y" stent installed in his seriously occluded coronary arteries. Because there were continuing issues with his heart and the need for additional stenting over a short period of time, I recommended the removal of his only root canal-treated tooth. His supplementation regimen was one of the best I had ever seen, yet it was not until his root canal came out that his chest pains stopped and his blockages stopped their rapid progression. It was only then that his high-quality supplementation, which included 9 grams of liposome-encapsulated vitamin C per day, were finally "allowed" to do their job. At his 5-year checkup, the cardiologists were totally flabbergasted that the stents were as "clean as the day they were placed!" Certainly I was pleased, but not at all surprised. They were clean because the vitamin C deficiency in his arteries had finally been resolved.

Cures result when root causes are eliminated, not when symptoms are treated or suppressed. In the same way that putting a new pipe around an old blocked pipe under your kitchen sink will not clear the blockage, treating arterial blockages without addressing the underlying cause — low vitamin C levels in the coronary arteries — will never provide a permanent resolution. The blockages will continue to worsen.

## Cholesterol and Vitamin C Deficiency

For decades "traditional" medicine has promoted cholesterol as a primary villain in coronary heart disease. Granted, multiple trials have shown that a decrease in cholesterol levels decreases the incidence of arterial blockages and heart attack.[28-35]

But additional studies show that:

- Arterial blockages will start and grow with a vitamin C deficiency *alone* — in the total absence of cholesterol elevations[36]

- Serum cholesterol levels increase with a vitamin C deficiency[37-43]

- Excessive cholesterol depletes vitamin C[44-45]

- Vitamin C supplementation lowers serum cholesterol — even with a high-cholesterol diet[46-51]

- Vitamin C supplementation protects arteries from plaque build-up, even in the presence of high serum cholesterol[52,53]

These studies add further proof that vitamin C is essential for maintaining the health of the coronary arteries. The build-up of cholesterol-containing plaque is simply part of the body's response to a weakening of the arterial wall initiated by a lack of vitamin C. In the presence of a continuing deficiency of vitamin C, a progressive arterial breakdown occurs that triggers further formation of vessel-narrowing plaque.

## High Blood Pressure and Vitamin C Deficiency

Although not assigned the primary role in the cause of coronary heart disease, high blood pressure is seen as a very significant risk factor in the development of arterial disease, and it is known to speed up the process.[54-56]

Additional studies show that:
- Vitamin C deficiency can cause and worsen high blood pressure[57-59]
- Vitamin C supplementation lowers blood pressure of hypertensive patients[60-65]
- Regular and sufficient vitamin C supplementation is required to maintain the optimal collagen content in blood vessels[66-68]
- Maintenance of arterial integrity in the presence of elevated (or even normal) blood pressure requires optimal quality and quantity of collagen in the artery[66-68]

High blood pressure is not something to ignore; it can be very dangerous when sustained over time. However, multiple studies show that adequate levels of vitamin C lower blood pressure and protect the coronary arteries from damage resulting from excessive pressure in these vessels.

## *Diabetes and Vitamin C Deficiency*

Studies show that diabetes is a well-established risk factor for coronary heart disease.[69-70] The relationship between diabetes and atherosclerosis is so strong that two out of every three diabetics will die from coronary heart disease or stroke.[71] Many other studies highlight the close interrelationship between vitamin C deficiency and diabetes. Here's a small sample:
- Vitamin C is involved in the synthesis of insulin[72]
- Vitamin C plays an essential role in regulating the release of insulin[73]
- Diabetics have greatly reduced plasma levels of vitamin C[74-78]
- High blood sugar limits cellular uptake of vitamin C[79-84]
- Low serum insulin limits cellular uptake of vitamin C[79-84]

- Diabetics have a much greater incidence of advanced periodontal disease — another risk factor for increased risk of heart attack[85] (A severe deficiency of vitamin C is always seen in the inflamed and infected gums of advanced periodontal disease)
- Regular and sufficient vitamin C supplementation is extremely important for the optimal treatment of diabetes[85]

The continual and severe vitamin C deficiency caused by diabetes is responsible for most of this disease's negative impact on the body. In combination with the increased inflammation and elevated blood fats (like cholesterol) typical in diabetes, this critical deficiency of vitamin C in blood vessels greatly accelerates the development of arterial blockages. The detrimental health impact of diabetes is not only compounded by a vitamin C deficiency, but the disease itself greatly adds to that deficiency in the blood and tissues. This reality underscores the diabetic's enhanced need for large doses of vitamin C every day.

## *Conclusion*

Consider the facts:
- Vitamin C deficiency in the coronary arteries is the ***SOLITARY ROOT CAUSE*** of all coronary heart disease
- Continuing vitamin C deficiency in the coronary arteries diminishes the quality and quantity of collagen in the arterial wall which causes further breakdown of the artery and facilitates the growth of plaque
- Vitamin C deficiency is associated with every known heart disease risk factor
- Vitamin C supplementation lowers cholesterol
- Vitamin C supplementation reduces high blood pressure

- Vitamin C supplementation is extremely important for the optimal treatment of diabetes
- Vitamin C, alone and in combination with other supplements, has reversed arterial blockages
- Vitamin C supplementation lowers the incidence and mortality risk of coronary heart disease
- "Traditional" therapies for treating arterial blockages are admittedly temporary and cannot be relied upon to reverse, stop, or even slow the growth of those blockages

The importance of high-dose vitamin C in maintaining healthy arteries and preventing atherosclerosis cannot be underestimated. If humans still had the capacity to synthesize vitamin C in quantities commensurate with their need, this disease might be totally non-existent. Since most of us (perhaps all of us) do not have that ability, the only reasonable option is to supplement based on our changing needs. This requires regular evaluation of our disease state, the degree of our exposure to toxins, and the status of the various coronary heart disease risk factors known to further reduce vitamin C levels in the body. The best vitamin C supplementation cannot be expected to prevent coronary heart disease when high daily toxin exposures are not also eliminated or severely curtailed.

Don't expect "traditional" medicine to embrace and promote vitamin C, however. Shiploads of ego and unimaginable quantities of money stand behind maintaining established heart disease treatment methods. In fact, the resistance will grow until an educated populace forces change. Yet, an even greater resistance — more money and greater ego — opposes the proper use of vitamin C against cancer, our next topic of discussion...

## Chapter Five

# Toxic tissues gone mad!

Since President Nixon declared war against cancer nearly 40 years ago, U.S. taxpayers have spent billions upon billions of dollars on cancer research. What has that bought us?

Cancer researchers tell us that survival rates are better now. That's good news, but the improvement cannot be attributed to superior treatment methods and drugs. A recent report from the Centers for Disease Control credits much of the positive change to early detection and lifestyle modifications.[1] In addition, there's a commonly misunderstood factor that further distorts the picture: a "cancer survivor" is defined as a patient who lives beyond the fifth year — even if death from cancer occurs a day later.

Fact is, cancer deaths are at an all-time high. Even by the most optimistic of appraisals we are not winning the war! Why?

### Perhaps we're fighting the wrong enemy...

Lesions and tumors are the visible evidence of cancer. They appear when normal cells go "mad" and begin to malfunction and multiply in a way that is detrimental to the body. Conventional protocols attack these malignant tissues with surgery, radiation, and/or chemotherapy. If and when these diseased tissues disappear, the cancer is said to be in remission. Frequently, to everyone's dismay, the cancer returns. This is why oncologists never use the word "cure."

Healthy cells, by definition, are not diseased; nor do healthy cells cause disease. All disease starts when healthy cells are damaged and cease to function normally. So why wouldn't we expect cancer to return if the factors that pushed normal cells into a malignant state are never addressed?

The real enemy then, is whatever causes the malignant change in the first place. Interestingly, the American Cancer Society has a realistic grip on what causes cancer, even though its purported pursuit of a cure has been completely futile.

Although the American Cancer Society asserts that "cancer is a complex group of diseases with many possible causes,"[2] it seems to understand that toxins and pathogens are always the root cause of cancer. It divides the risk factors into five areas: genetics, tobacco, diet and physical activity, sun and UV exposure, and other carcinogens.[3] This is hardly an exhaustive list, yet an effective treatment would certainly need to address all of these areas, and more. Interestingly, most of these causes are related to toxins and/or pathogens. Of course, toxins and pathogens are both best treated with high-dose vitamin C. Let's examine some of these causes a little further:

*Genetics.* A predisposition to develop certain cancers can be passed on genetically. However, the actual disease is not inherited. Although not a direct cause, an inherited propensity weakens the body's ability to defend against cancer-causing agents. For example, an individual may be lacking in an enzyme that helps to naturally neutralize a significant toxin.

*Tobacco.* This substance, along with many other legal and illicit drugs, contains multiple *toxins* and is clearly linked to the development of cancer.

*Diet and Physical Activity.* The American Cancer Society proposes that poor lifestyle choices contribute to cancer risk. As the lifestyle issues are examined it becomes clear that *toxins* and *pathogens* are the final common denominator of that risk. Some dietary choices introduce *toxins,* such as pesticides or food additives, into the body. As well, wrong food choices can inhibit the body's ability to neutralize and/or eliminate *toxins* and it's ability to keep *pathogens* at bay, primarily through immune system-damaging nutrient deficiencies. A lack of exercise also suppresses the body's defense system against *toxins* and *pathogens.*

*Sun and UV Exposure.* All radiation — whether from the sun, tanning beds, diagnostic equipment, radioactive contamination, or other sources — is a known carcinogen. Although radiation may not look like one, it still damages cells and tissues just like a *toxin*, depleting electrons from vital biomolecules *(see Resource H: Radiation).*

*Other Carcinogens.* The American Cancer Society rightly identifies *toxins* and certain *pathogens* as cancer-causing agents.

*Metastasis.* One of the causes not mentioned by the American Cancer Society is cancer itself. Oncologists call it "metastasis." This process occurs as cancer cells from one tissue break into the blood or lymphatic vessels and move to a new site and initiate cancer there.

Since most, if not all, cancers begin through *toxic* exposure, *pathogenic* challenges, or *metastasis*, it follows that a "cure" would have to address all three causes. In addition to removing all known pathogen and toxic exposures where possible, the strategy must administer a safe and effective:

1. Universal antimicrobial *(pathogenic causes)*

2. Ultimate antidote *(toxic causes)*

3. Agent that strengthens blood and lymphatic vessels *(metastatic causes)*

4. Agent that selectively kills cancer cells *(metastatic causes)*

5. Agent that selectively strengthens healthy cells *(all causes)*

Vitamin C has already been shown to be a universal antimicrobial *(Chapter One)*, and the ultimate antidote *(Chapter Two)*. It is required to keep blood vessel walls strong and healthy *(Chapter Four)*. Studies that will be discussed in this chapter also show that vitamin C selectively kills cancer cells and simultaneously strengthens healthy cells. No other substance can make these claims, thus proving that....

## *Nature's Powerful Cancer Answer is High-Dose Vitamin C*

### Cancer Prevention

Previously, the Cambridge study that measured blood levels of vitamin C and correlated the results to mortality rates was cited. This study found that the number of deaths — including cancer deaths — in the group with the highest vitamin C blood levels was 50% less than the mortality rate in the group with the lowest levels.[4]

An earlier study found similar results. Those researchers concluded that death from cancer was 45% less in the group with the highest blood levels of vitamin C. Such findings strongly demonstrate that increasing blood levels of vitamin C provides significant anti-cancer protection.[5]

In addition, there is every reason to believe that vitamin C blood levels even higher than those measured in the healthiest group in each study would provide even greater protection.

## Cancer Treatment with Vitamin C

In the United States, the government only authorizes surgery, radiation, and FDA-approved chemotherapy drugs for the treatment of cancer. Those providing alternative treatments risk fines, imprisonment, persistent investigation, and/or loss of license if they prescribe or utilize anything outside of these approved protocols. Not only does this totalitarian structure block progress in the war against cancer, it effectively keeps those who are making progress from publishing their findings in peer-reviewed journals.

Even so, some are courageous enough to step forward. Here are recaps of three such cases where vitamin C therapy was used:

*Renal Cell Carcinoma.* The right kidney of a 70 year-old male was removed after it was found to be cancerous. During the surgery doctors discovered that the patient's cancer had spread to the liver and lung. Neither radiation nor chemotherapy was used. Instead, intravenous vitamin C treatment was started at 30 grams twice a week. After six weeks of therapy, the patient stated that he felt good and an exam confirmed that his cancer lesions were shrinking. Fifteen months after starting therapy, there were no signs of progressive cancer. He remained cancer-free for 14 years until he finally died of congestive heart failure.[6]

*Non-Hodgkin's Lymphoma.* A lymphatic tumor around the spine of a 66 year-old female was treated with localized radiation therapy five days per week for five weeks. Simultaneously, she was started on intravenous vitamin C twice per week. After the radiation therapy, chemotherapy was recommended which the patient refused. The vitamin C therapy was continued, however, and she also added several oral supplements after lab tests indicated specific deficiencies.

About five months after the start of treatment, the patient reported pain and swelling of the lymph nodes at the base of her neck just above the collarbone. One of the nodes was surgically removed. A pathology report indicated the presence of malignant lymphoma cells. Her oncologist recommended more radiation and chemotherapy, which she refused. Instead, the intravenous vitamin C and oral supplementation were continued for another 19 months. The cancer finally disappeared, and eight years later, when the study was published, the patient was still cancer-free.[7]

***Colon Cancer.*** A 51 year-old man developed bright red rectal bleeding. Examination found a malignancy in the colon. Surgeons discovered that his tumor had penetrated through the bowel and into surrounding fatty tissue. They also found that the cancer had spread to his liver. Following surgery, chemotherapy was started. The patient and his wife asked the oncologist about vitamin C therapy. He assured them that vitamin C would be of no value.

Subsequent examination and surgery determined that his cancer had continued to spread and had moved to his stomach. Although he was told his prospects for survival were slim, another round of chemotherapy was prescribed. Again the patient asked about vitamin C therapy. The oncologist responded, "I know of no studies which show that this [vitamin C therapy] would eradicate or delay progression of cancer."

Despite the two recommendations against it, the patient found an independent clinic to administer intravenous vitamin C at 100 grams twice per week while he continued the prescribed chemotherapy. A little later oral supplementation of vitamins and minerals was added to the regimen of vitamin C. After about five months the patient went on a two-week vacation. During this time he continued chemotherapy but discontinued the intravenous vitamin C. Almost immediately he began to experience, for the first time, the typical chemotherapy side effects of nausea, diarrhea, stomach pain, and inflammation of the mucous membranes of the mouth and throat.

Upon returning from vacation, vitamin C therapy was resumed. The side effects stopped immediately. A CAT scan over a year later showed no evidence of cancer. In an interview afterwards, he described himself as "perfectly healthy."[8]

Undoubtedly, many will assert that the three preceding case studies are only anecdotal and that it does not prove that vitamin C is effective in treating cancer. The tobacco industry used the same kind of self-serving "logic" for decades. "The much higher incidence of lung cancer among those who smoke doesn't prove that smoking causes cancer."

From a philosophical position it may be true that case studies don't provide the same quality of proof as a large, randomized, double-blind, placebo-controlled study. But from a practical position, these people — and many others[9-14] — were very sick and now are well. Coincidence? I don't think so.

***More Evidence.*** At the Oasis of Hope, a cancer treatment hospital outside the U.S., a new high-dose intra-venous vitamin C protocol without chemotherapy is being employed. They've been using it for just over two years. Even so, their published 2-year survival rates for Stage IV cancers are impressively better than those achieved with conventional therapies:[15]

- Breast cancer — 75% more survivors
- Lung cancer — 887% more survivors
- Colorectal cancer — 107% more survivors

To be complete, it should be noted that treatments at the Oasis of Hope include several aspects not associated with conventional therapies in the U.S. These include:

- Lifestyle changes including exercise and a diet rich in raw, organic foods (reducing toxic exposure) and avoidance of refined sugars *(improving vitamin C uptake and eliminating cancer's favorite food)*[16]

- Emotional and spiritual counseling[17]

The Oasis of Hope, which also offers conventional therapies, says this about their alternative vitamin C therapy (IRT-C):

> "The very good news about the IRT-C approach is that it does not harm normal healthy tissues, which have adequate antioxidant defenses; thus, IRT-C is virtually free of side effects."[18]

Every month thousands of hospital patients die from reactions to drugs — drugs that have been prescribed and properly administered according to FDA-approved protocols. Not a single FDA-approved cancer drug has ever come remotely close to being free of hazardous side effects. A very unacceptable percentage of people treated with FDA-approved cancer drugs still die from cancer. And yet a physician in the U.S. who gets caught using non-FDA-approved protocols on cancer patients can go to prison. And it doesn't matter how often or how many of the cancers disappear.

## *Specific Anti-Metastatic Mechanisms of Vitamin C*

### *Vitamin C Inhibits Both Tumor Growth and Cancer Spread*

In the same way an optimum level of vitamin C in the coronary arteries keeps the cellular glue *(ground substance)* in blood vessels firm and healthy, it is also responsible for the formation of a strong, supportive, extracellular matrix in other tissues throughout the body.[19-25] A deficiency of vitamin C allows this ground substance, or matrix, to become weak and watery. When this deficient state becomes continuous, tumor growth can be both initiated and facilitated because the external support grid that would normally restrain cellular proliferation can no longer do so.

When ground substance loses its firm gelatinous consistency and becomes watery, the door is open for malignant cells to break through lymphatic and blood vessel walls and migrate to other areas of the body.

High-dose vitamin C keeps ground substance strong and provides optimum anti-cancer protection for healthy cells — including those directly adjacent to an already existing tumor or lesion.

## High-Dose Vitamin C Kills Cancer Cells

One of the amazing properties of vitamin C is that it can protect healthy cells while simultaneously and selectively causing rapid cell death in cancer cells. Until recently the mechanism for this seemingly contradictory function was a mystery. But now we know how. Here's the secret...

Cancer cells differ from healthy cells in several ways that make them vulnerable to vitamin C-initiated death. Here are two of the most significant:

1) Cancer cells *(and many pathogens as well)* accumulate very high levels of free iron.

2) Cancer cells do not produce significant amounts of a protective enzyme *(catalase)*, which permits accumulation of intracelluar hydrogen peroxide.

In the presence of vitamin C, free iron produces a powerful pro-oxidant substance from hydrogen peroxide — called the hydroxyl radical *(via a biochemical pathway known as the Fenton reaction)*.[26] This aggressive pro-oxidant is the **most toxic substance** known to man because it will destroy any molecule to which it is exposed. Fortunately, in healthy cells there is little Fenton reaction activity, since normal catalase levels keep hydrogen peroxide levels very low, and very little free iron is ever present as well.

If, however, there is sufficient vitamin C in a cancer cell, large quantities of hydroxyl radicals are produced because of the high levels of free iron and hydrogen peroxide inside the cancer cell. With enough Fenton reaction activity, many newly created hydroxyl radicals vigorously attack and ultimately destroy the contents of the cancer cell, and then the cancer cell itself.[27-28] In this way...

## Vitamin C is the ultimate chemotherapeutic agent: It improves and protects the health of normal cells while producing the most toxic of substances inside cancer cells!

### Vitamin C Does Not Hinder, But Supports Traditional Chemotherapy

Most, if not all, oncologists realize that vitamin C is a powerful antioxidant. They also know that radiation and chemotherapeutic drugs are highly pro-oxidant, or highly toxic due to their pro-oxidant nature. That is why most cancer doctors will recommend against the concurrent use of vitamin C and radiation/chemo. Their argument suggests that vitamin C will powerfully neutralize their highly toxic therapies, thereby rendering them ineffective. And, in fact, if the vitamin C and radiation/chemo were administered simultaneously, they would be correct.

When administration of vitamin C is appropriately staggered from the administration of radiation and/or chemotherapy, the damaging aspects of conventional therapies can be minimized while the cancer-killing properties are optimized. Consider the following points:

- Radiation/Chemotherapeutic drugs weaken all cells exposed to it — yet the desire is to inflict damage on cancer cells alone

- Vitamin C enters already weakened cancer cells and facilitates cell death via the Fenton reaction discussed previously
- Vitamin C helps weakened healthy cells, including immune system cells, to repair damage to them caused by the traditional therapies, thereby greatly lessening side effects and improving immune function

Vitamin C, in fact, is so good at lessening side effects that oncologists often conclude their prescribed radiation or chemotherapy is being neutralized and therefore not effective. However, studies have shown that vitamin C not only has its own cancer cell-killing abilities, but that it actually enhances the effectiveness of chemotherapy.[29-31]

## Adverse Studies Regarding Vitamin C and Cancer

A few studies have failed to confirm earlier findings of vitamin C's efficacy in the treatment of cancer. However, all of these studies used inadequate doses of vitamin C, and some used oral rather than intravenous administration. Of course, it is well-known that every medication is more potent when given by vein rather than by mouth.

Furthermore, it is well-established that intravenous infusions produce much higher blood levels of vitamin C than oral supplementation of an identical dose. This is especially true when the oral vitamin C is in a water-soluble form. Research shows that as an oral dose increases, the actual percentage of C entering the bloodstream dramatically decreases. Most physicians who utilize vitamin C in their cancer treatments state that doses between 50 to 100 grams per treatment are required. Therefore, it is unlikely that a therapy using only oral supplementation therapy would be effective in treating cancer. Some researchers, however, maintain that oral supplementation can actually improve the efficacy of intravenous vitamin C when used together.

As in the treatment of infectious diseases and serious toxin exposures, a dose size that is too small will guarantee unsatisfactory results. Since vitamin C is inexpensive and completely safe — even at intravenous doses of 300 grams *(see Chapter Seven)* — there is absolutely no reason to skimp. That is, unless one wants the therapy to fail, as in the Allan Smith case discussed earlier.

## Conclusion

The "cure" for cancer has eluded researchers for half a century. Strategies that rely entirely on the use of radiation and chemotherapy drugs — both known to cause cancer and damage or kill normal cells — have not, and dare I say, **will never** produce anything approaching a victory in this war. What's more, as long as surgery, radiation, and chemo-therapy are the only approved modes of treatment, cancer survival statistics will never be acceptable.

Vitamin C has been shown to prevent cancer and to selectively kill cancer in both the laboratory and the body. Although I'm not suggesting that vitamin C on its own will prevent or cure all cancers, it does have a track record that shows it is significantly more effective than conventional therapies. If the Food and Drug Administration would lift its "unapproved drug" restrictions, vitamin C will become a foundational part of many powerful, and exceptionally suc-cessful protocols used to fight this disease.

Vitamin C is safe, inexpensive, easy to use, and pre-vents, mitigates, and even cures a mind-numbing list of diseases and conditions. Based upon the Cambridge study and my own clinical experiences, I believe that people who reduce their exposure to toxins (particularly dental toxicity), eat a healthy diet, and regularly supplement with high-dose vitamin C, would profoundly lower their risk of cancer and heart disease. By this time, it should be easier to appreciate the power of this unmatched Primal Panacea. And, yet, there is still more...

# Deliverance from dreaded deterioration

It's a law of nature and a law of science that all things lose energy and eventually disintegrate. When it happens to iron-containing metals it's called rust; as it becomes visible in humans we call it *aging*. The primary force in the aging process — and all the degenerative diseases associated with aging — is a process called *oxidation.*

By direct and indirect mechanisms all of vitamin C's ability to prevent and control degenerative diseases — as well as infectious diseases and toxic exposures — is tied to its powerful ability to counteract oxidation. To fully appreciate the value of vitamin C, then, requires a foundational under-standing of the oxidation process. The next four paragraphs will attempt to provide that understanding by taking a tiny detour into some basic science *(for any who want a more complete and more technical explanation, see Resource A).*

We must start with a quick review of chemistry:

- Physical matter is composed of atoms consisting of a nucleus circled by one or more electrons
- Electrons are small negatively charged particles that orbit the nucleus like planets circle the sun

- Molecules consist of two or more atoms held together through a sharing of their electrons

In simple terms, *oxidation* occurs when a molecule loses one or more of its shared electrons. In the same way that pulling a brick out of a brick wall would weaken the wall, most molecules become unstable with the loss of electrons. This electron deficit is so destabilizing to some molecules that they initiate a vigorous chain reaction of stealing electrons from all the molecules around them. These highly reactive electron thieves are called *free radicals* and they inflict damage via what is called *oxidative stress.*

Ultimately, all pathogens and all toxins cause their damage by initiating and increasing *oxidative stress* within the cells of the body. And at a minimum, *oxidative stress* is a major factor in every degenerative disease known to man.

On the other hand, molecules that can donate electrons without losing stability themselves are called *antioxidants.* By contributing electrons to unstable, electron-depleted free radicals, antioxidants can neutralize them, defuse the attack, and often reverse the damage that had already been inflicted. When an antioxidant has its full complement of electrons, it is said to be in the *reduced* form. When an antioxidant has lost its free electrons, it is in the *oxidized* form. Although considered "spent" while in the oxidized state, antioxidants can be recharged from a new source of electrons — typically received from quality nutrients.

## The Role of Oxidative Stress in Degenerative Disease

Unaddressed oxidative stress unravels tissues, rips through membranes, distorts DNA, interrupts normal metabolism, sets off destructive chemical reactions, and creates cellular debris that disrupts normal bodily functions. A "PubMed" search for oxidative stress and its synonyms yields over a half million studies. It is scientifically established that oxidative stress initiates many but worsens **all** chronic degenerative diseases.[1]

Here's just a short list of some of these degenerative diseases:

- ALS (Lou Gehrig's Disease)
- Alzheimer's Disease and other dementia-causing disorders
- Arthritis
- Cancer
- Cataracts
- COPD (Chronic Obstructive Pulmonary Disease)
- Diabetes
- Glaucoma
- Gout
- Heart Disease
- Lupus
- Macular Degeneration
- Multiple Sclerosis
- Osteoporosis

Three major factors determine which degenerative diseases manifest in an individual:

1) pro-oxidant (toxin) source and type
2) oxidation location (site of toxin accumulation)
3) genetic predisposition

***Pro-Oxidant Source.*** There are countless sources of oxidizing agents. The agent could be a toxin like mercury, a pathogen such as strep, or a free radical generated by an earlier oxidizing process — including the necessary metabolic functions such as breathing or the cellular conversion of glucose into energy.

***Oxidation Location.*** Degenerative diseases are typically concentrated in specific organs: Alzheimer's disease and Parkinson's disease in the brain, arthritis in the joints, macular degeneration and cataracts in the eye, and osteoporosis in the bones. Even in these diseases the actual target narrows to certain cellular structures like DNA, cell membranes, or the energy-producing factories within each cell (mitochondria).

*Genetic Predisposition.* A predisposition is not the cause or a guarantee of disease development but rather a genetically-passed weakness in the specific tissues, organs, or cellular structures. Certain toxins or pro-oxidants might cause a disease in one genetically-prone individual while having no effect in a genetically normal individual.

The body has an elaborate defense system for neutralizing oxidative stress by synthesizing an antioxidant like glutathione and an antioxidant enzyme like sodium superoxide dismutase. Most of us who are getting even small amounts of antioxidants in our diets are usually protected from the minimal level of pro-oxidants produced by normal bodily functions — like breathing, digestion, and energy production. A continuous exposure to certain toxins or pathogens, however, can overwhelm our natural antioxidant defenses, ultimately resulting in a chronic, degenerative disease. As the body grows older, its production of antioxidants diminishes, thereby further increasing the risk of damage through oxidative stress and inadequate antioxidant intake.

## A Logical Strategy for Fighting Degenerative Diseases

The pill-for-every-ill, lessen-the-symptoms-until-the-patient-dies protocol promoted by the medical establishment unashamedly admits defeat from the start. Instead of prevention or cure, we're given a handful of prescriptions for expensive maintenance drugs. These non-nutritive, foreign substances supply their own toxic, disease-promoting effects.

It's time for a better approach to medicine. The fact that the causes and promoters of degenerative disease are directly tied to oxidative stress is well-established. It logically follows that these diseases can be more effectively treated and often prevented by maintaining sufficient antioxidant levels throughout the body.

Vitamin C is not only a universal antimicrobial and the ultimate antidote, it is also a particularly important antioxidant. That's because vitamin C...

- Has double antioxidation power — it can donate not just one, but *two* electrons per molecule
- Is the safest antioxidant — no toxic effects even at very high levels
- Provides universal protection due to universal access — unlike some antioxidants, it can protect the brain because it can cross the blood-brain barrier
- Can "recharge" (reduce) previously "spent" (oxidized) antioxidants — including those synthesized by the body

## Proof of Vitamin C's Power Against Degenerative Diseases

The scientific evidence documenting the role oxidative stress plays in the development of degenerative diseases logically indicates vitamin C should be a powerful weapon in their treatment. In fact, the medical literature provides substantial evidence that vitamin C can prevent, lessen, and even reverse the damage inflicted by these diseases.

Six of the most prevalent degenerative diseases are heart disease, diabetes, cancer, osteoporosis, arthritis, and Alzheimer's disease. The first three — heart disease, diabetes, and cancer — were discussed in the previous two chapters. What follows is a very quick review of the other three.

88


## Osteoporosis

Vitamin C's involvement with the formation and maintenance of bone mineral structure and density is well-established in the scientific literature, although probably not that well-recognized. Our appreciation of C's importance in bone formation continues to evolve as scientists further explore this issue. Contrary to popular opinion, osteoporosis almost never results from a chronically poor dietary intake of calcium. This condition stems from an inability to transform the calcium salts circulating in the blood into a healthy, calcium-dense bone matrix.

Vitamin C is critically important in the three most significant factors involved in forming and maintaining quality bone.[2,3] These factors are:

1) Mineralization (assimilation) of calcium into the bone

2) Resorption — calcium being leached from the bone and reentering the bloodstream

3) Oxidative stress which inhibits mineralization and increases resorption

These mechanisms of bone biology are controlled by two kinds of bone cells: osteoblasts (mineralizing cells) responsible for bone formation and osteoclasts (resorbing cells) that actually pull calcium out of the bone.

The presence of vitamin C stimulates bone precursor cells to develop into osteoblasts. At the same time, vitamin C inhibits the creation of osteoclasts. On the other hand, in the presence of a C-deficiency, these calcium-dissolving osteoclasts proliferate in an uncontrolled manner, resulting in a detrimental mineral loss from the bone tissue.[4,5]

These biological factors alone are enough to justify copious vitamin C supplementation for osteoporosis patients. And yet, the other major factor in bone density loss — oxidative stress — provides additional sound justification for maintaining high blood levels of this powerful antioxidant.[6]

Almost as important, a ready supply of vitamin C is essential for the collagen cross-link formation needed to optimize the physical strength of the bones.[7,8] Conversely, a vitamin C deficiency results in weaker bones.[9]

Several clinical studies demonstrate the importance of vitamin C supplementation in the prevention of bone loss[10-15] — even though most of the supplementation dosages employed were woefully small. A profoundly significant study monitored bone fractures in relation to the dietary and supplemental intake of vitamin C of nearly 1,000 subjects between the ages of 70 and 80 during a 17-year period. The researchers found that dietary C intake alone, without additional supplementation, provided *no* protection from fracture risk. However, they also discovered that there was a *significant* lowering of risk in subjects who *supplemented* with vitamin C — the higher the dose, the lower the risk of fractures.[16]

As a more general correlation, researchers found that elderly patients who fractured their hips had a "significantly lower" level of vitamin C in their blood than elderly patients who had not sustained such a fracture.[17]

A lessening of calcium deposition in bone tissues appears in scurvy — the ultimate state of vitamin C deficiency. An increasing amount of calcium is excreted and/or finds its way into various tissues, similar to the deposits found in atherosclerosis when C is profoundly depleted.[18]

On the other hand, postmenopausal women who took vitamin C supplements had greater bone mineral density.[19] In a similar study, women between the ages of 55 and 64 years of age who had taken vitamin C supplements for 10 years or more — and had NOT taken estrogens — had a higher bone mineral density than those who did not.[20]

**The bottom line**: Proper blood levels of vitamin C are essential to bone health. It is so important that I believe existing research could easily conclude that osteoporosis is a focal scurvy of the bones.

## Arthritis

There is no credible argument disputing that oxidative stress is the major culprit in the development of
osteoarthritis, polyarthritis, and rheumatoid arthritis.[21,22]
Aside from the fact that joints are constructed from
vitamin C-dependent collagen and collagen-containing
cartilage — a fact that seems to have remained unappreciated in most research studies — the relationship between
vitamin C deficiency and arthritis is clear-cut. In fact, in the
literature five different cases of scurvy were initially diagnosed as arthritis. This clearly demonstrates that a severe
vitamin C deficiency can manifest itself in a breakdown of
bone and joint tissues themselves, as well as in the antioxidant defenses around those tissues.[23-26]

In addition, researchers often cite low vitamin C intake
as a risk factor in the development of arthritis and vitamin C
deficiency as a nearly universal finding in those diagnosed
with the disease.[27-29] Even though no high-dose vitamin C
studies treating arthritis could be found, there are several
low-dose studies that provide significant evidence of C's
helpful role in the prevention and treatment of this disease.
In one such study, vitamin C supplementation was found to
reduce the size and number of bone marrow lesions. These
lesions are known to be instrumental in the development of
osteoarthritis.[30]

Further evidence of high-dose vitamin C's potential in
the prevention and treatment of arthritis comes from animal
studies. In one such investigation, high-dose vitamin C was
shown to significantly reduce arthritic swelling, arthritic
inflammation, and the migration of inflammatory cells into
the synovial tissues around the joint.[31]

## Alzheimer's Disease

The incidence of degenerative brain diseases is growing
very rapidly. Reasons abound for this disturbing reality, but

it is very clear that oxidative stress in the brain plays a major role in the initiation and development of these mind-killers.

Considering the half million studies found in "PubMed" on oxidative stress, relatively few address the role of anti-oxidants in the prevention and treatment of Alzheimer's and similar diseases. Even so, there are some that demonstrate the importance of vitamin C in their treatment. Unfortunately, none of the studies investigate the use of *high-dose* vitamin C. In the mix of studies, however, are a few that attempt to discourage vitamin C's use in prevention or treatment. These are poorly designed studies that use broad-stroke generalizations. It's not hard to conclude that researchers exploit this anti-vitamin C bias to promote their sponsor's costly prescription drugs.

One such study claims, "the use of supplemental vitamin E and C, alone or in combination, did not reduce risk of AD (Alzheimer's disease) or overall dementia over 5.5 years of follow-up."[32]

Certainly this is ammunition for those who want to discredit vitamin C or vitamin E... until one examines the methods the researchers employed to arrive at this conclusion!

First, 2,969 subjects were recruited. These people had to be age 65 or older without cognitive impairment (determined by testing). Then the population was divided into four groups based on their **self-reported** supplementation regimens.[32]

On the day of initial testing — and at that time alone — the subjects were asked about their supplement use for the previous month ONLY:

- The **No Supplement Group** reported no vitamin C or vitamin E supplementation *one month prior* to the start of the study.
- The **Vitamin E Group** reported using some (*any dose no matter how small*) vitamin E without vitamin C for a minimum of one week during the *previous month*.

- The **Vitamin C Group** reported using some (***any*** *dose no matter how small*) vitamin C without vitamin E for a minimum of one week during the *previous month.*
- The **Vitamins C & E Group** reported using both (***any*** *dose no matter how small*) vitamin C and vitamin E for a minimum of one week during the *previous month.*

No dosage information or supplementation history before the baseline month (the month just prior to subjects' initial testing), during, or after the study period was reported for any of the subjects. Although the subjects were tested for dementia twice a year for the next 5.5 years, vitamin supplementation was not monitored.

At the end of the study, 405 subjects had been diagnosed with dementia (289 of them with Alzheimer's disease). Statisticians then did their math by determining the percentage of each group that developed dementia. Since there was no "significant" difference between the groups, the researchers concluded that vitamin C, or vitamin E, or the two used together had no preventive impact on the development of dementia.

Based on the selection criteria, subjects who had only supplemented a total of one week with as little as 100 mg of vitamin C could have made their way into the supplementing groups. With all the uncontrolled variables, self-reporting, and lack of measurements, even a high-school science student would be able to detect the flawed design of this study. Unfortunately, peer-reviewed medical journals are littered with this kind of pseudo-scientific rubbish where vitamin C is concerned. Sadly, such loose-dose studies are the rule rather than the exception.

In contrast, a different study found that a combination of vitamin C, vitamin E, and non-steroidal anti-inflammatory drugs had a positive effect in slowing the cognitive decline of Alzheimer's disease.[33] Another study, one that was randomized, double-blind, and placebo-controlled, concluded that Alzheimer's patients who received an anti-oxidant formula, including vitamin C, demonstrated significantly improved cognitive scores.[34] Several animal studies have also validated a preventative and restorative role for vitamin C in combating oxidative stress in models of neuro-degenerative diseases.[35-37]

Unfortunately, at this writing, there just are no *high-dose* vitamin C studies with degenerative brain diseases, period! However, there are well-designed studies that do show us that Alzheimer's disease and the other dementia-related diseases involve high levels of oxidative stress.[38] There are three other important facts that have also been well-established:

1) Vitamin C is highly concentrated in the brain[34]

2) Vitamin C is a safe and powerful antioxidant

3) Antioxidants *do* make a big difference in preventing and slowing the development of Alzheimer's

At this point, it is also helpful to remember the two large population studies cited previously that monitored blood levels of vitamin C in relation to mortality. These studies tied a 50% drop in mortality — from all causes, including degenerative diseases of the brain — to high blood levels of vitamin C. This provides additional evidence to support vitamin C's powerful contribution in preventing and fighting these neurological diseases.

## Conclusion

Excess oxidative stress exerts a pathological effect wherever it is found in the body. Left unchecked, it results in degenerative disease. Nature has provided a universally effective remedy to combat these increasing concentrations of pro-oxidants: vitamin C, the primary anti-aging antioxidant!

And, without a doubt, the powerful antioxidant capacity of vitamin C is the main reason that it can prevent and often reverse the oxidative damage characteristic of ALL degenerative diseases. But, as we have seen, vitamin C has multiple mechanisms for fighting degenerative diseases that extend beyond its antioxidant abilities (such as collagen formation, osteoblast formation, maintenance of the ground substance, and others). This is also true for all of the other degenerative diseases not specifically addressed here. Vitamin C plays a crucial role in maintaining normal biochemistry everywhere in the body.

To summarize: vitamin C has always been the universal antimicrobial, the ultimate antidote, the prime protector of arteries, nature's cancer answer, and primary anti-aging antioxidant. In other words: *Vitamin C is the Primal Panacea*. What would it be like if humans still synthesized vitamin C in response to their level of oxidative stress, toxic exposure, and pathogen load, as do so many of the animals in the wild?

The exciting news is: Intelligent, high-dose supplementation can come close to achieving the same level of health seen in wild animals that synthesize whatever vitamin C they need.

Unfortunately, some who profit from the big business of "treating" diseases work to keep the truth about high-dose vitamin C little-appreciated and little-utilized. This is accomplished in several ways. The first way involves the propagation of lies — lies that keep people sick, lies that doom people to a premature death. In fact, there are seven widely circulated, death-promoting lies that need to be debunked right now...

## Chapter Seven

High-Dose Vitamin C: Spin Doctors Lie

# 7 medical
# lies that kill!

It is surprising what a simple Google™ search for "urban legends" brings to your computer. Without a doubt, vitamin C lies — like urban legends — are sincerely believed by most of those who pass them along. But, unlike relatively harmless urban legends, vitamin C lies are responsible for much sickness and death because doctors continue to refuse to administer vitamin C correctly, or at all. As a result, patients are far too often denied optimal health and even life because their physician believes one or more of the following vitamin C lies...

## *Lie #1: There Are No Vitamin C Studies*

Medical professionals are quick to justify their disinterest in high-dose vitamin C with this fable. This statement, or any like it, is so absurdly false, and so easy to disprove, that it boggles the mind why any educated medical practitioner would repeat it! If a mechanic or stonemason said there were no studies on vitamin C, it would be forgivable. That's not their line of expertise. But for a person trained in the healing sciences... this degree of ignorance — or dishonesty — borders on the criminal! It is undoubtedly the most flagrant display of medical malpractice.

Here's a scientific study you can perform at home:

1) Log onto the internet.

2) Type "pubmed" into your browser search box.

3) Click on the "PubMed" home link when it appears *(PubMed is a U.S. government website run by the National Institutes of Health. This site catalogs all the studies from thousands of peer-reviewed medical journals around the world — in other words, scientific journals specifically published for medical doctors and researchers.)*

4) Type the phrase "vitamin C or ascorbate or ascorbic" in the "PubMed" search box and click the "Search" button *(This calls up all the studies that discuss vitamin C — ascorbate and ascorbic are scientific names for vitamin C).*

5) Note the number of studies retrieved directly under the "PubMed" logo.

As of this writing the number was: 51,027! This number is always growing. To put this in perspective: if a doctor were to read one vitamin C study per day for the next 40 years, he would still have reviewed less than 30% of the studies published to date. This literal flood of research actually makes it easier for so many incredible vitamin C findings to be "hidden in plain sight."

Undoubtedly, the question will be raised, "How can the medical community possibly justify their claim of 'no studies'?" Here's how. They define the word "study" very narrowly. By their clever definition, a published, peer-reviewed finding only counts as a study when it is a large, randomized, placebo-controlled, and double-blind clinical trial. Here's what that means:

In order to qualify, a significantly-sized group of qualified subjects must be divided into two groups using a statistically valid method of random selection. Then, one group has to be given a placebo (like a simple saline solution) and the other the ingredient to be tested (such as vitamin C). Neither the subjects nor those administering the test are allowed to know what is being given. At the end, the results are compared to determine if there is a significant difference between those receiving the placebo versus those receiving the agent to be tested.

For example, if 500 people have a confirmed case of herpes, all are given large IV drips of vitamin C in a hospital, all are closely monitored, and all are cured within 72 hours, the data **does not count as a study** for many doctors. The fact that there's not a drug anywhere that has ever cured any case of herpes in any amount of time does not appear to be relevant to the general medical community. As a doctor in the *60 Minutes* documentary, "Living Proof?" suggested, there's no proof that the vitamin C worked, it could just as easily been cured by a passing bus. Such a stunningly stupid comment is probably the best example as to how vigorously medicine resists and blocks change that does not come from its traditional channels.

This tight definition of "study" eliminates all but a tiny portion of scientifically valid research. Never mind the fact that large, randomized, placebo-controlled, double-blind clinical trials rarely exist to justify the use of many, if not most, prescription drugs. The fact remains: there are over 50,000 studies in the medical literature indexed by the U.S. government's "PubMed" medical library on the impressive qualities of vitamin C. Even if all the studies were unimpressive — and they're not by even the most perverse stretching of the truth — it remains a boldfaced lie to say there are no studies concerning vitamin C. The claims in this book are backed by well over a thousand published, peer-reviewed studies.

Vitamin C is held to a much higher standard than all of the prescription drugs. And even when that standard is met, the results are largely ignored, with the ever recurring refrain of "more studies are needed" punctuating the end of so many dramatic studies.

The number of heart attacks and strokes that could have been averted... the cases of cancer that would never have materialized... amputations avoided... infections and diseases cured... poisonings reversed... with the proper administration and/or supplementation of vitamin C is depressingly huge.

In Chapter Three a study published in one of the most prestigious journals in the world, *The Lancet*, was cited. This large population study conducted at Cambridge University monitored blood levels of vitamin C in nearly 20,000 people over time and found that those with the highest levels experienced half the mortality of those with the lowest levels. This suggests that millions upon millions of lives could have been spared and hundreds of billions, or even trillions of dollars saved if the population was supplementing with adequate doses of vitamin C and doctors were using it in their treatment protocols. But, sadly, I believe this is exactly why vitamin C is yet to be properly embraced, and may never be. In a nutshell, it would ruin the big business of medicine.

### Lie #2: No Evidence that Vitamin C Works

Are they totally blind? Yes! Even when doctors see a miraculous cure, as in the Allan Smith case in New Zealand — documented by *60 Minutes* in and referenced in Chapter One — they refuse to see what they have actually witnessed.

How can any health professional say, "No evidence," when studies published in medical journals show vitamin C cured *60* out of *60* polio victims without any lingering complications within five days... resolved *327* out of *327* cases of shingles in three days... cured **7** of **7** cases of rheumatic fever just as quickly... and on and on?

This is only three of many instances of a 100% success rate. Shouldn't these studies merit — at a minimum — a second look? As far as I can tell, none of these particular results have been retested or challenged in a published study. In the drug-approval realm, a demonstration of a very slight improvement is enough for rave reviews.

But a 100% cure rate gets no attention... no questions... no follow-up studies. The one thing that is consistently given is a seemingly obligatory statement at the bottom of the article: "but more research is needed." This instead of a recommendation for the use of a completely nontoxic substance — one that has cured disfiguring diseases still considered incurable, or at best, diseases that are minimally responsive to accepted mainstream therapies.

After thousands of studies, why do researchers continue to investigate vitamin C with such vigor if there is no evidence... if it's a hoax? If there is no evidence, why are clinics offering intravenous vitamin C therapies (often run by medical doctors who have the training and credentials to administer "traditional" medicine) continually busy? And why are more of these clinics continuing to open all over the U.S., Mexico, Europe, New Zealand, Australia, and Asia? Perhaps some can find "no evidence" because it's easier to travel with the herd — to accept and repeat a lie — than it is to search for the truth. Myths and lies eventually become accepted as truth when repeated often enough.

I've personally witnessed hundreds of "medical miracles" as a response to high-dose vitamin C. Doctors all over the globe have told me of similar experiences. This book references hundreds of studies that show vitamin C works. Truth is, there is plenty of evidence for anyone who is willing to see it!

## Lie #3: Vitamin C is Not Safe

The evidence says, "vitamin C is safer than drinking water." Researchers have documented lethal overdoses of water,[1] yet no lethal dose has been found for vitamin C.[2] There's not a single drug — prescription or over-the-counter — that can claim that level of safety. As well, there are few other nutritive supplements that can even approach the safety of any amount of vitamin C.

According to an article published in the *Journal of the American Medical Association*, 106,000 patients died in hospitals in 1994 from drug reactions. The authors further stated that the number of hospital drug deaths per year had remained unchanged for 30 years.[3] That's shocking: over 3 million people were killed in the hospital, under strict supervision, with prescription drugs from 1965 to 1994! What incredible hypocrisy from those who are the first to broadcast the "vitamin C is not safe" lie — the very people who make or prescribe dangerous drugs.

In contrast, high-dose vitamin C has been widely used since the late 1940s without a confirmed report of *any* dosage level that will result in serious adverse effects.

Terminal cancer patients, a segment of the population that is arguably the sickest and most sensitive to toxins, have been given daily intravenous doses of 50,000 mg for up to eight weeks without any evidence of toxicity or side effects.[4] A study in Australia reports that some 100 physicians have administered as much as 300,000 mg of vitamin C per day to their patients. The researchers state that "in most cases the results have been spectacular, the only side effect is 'chronic good health.'"[5] Robert Cathcart, MD, asserted that he treated over 20,000 patients during a 21-year period with as much as 200,000 mg per day with no incidence of major side effects. Interestingly, most of the side effects — of the few that did appear — were minor and were eliminated by *increasing* the dose of vitamin C.[6-9]

In a double-blind clinical trial with 123 terminal cancer patients who were felt to be "unsuitable" for chemotherapy, a daily dose of 10,000 mg of vitamin C was tested against a placebo. These patients were very ill, with an average survival time of seven weeks. Nevertheless, the vitamin C was very well-tolerated, producing only mild nausea and vomiting with the *same frequency as the placebo*.[10] Several years later a similar study was conducted with 100 colorectal cancer patients. These researchers noted that a slightly greater number of those receiving the 10,000 mg daily dose of vitamin C reported heartburn. They also stated that the difference in heartburn occurrence between those who received vitamin C and those who took the placebo was "not statistically significant."[11]

In eleven other studies with high-dose vitamin C — five of these were placebo-controlled — no side effects were reported.[12-22] Even a double-blind, placebo-controlled trial with premature babies concluded that vitamin C administration is very safe.[23]

Regardless of any claims to the contrary, no one who has done a critical appraisal of the scientific literature can say anything other than, "Vitamin C is one of the *safest* substances on earth."

## Lie #4: Vitamin C Supplementation Causes Kidney Stones

The "vitamin C causes kidney stones" myth is a much more specific version of the "vitamin C is not safe" fable. As with most legends, there is a sliver of truth here. Most kidney stones are made when oxalate in the urine becomes overly concentrated, hooks up with calcium, and starts to crystallize. It is true that vitamin C, in certain forms and under certain conditions, can contribute to oxalate production. But here's what the proponents of this myth fail to disclose:

*The presence of high oxalate concentrations ALONE is NOT sufficient to create kidney stones.*

In addition, they also fail to mention that there are well over 50 different documented risk factors that also contribute to increased oxalate formation *(see Resource E for a list)*.

But the quantity of oxalate generated by a given substance or health condition is ***not*** the issue. The real question is whether there is a genuine risk of *kidney stone formation* from vitamin C intake.  Several small studies say the risk is real. However, this conclusion is typically reached by comparing the amount of oxalate excretion in the urine with and without vitamin C supplementation.

Although at first glance this approach may seem logical, it is greatly flawed! That's because oxalate excretion and kidney stone formation are not equivalent. For example, pregnant women in their third trimester maintain ***supersaturated*** levels of oxalate in the urine and yet the incidence of kidney stones is the ***same*** as in the general population.[24]

What was needed was a large-scale study that actually measured the incidence of kidney stones — not excreted oxalates — in relation to ingested vitamin C. Fortunately, such a study was conducted by Harvard Medical School, keeping it from being automatically undermined and discredited. A large population of women (85,557 to be exact) with no history of kidney stones was monitored for 14 years. The researchers concluded that "***vitamin C intake was not associated with risk***" of kidney stone formation and advised "***routine restriction of vitamin C to prevent stone formation appears unwarranted.***"[25]

Previously, another large-scale study found that "the intake of high doses of vitamin C does not increase the risk of calcium oxalate kidney stones." In fact, the members of the group with the highest vitamin C intake "***had a lower risk of kidney stones***" than those with the lowest intake.[26]

Finally, high-dose vitamin C has been administered all over the globe for decades with no noticeable increase in the incidence of kidney stones.[27]

## Lie #5: Vitamin C Needs Are Met with Normal Dietary Intake

Since the medical community defines vitamin C as the trace nutrient that prevents the deficiency disease known as scurvy, it is easy for them to accept and perpetuate this myth. Indeed, 75 to 90 mg of vitamin C per day will prevent the development of overt scurvy in most people. Since scurvy is extremely rare in this country it is presumed that the general population — most of which does not supplement with vitamin C — is getting enough of this substance in their daily food intake.

For a person in their early 20s with

- A diet free from fried, sugary, refined, or processed foods, or food tainted with pesticides, herbicides, hormones, antibiotics, artificial sweeteners, artificial colors, etc.

- Healthy teeth and gums with no fillings or root canals

- No exposure to lead, cadmium, mercury or other toxic metals

- No exposure to poisonous chemicals or vapors from paint, solvents, petroleum fuels, or vehicular emissions

- No ingestion of drugs (prescription, over-the-counter, legal or illegal)

- No tobacco use or alcohol intake

- Freedom from infection, acute and chronic (including colds, flu, acne, yeast)

- No wounds or scars

the case might be made that 75 to 90 mg is sufficient.

But each of these and other factors consume serum and tissue levels of vitamin C at a very fast rate. In addition, the body also needs vitamin C for many metabolic processes, maintenance of the immune system, proper collagen formation, and for keeping the "glue" (ground substance) intact that holds the cells of the body together.

No evidence exists indicating someone who lived in a nontoxic utopia free of infections would be protected from developing chronic, degenerative disease by a 75 to 90 mg daily intake of vitamin C. However, much evidence indicates that multi-gram daily doses of vitamin C can do exactly this, even in the highly toxic world of today.

Vitamin C will prevent, mitigate, and/or cure a myriad of infectious diseases, toxic poisonings, coronary heart disease, cancer, and a host of chronic degenerative diseases — as shown by the hundreds of studies referenced in this book. If the evidence has merit, then the real proof of vitamin C sufficiency would be a pronounced lack of all these diseases and conditions. I contend that the pandemic incidence of heart disease, cancer, diabetes, Alzheimer's disease, cataracts, periodontal disease, pneumonia, staph infections, strep infections, etc... is evidence that the world population is dangerously deficient in vitamin C. Since everyone seems to have a chronic illness, it must be normal, right?

## Lie #6: High Doses of Vitamin C Only Make Expensive Urine

This untruth is similar to the previous myth. It attempts to make people feel foolish for supplementing with vitamin C. In other words, "the vitamin C you just excreted into the toilet is proof that your body didn't need it!"

This is more flawed logic. The argument falsely assumes several things:

- Kidneys only excrete substances when their concentration exceeds the body's need
- Supply of a diet- or supplement-delivered substance is distributed throughout the body in accordance with need

- Nutrient deficiencies occur evenly throughout the body and are never localized in a particular area
- Vitamin C is expensive

Each of these assumptions will be addressed separately...

**Assumption:** *Kidneys only excrete substances when their concentration exceeds the body's need.*

**Rebuttal:** This would be convenient for clinicians if true. But it is not. Even healthy kidneys will continue to waste some essential electrolytes (sodium, calcium, magnesium) when the tissue and blood concentrations of these minerals are dangerously low. Diabetics know that glucose often spills into their urine — even as their cells are starving for it. This certainly does not mean the cells have all the glucose they need.

**Assumption:** *Supply of a diet- or supplement-delivered substance is distributed throughout the body in accordance with need.*

**Rebuttal:** All substances, regardless of the method of administration (*sublingual, oral, intramuscular, intravenous, etc.*), enter the body at specific points and circulate to other areas from there. Depending on factors like the distance from the entry point, the substance's access to receptor sites, and the ability of particular cells to absorb the substance (regardless of need), some areas may get enough and others may remain deficient. For example, in chronic periodontal disease, a localized vitamin C deficiency in the gums exists even when other areas of the body do not share that deficiency.

**Assumption:** *Nutrient deficiencies occur evenly throughout the body and are never localized in a particular area.*

**Rebuttal:** It is almost too obvious to mention, but the brain and liver need lots of essential fatty acids; the bones do not. Muscles have much different nutrient needs than nerves. Eyes have a greater need for vitamin A than ears. In addition, an infected, ingrown toenail has a greater need for vitamin C than any non-infected tissue. Because the general needs for each substance in the body vary and because the specific needs change with the dynamic nature of different disease and toxin challenges, nutrient deficiencies can often have a very localized nature.

**Assumption:** *Vitamin C is expensive.*

**Rebuttal:** Are you kidding? Compared to what? A round of chemotherapy... open-heart surgery... amputating your foot... blood pressure medication... Is ten cents of vitamin C in my urine expensive?

## Lie #7: If Vitamin C Worked, We Would All Be Using It

Yet another dose of circular nonsense! In other words, those who spew this foolishness are saying, "Here's proof it doesn't work — the doctors in my physician fraternity don't use it."

When asked "how many vitamin C infusions have you administered?" the reply is "none!"

"Why?" we ask.

"It doesn't work!" they retort.

"How do you know it doesn't work if you haven't tried it?" we query.

"If it worked, we would all be using it!" they exclaim.

"Did you see the miraculous response to vitamin C in the Allan Smith case?"

"That wasn't vitamin C!" they say.

"How do you know?"

"Because vitamin C doesn't work, if it did, we'd all be using it!"

No they wouldn't! Even when they see results with their own eyes, they can't accept it! The evidence is overwhelming to anyone who looks at it with an open mind. The medical community has continued to stonewall the use of vitamin C for decades because it doesn't fit into their "treat but don't cure" model. That will change only when patients begin to push for an honest appraisal of vitamin C and its unequalled benefits. The new age of information access on the internet prevents anyone, including doctors, from controlling who reads what. The truth eventually becomes known.

If the reader has any doubts about the veracity of the preceding dialogue, it is recommended that he obtain and watch the *60 Minutes* DVD, "Living Proof!" (see the last page of this book for details on how to obtain the DVD).

## What About Negative Studies?

With over 50,000 published studies and counting, it's no surprise that some reach conclusions other than what has been presented thus far.

However, the vast majority of "negative" studies are only negative in the sense that vitamin C was determined to be ineffective. Often conclusions are so broad they leave out important facts. Instead of conveying a dose-specific truth such as, "A daily vitamin C dose of 50 mg was found to be ineffective in the treatment of lung cancer," the researchers and media will convey what is effectively a lie by saying, "Vitamin C is ineffective in the treatment of lung cancer."

Since successful treatment is ALWAYS dose-dependent, this omission of dose in the conclusion is misleading at best, and basically dishonest. Let's say a study shows 500 mg of aspirin is successful at abating a headache for 100 adult women. What if the makers of acetaminophen decided to discredit the study by testing 15 mg of aspirin with 20,000 women? The larger study would be more impressive and would get more media attention. The headline would read "Study with 20,000 women shows aspirin ineffective for headache treatment." The unethical nature of this strategy is obvious. Does this happen? Yes! And frequently.

Research can be defective in another way. In one study, in an effort to "prove" vitamin C reduces the effectiveness of chemotherapeutic drugs in cancer treatment,[28] the researchers did not even use a legitimate form of vitamin C! A reviewer of the study pointed out that dehydroascorbic acid was used instead of vitamin C.[29] Dehydroascorbic acid is the oxidized (expended) form of vitamin C just as rust is the oxidized form of iron. Anyone familiar with the chemical structure of vitamin C should have known this. One can only speculate as to whether the researchers were intellectually challenged, ethically challenged, or both.

Although I am not directly making an accusation of malicious activity, the Allan Smith case gives a great deal of reason to wonder. The attending physicians recommended Allan "be allowed to die." These doctors were also in "unanimous agreement vitamin C would be of no benefit." Even so, they agreed to placate the family with a 2-day trial. Allan was given 100 grams per day and "miraculously" recovered to the point of removing him from the ECMO external lung machine.

Then, without explanation, the vitamin C was discontinued. Upon protest from the family, the treatment was resumed, but at only *two grams per day*. Why resume the vitamin C at such a low dose? Is it really possible the doctors wanted Mr. Smith to resume his downward spiral so that it could be said he died in spite of receiving vitamin C, without reference to the tiny size of the dose?

From my own experience, exhaustive research in the medical literature, and through consultation with doctors in this country and throughout the world, I am absolutely convinced of one thing — when enough vitamin C is given, in the right form, and for a long enough time, vitamin C helps virtually every condition, resolves many of them, and prevents still others. Although I have not personally analyzed every negative study, the ones that I have reviewed use very inadequate quantities of vitamin C, or they are clearly flawed in some other way. Furthermore, I have never found a single article showing properly dosed and administered vitamin C to fail to improve the status of a toxic or infected patient.

## Conclusion

All the objections against using vitamin C are clearly myths that are easily debunked. The resistance from the "traditional" medical community against vitamin C will not be so easily thwarted. Trillions of dollars per year are dependent upon maintenance of the status quo. Decades of propaganda have blinded physicians and patients to the truth. Unfortunately, millions of lives — and even the financial solvency of our nation — are in the balance. The time has come for people to insist on science-based medicine structured to improve the health of patients rather than a "tradition-based" medicine intent on boosting the bottom line of huge, multi-national pharmaceutical corporations. If you still believe that the primary focus of "traditional" medicine is patient-centered, read on...

## Chapter Eight

## High-Dose Vitamin C: Revolution Required

# Are profits more important than people?

It is a dangerous fantasy to believe that the U.S. Food and Drug Administration (FDA) vigilantly watches for, and effectively protects us from, the threat of unsafe foods and drugs. The actual record shows a much different reality — either the FDA is grossly incompetent or it has another agenda. Or maybe some of both?

The Fact is: FDA-approved drugs kill! Even when used as directed, adverse reactions to FDA-approved drugs was the **4th leading cause of death** in the United States in 1998.[1] In that same year, 2.2 million Americans were hospitalized for adverse drug reactions.[2]

By law, all adverse drug reactions must be reported to the FDA *(Code of Federal Regulations, Title 21)*, but for some reason summary statistics are conspicuously absent from the public record— my exhaustive search for this data found nothing after 1998. Rest assured, this lack of visibility is not because these deaths have diminished.

From 1994 to 2005 prescription use in the United States rose nearly 71%.[3] Deaths from adverse reactions have increased as well. Consider the multiple warnings receiving national media attention over drugs like Vioxx, Darvon, Darvocet, and Avandia — as well as the many advertisements recruiting victims for class action suits against drug companies. So again, why this lack of visibility? Is the FDA protecting the public or the pharmaceutical industry by not fully informing the public about the many adverse reactions to so many toxic prescription drugs?

Compare this with official statistics concerning the safety of nutritional supplements. The last five annual reports from the Centers for Disease Control show *NO DEATHS* attributed to vitamin supplements.[4-8] In fact, the safety record of vitamin C in particular is so impeccable that it is impossible to find statistical data that justifies *any* suggestion of health risk. And yet, in spite of its stellar safety record, the FDA aggressively restricts and/or prevents its use for the treatment of disease. For example, it is against the law for a vitamin C seller to make even minimally suggestive health claims like "vitamin C may help reduce symptoms of the flu."

This all begs the question: Why does the FDA approve numerous toxic drugs that kill patients while it bans the medical use of completely nontoxic nutrients that heal them?

## Massive Conflicts of Interest

In theory, the FDA was established to protect the public from unsafe food and dangerous drugs. At its inception, the FDA's sole employer — the public — paid for its services through taxes. Although conflicts of interest have existed from the beginning, Congress opened up what has turned out to be a huge channel for corruption when it passed the **Prescription Drug User Fee Act** in 1992.

Until that time the FDA was presumably shielding us from overly aggressive, profit-driven, pharmaceutical companies. But this new law (instigated and backed by the companies posing the danger) established drug companies as the FDA's best customers.

Because of this Act, deep-pocketed pharmaceutical companies were able to put their new drug applications on the approval "fast track" for a small "user fee." In fiscal year

2010, the established "user fee" for drugs requiring clinical data was $1,405,500 per application. The total in "user fees" collected by the FDA from pharmaceutical companies in 2010 was $569,207,000![9]

If a company finds that the FDA is not providing favorable service, it can avoid paying the "user fee" altogether by simply avoiding the "fast track" submission. This structure compels the FDA to provide favorable rulings to those paying "user fees" or risk losing a massive portion of its funding. The sheer volume of this Big Pharma stipend has the FDA addicted to "user fees."

Anyone who says that a "fast track" drug approval application — with a $1.4 million check attached — *doesn't* receive a more favorable ruling is just not paying attention. Yet as outrageous as this is, the corrupt dealings between the FDA and drug companies go far beyond "user fees."

Sales of food and drugs account for about 25% of the entire U.S. economy, underscoring the incredible financial impact that the FDA wields with its virtually unrestricted regulatory control. What strategies might a profit-hungry company executive employ to obtain the sole marketing rights for a billion-dollar drug? Thieves steal and kill for paltry sums of money every day. It is not hard to see how the potential for billions could minimize the attention paid to serious drug-induced side effects. One thing is for sure, billions of dollars continue to fill pharmaceutical coffers while hundreds of thousands of Americans needlessly suffer and die to generate that money.

Because there are men who might be tempted to overlook adverse drug reactions with the lure of huge profits, how unfortunate is it that the FDA's drug approval protocol provides a perfect cover for this criminal activity? At first glance it makes sense that the FDA would employ "experts" to help make policy and approve drugs. Perhaps, it's even understandable that these advisors are recruited from pharmaceutical researchers, pharmaceutical consultants, and even former pharmaceutical executives.

The real problem is that official FDA policy allows these advisors to have a continuing financial interest (consulting fees, stock ownership, etc.) in the companies that are submitting new drugs for approval. Any way you look at it, this arrangement cannot be considered anything other than a classical conflict of interest, regardless of the motives of the people involved.

## How Prevalent are these "Conflicts of Interest"?

A *USA Today* analysis of financial conflicts at FDA advisory committee meetings for an 18-month period provides a shocking picture. Out of 159 meetings covered, the following financial conflicts of interest were discovered:

- 146 meetings (92%) — at least one of the advisors had a conflict[10]
- 57 meetings (36%) — over 90% of the advisors present had a conflict of interest[10]
- 102 meetings (64%) — 33% of the advisors had a conflict and they determined the fate of a particular drug[10]

Imagine that a pharmaceutical company is presenting a new chemotherapy drug to a panel of experts and a third of them are either paid consultants or own stock in the presenting company or a close competitor. Is it even possible that such a "panel" of experts with a considerable financial interest in the decision is going to render a totally unbiased opinion?

This unholy FDA/pharmaceutical alliance has absolutely nothing to do with protecting the public, which is purportedly the primary reason that the FDA exists. Purposely allowing such a biased jury of investors to reign supreme when the decisions involve billions of dollars and affect the health and lives of millions, crosses all moral boundaries. The dismissive attitude toward the high death rate from adverse drug reactions is not so hard to understand after all!

## Why the FDA and Their Drug Company Clients Hate Food Supplements

Pharmaceutical companies reap profits that would make anyone, including oil companies, jealous. That's because they enjoy a monopoly that is unique to the drug industry. Here's how it works:

1) Find a natural substance that provides health benefits

2) Chemically alter the substance so that it can qualify for a patent (This is because natural substances cannot be patented — and often it is this altering process that makes drugs toxic)

3) Patent the new drug and get it approved by the FDA

4) Create demand by advertising your new drug to doctors and patients

5) Charge whatever price you feel the market will bear because no one else can sell the newly patented drug for a full 20 years

It is quite true that this drug development/approval process takes years and millions of dollars. But the prize of a 20-year run of annual sales in the hundreds of millions makes the effort worthwhile.

On the other hand, a substance like vitamin C that can render better results — without side effects — for a fraction of the cost puts the whole drug/money-making monopoly in jeopardy. Studies cited in previous chapters clearly indicate that the incidence of heart disease, strokes, cancer, and chronic degenerative diseases could drop by 50% or more if the entire population was taking high-dose vitamin C. It is extremely doubtful that the current pharmaceutical industry could survive such a bitter pill.

So, when a nutrient, like high-dose vitamin C, clearly has the potential to eliminate much of the enormous revenues of a whole host of drugs, wouldn't there be a tremendous temptation to discredit, disparage, and even destroy such a threat? Certainly the spawning and spreading of "Lies that Kill" (*see Chapter Seven*) would be a powerful strategy.

Because Big Pharma has huge amounts of money at its fingertips, they fight the war on many fronts, including influencing public opinion. Drug companies spend billions on medical school scholarships and research grants. Billions are also spent on advertising (TV, newspaper, magazines, as well as ads in peer-reviewed journals). No matter how benevolent the advertising appears, this money directly and indirectly influences medical school curricula, health news content, researchers and research directions, popular opinion, the way doctors practice medicine, and the way the FDA processes new drug applications.

Might this huge pharmaceutical industry influence explain why medical school students get almost no training in nutrition? Might it also explain why thousands of studies showing the effectiveness of vitamin C are totally ignored by the "gold standards" of medical information for physicians, like the primary textbooks of medicine, *Cecil Medicine* and *Harrison's Principles of Internal Medicine*?

In a world where money talks, the drug propaganda machine is understandable but never forgivable. Real abuse of power with criminal intent is evident as one considers that FDA officials have been charged and gone to jail for the commission of felonies in the granting of approvals for drugs or medical devices for monetary gain. A simple Yahoo!® or Google® search for "FDA conflicts of interest" will provide examples of these approval-for-sale wrongdoings by the FDA.

However, conflict of interest misdeeds don't stop or even slow at simple bribery. The Big Pharma-controlled FDA has a history of blatant Gestapo-style "enforcement" activities that occurs purely for the protection of Big Pharma's turf. Some of these actions of our pro-pharmaceutical government against the public are so terrifying that it is hard to believe that they still occur in freedom-loving America.

Although it does not involve vitamin C in any way, the following well-documented account reveals just one of the covert operations deployed by the Big Pharma-FDA alliance. The actions taken against a brilliant physician and the American people by the FDA, the National Cancer Institute, a huge drug company, and the Texas Medical Board of Examiners are downright wicked. The following account is fully documented in official government records — it is frightening, but completely true!

## *The Unholy War Against a Nontoxic Cancer Cure that Actually Works*

Stanislaw Burzynski, MD, PhD, is a doctor and biochemist who was able to do what over $5 billion per year in taxes — carelessly tossed to the National Cancer Institute — was unable to do: find a cure for cancer.

As he was earning his doctorate in biochemistry, Dr. Burzynski discovered that there were some proteins and amino acids absent in the urine and blood of people with cancer that were present in healthy people. He theorized that cancer patients might be helped through the administration of the compounds he calls *antineoplastons*. Over time, he was able to test his theory.

Truly miraculous results followed. So miraculous in fact, that in 1977 he retained legal council in his home state of Texas to determine if he could establish his own cancer research institute. The lawyers determined and the state courts confirmed that as long as he performed his research within Texas state lines the federal government, including the FDA, had no jurisdiction. It is more than revealing in itself that Dr. Burzynski sought to avoid future legal intrusions into his clinic before they ever occurred.

With that assurance and understanding, Burzynski set up a clinic and began to treat patients with his antineoplastons. People with incurable cancers were going into remission, quickly, thoroughly, and without side effects. As his fame grew, people started coming from all over the globe to receive treatment. Many cancer patients who were deemed terminal and incurable were often cured. Then the most incredible nightmare for Dr. Burzynski began.

In 1983, the FDA filed a civil action against Dr. Burzynski demanding that his activities be curtailed. Prior to the end of the trial the FDA sent a threatening letter to the judge stating the FDA would be forced to use "more severe and less efficient remedies" to stop him if the court failed to do so. Even though the court ruled in Burzynski's favor, FDA attorneys boasted, "we have other ways to get him."

With obvious pressure from the FDA, the Texas State Board of Medical Examiners began to send investigators to the homes of Burzynski's former patients — even as far away as California — in an attempt to get them to file complaints against him. In spite of the huge number of patients visited, their efforts failed.

In 1985, any inquirers asking the FDA about Dr. Burzynski were told that he was under criminal investigation. Eventually a judge issued a cease and desist order against the FDA along with a firm reprimand for this obvious attempt to destroy Dr. Burzynski's reputation. Later that year, the FDA raided Dr. Burzynski's clinic and seized over 200,000 pages of research documents, along with all of his patient records. A few months later, the FDA convened a grand jury in an attempt to bring an indictment against Dr. Burzynski. The grand jury found no wrongdoing and refused to permit the filing of any formal charges against him.

A year later, the FDA conducted another raid on the clinic and seized another 100,000 pages of research documents and patient records. Soon after, the FDA convened another grand jury. The jury again found no wrongdoing and refused to indict Burzynski.

In May of 1986, due to outside pressure (most believe from the FDA), the Texas State Board of Medical Examiners informed Dr. Burzynski that, although there had been *no complaints*, they were starting an investigation and he might want to retain legal council. Subsequently, the Board called him in and tried to persuade him to cease his activities. In November, the Board requested patient records to show efficacy of his treatments. They promised to leave him alone if a board of oncologists found that his therapies were helping people. In good faith, Dr. Burzynski agreed and submitted more than double the documentation requested.

Nearly two years later, in 1988, the Texas State Board of Medical Examiners disallowed all Dr. Burzynski's documentation and filed a charge that he was in violation of Section 3.08, Paragraph (4)(A) of the law stating it was "grounds to cancel, revoke or suspend" his medical license. Two years later, in 1990, the Board filed an amended complaint with virtually *identical* charges. Again the court found no wrongdoing, and no action against his medical license was taken.

In the same year, the FDA convened a third grand jury. At the same time, the FDA began to contact suppliers and others associated with the clinic stating that Dr. Burzynski was under grand jury investigation. No wrongdoing was found, and still no formal charges were filed. Nevertheless, the FDA continued to investigate and harass Burzynski for the next two years.

The Texas State Board of Medical Examiners filed a second amended complaint against Dr. Burzynski on August 14, 1992. Again the court found him not guilty. In January of the following year, 60 of Dr. Burzynski's patients petitioned the Texas State Board of Medical Examiners to stop harassing him. Almost immediately, the Board requested that the patients' petitions be stricken from the record.

A few months later the case went to trial. During this trial Nicholas J. Patronas, M.D., a board-certified radiologist, professor of radiology at Georgetown University, and both Founder and Chief of Neuroradiology at the National Cancer Institute voluntarily flew to Texas to testify on the doctor's behalf. Under oath he stated that Dr. Burzynski's antineoplaston therapy was *safe and effective* against brain cancer. At the conclusion of the trial the judge ruled in Dr. Burzynski's favor finding that the Board did not introduce any competent or substantial evidence that his therapy was not safe or effective.

The FDA convened a fourth grand jury in 1994! Once again, no credible basis for formal charges could be found.

Because Dr. Burzynski was now getting national attention, "CBS This Morning" invited the doctor and three of his patients on the program to tell their stories. That same afternoon the FDA again raided Dr. Burzynski's office, took more documents, and issued more subpoenas. A few days later, the FDA subpoenaed medical records of all patients who had appeared on TV regarding Dr. Burzynski's treatments.

At about this same time the Texas State Board of Medical Examiners appealed the earlier decision. The judge again ruled in Dr. Burzynski's favor.

Finally, due to much public outcry on Dr. Burzynski's behalf, a Congressional Subcommittee Hearing convened to review his case. During the hearing, dozens of Dr. Burzynski's patients testified of cures they had received and pleaded against the FDA's continued harassment. The committee members could not understand why the FDA had called so many grand juries and even suggested that the FDA had a vendetta against Dr. Burzynski.

Undeterred, the FDA convened a *fifth* grand jury in March of 1995. At no point did the FDA claim that Dr. Burzynski's cancer treatments were not safe or that they did not work. The only complaint was that the treatments were **unapproved**. At this point, they were able to get the judge to agree that the jury would not be allowed to hear any testimony about the safety of antineoplastons and that no evidence of their ability to cure cancer could be presented.

With these restrictions, the grand jury finally issued indictments for 75 counts of violating federal law and fraud. If convicted, the law would slap Dr. Burzynski with a maximum of 290 years in a federal prison and $18,500,000 in fines.

At the same time, the Texas State Board of Medical Examiners appealed their complaint to the Texas Supreme Court. Although no wrongdoing was cited, the judges put Dr. Burzynski on a 10-year probation.

Later in 1996 Congress convened another subcommittee hearing and asked the FDA to accept all of Burzynski's patients into a series of FDA-supervised Phase II clinical trials. The FDA agreed. Even so, the FDA continued its prosecution of Dr. Burzynski on the basis of the previous grand jury indictment. And again, an attorney for the FDA stated that, "Whether antineoplastons do or do not work is not an issue... and the jury should not be asked to decide the question." The judge caved.

In spite of the unfair stipulations of the trial, Dr. Burzynski was acquitted on 42 of the 75 charges against him. A mistrial was called for the remaining counts. Shortly thereafter, pressure from Congress and the public forced the FDA to drop all but one of the remaining charges. Later that year, Dr. Burzynski was acquitted of the final charge against him.

Unfortunately, this Gestapo-like campaign cost the American taxpayer (at least what the FDA reported) $60 million and piled $2.2 million in legal fees on Burzynski. Thankfully, an outraged public helped cover his legal fees. All of this money would have been much better spent in a grant to further Burzynski's research.

And yet, the story doesn't end here. In fact, it gets *more* horrifying...

During this entire ordeal, the National Cancer Institute (NCI), (*like the FDA, the National Cancer Institute is part of the U.S. Department of Health and Human Services*) had established an agreement with Dr. Burzynski to test his antineoplaston therapies. In an apparent attempt to discredit the treatment, the NCI altered the protocols by using doses that were much too small and by enlisting patients who had cancers that were far worse than the testing protocol specified. Logic would dictate that this was done *intentionally* in order to destroy Dr. Burzynski's credibility, as the tiny doses employed were clearly unable to prevent the death of any of the patients in the trial.

Unfortunately, there is even more perverse intrigue and corruption that won't be disclosed here. The entire story has been recorded in a movie-length documentary called *Burzynski*. Interested readers are encouraged to see the complete documentation of what has been reported thus far and the rest of the story at www.burzynskimovie.com.

The truth is, Burzynski's antineoplastons cured many cancers, even those considered untreatable by their oncologists! Not even the federal government disputes that fact. It is also true that chemotherapy drugs have collectively generated **trillions** of dollars in revenue since their inception. In general, they do not cure cancer, and they have terrible side effects. To maintain their lucrative monopolies, Big Pharma, the FDA, and the National Cancer Institute simply have to protect the cancer drug business. As shown in the preceding story, they will go to very great lengths to keep a legitimate cancer cure away from the public.

Millions upon millions have died who could have been cured during the 28 years that the FDA — in an attempt to protect the pharmaceutical industry's wildly profitable cancer cartel — tried to lock Dr. Burzynski away forever. This is far beyond criminal. In any other context, causing the death of millions of people is called *GENOCIDE*!

In spite of all this and against all odds, antineoplastons successfully completed the FDA Phase II Clinical Trials and have now entered the final set of trials before gaining approval. If the FDA, National Cancer Institute, and Big Pharma can be kept under control, most radiation and chemotherapy, with all of their toxic side effects, will be replaced by real cures such as antineoplastons and vitamin C.

Unfortunately the battle is far from over. An international treaty, already ratified, is working against natural medicine and causing the federal government to give the FDA even more money and much more power.

## Codex Alimentarius: High-Dose Vitamin C Banned via International Treaty

In December of 2009 the United States became a member of Codex Alimentarius (Latin for "food law"). This treaty was conceived, drafted, and pushed by international pharmaceutical companies and agricultural chemical conglomerates through the World Trade Organization (WTO), which is a part of the United Nations. The stated purpose for the law is to standardize the "farm-to-fork" production — growing, pesticide residues, veterinary drugs, contaminants, food harvesting, food hygiene, food preparation, packaging, labeling, presentation, and marketing rules — for *all* food, food additives, drugs, herbs, and food supplements worldwide.

According to the U.S. Constitution, treaties take precedence over any and all national, state, county, or municipal laws. As a member of this treaty, the United States must "harmonize" its laws to comply with the standards established by Codex Alimentarius (Codex) or face fines and penalties payable to the WTO.

Among many other frightening standards to be imposed through Codex, the treaty will control supplement dosage sizes. For example, the dosage size of vitamin C will not be allowed to exceed 200 mg. A vitamin C supplement that delivers more than the stated dosage will be considered to be a drug, and assuming that it can eventually receive FDA drug approval, will have to be prescribed by a doctor and purchased at a pharmacy. All of these legal manipulations decrease the availability while increasing the price of vitamin C or any other targeted nutrient.

On January 4, 2011, in a move toward U.S. compliance with Codex, President Obama signed one of dozens of laws headed our way: The FDA Food Safety Modernization Act. This law gives the FDA *more* authority. And, in response, the FDA has already called for $100,000,000 in "user fees" (*a.k.a., bribes?*) to fund its enforcement.

Remember, this is just the first of many laws — each one awarding the corrupt and metastasizing FDA more regulatory and enforcement power — that the U.S. must establish in order to "harmonize" with Codex.

Although the FDA Food Safety Modernization Act does not address food supplements specifically, in the near future laws will need to be implemented that do match the Codex standard. ***This means that ultimately vitamin C supplements over 200 mg will be illegal.*** This is already the case in several European countries.

For those who think it can't happen here, consider this...

## *Living Proof, Vitamin C, McGuff, and the FDA*

As referenced in Chapter One, *60 Minutes* in New Zealand produced a documentary about the miraculous recovery of Allan Smith from swine flu, white-out pneumonia, and hairy cell leukemia. "Living Proof?" was first aired in the summer of 2010.

The news program revealed the decision by the hospital staff to allow Mr. Smith to die upon removal from life support. Caving to intense pressure from the family, the hospital reluctantly agreed to administer high-dose intravenous vitamin C. As part of the documentary, the scene cut to a picture of a vial of vitamin C — the same brand that the hospital used in the treatment. The manufacturer's name, McGuff Pharmaceuticals, Inc., was clearly evident on the vial. After many battles with doctors and hospitals to continue the vitamin C therapy, the man who was supposed to be dead totally recovered from all of his illnesses and resumed normal life.

This revealing and moving documentary was so popular that it soon appeared on several internet sites. Links on many more sites sent people to places where "Living Proof?" could be viewed — and millions of people did.

Then, in a letter to McGuff dated December 28, 2010, the FDA banned any further mass production of its vitamin C formulations. Why? Was it to protect all the patients who might be at risk of being cured or to protect Big Pharma from a potential loss of revenue? Or was it to "protect" so many patients from the benefits of high-dose vitamin C?

## New Zealand: First Victory in the High-Dose Vitamin C Revolution

Regardless of its complicity in stopping the intravenous vitamin C therapy on Allan Smith after a dramatic improvement had already been seen, the treating hospital in New Zealand deserves some credit. It actually allowed the vitamin C to be given in the first place! To my knowledge, the administration of high-dose intravenous vitamin C still has not occurred in a *single* hospital in the United States. Many private clinics, yes; a single hospital, no.

Because of the *60 Minutes* documentary, "Living Proof?," New Zealand patients can now request its use in their treatments. Nevertheless, a great deal of fighting with doctors and hospitals still must precede all such vitamin C infusions. In September of 2010, a New Zealand citizens group, "Vitamin C Can Cure," invited me to speak to them about vitamin C, the massive evidence for its efficacy, and their legal rights in its application.

The groundswell is building and a similar movement is now spreading in Australia. However these important advances only happen when enough people demand it. Massive pressure needs to be brought to bear on politicians by informed citizens. Otherwise, vitamin C will remain just another trace ingredient in your morning cereal and other processed foods. You won't get scurvy, but you will still be at risk for scores of other diseases.

The U.S. Congress needs to hear from an electorate that will not tolerate the current direction of health law. Here are some suggestions:

- Experts with ANY conflict of interest should not be allowed to participate in related FDA approvals or policy-making at any time

- The FDA should not be able to arbitrarily and capriciously search and seize supplements and office records without well-defined due process and a warrant

- The FDA should be prevented from legal harassment (for example, one grand jury acquittal should be the end of the matter)

- Funds should be diverted from the National Cancer Institute and the FDA to establish an Institute of Natural Health that would be directed by science-based physicians who can cite the evidence establishing that natural foods and supplements can heal

- The safety and use of natural medicines and supplements should be regulated by this Institute of Natural Health

- The Institute of Natural Health would appropriate grants and establish reasonable protocols for determining the safety and efficacy of natural substances and therapies and approve them for medical use

Hopefully this book, and especially this chapter, is opening your eyes, giving you hope, and making you angry enough to tell others. For resources that can help in such a campaign, see the final page of this book.

With your help, we can make a difference and protect our rights to inexpensive and nontoxic therapies, like vitamin C.

Now let's discuss how to most effectively supplement with vitamin C...

## Chapter Nine

# Where do we go from here?

Vitamin C is uniquely suited to kill pathogens, neutralize toxins, and supercharge the immune system. It serves well in not only preventing cancer and heart disease, but also in treating, arresting, and even resolving pre-existing heart disease and cancer. Even when diseases are beyond the point of reversal and cure, vitamin C will always reduce symptomatology and improve the quality of life. It usually extends the length of life as well. Its antioxidant capabilities fight oxidative stress and the degenerative diseases caused by that stress in ways that put it in a class by itself. We know that people who have the highest levels of vitamin C have much lower mortality rates because it keeps them from getting sick in the first place.

## *Why is this One Substance so Effective and Important?*

Because the intended role of vitamin C has always been the *Primal Panacea*! Man's body was designed to function best with high blood and cellular levels of vitamin C — synthesized as needed by the liver. Due to an inborn error of metabolism, the vast majority of us no longer have the ability to make it, but that does not lessen our need for vitamin C or the benefits derived from it.

Unfortunately, the use of high-dose vitamin C is at cross-purposes with an industry that CANNOT EXIST without a chronically ill population.

Don't be fooled! The government and the traditional medical industry are looking for cures about as diligently as crack dealers search for a non-addictive form of cocaine. Even though the traditional medical world is starting to give lip service to "health and wellness," the truth is that sickness and disease pay the bills.

Think about it... what would happen if by some twist of fate the entire population suddenly became well for a period of time? Worker and student productivity would be at top levels because people would be healthy and feeling better than they have in years. But wait... all the hospital beds would be empty, the surgical suites dark, the pharmacy free of prescriptions, doctors idly sitting in their offices, and insurance clerks with nothing to do.

Yes, that's far-fetched and unrealistic. Yet, what if just 25% of the population was significantly healthier? How would that impact the medical system? One would hope it would rejoice — but it couldn't! Would any pharmaceutical company embrace a cure for heart disease or cancer when their financial existence depends on selling heart and cancer drugs?

How could the current medical establishment not see the *Primal Panacea* as a threat?

Fortunately for them, many people will never know about the power of high-dose vitamin C, and they will never avail themselves of its benefits. The myths will continue to circulate and the masses will continue to believe. But what about those of us who do know? We need to protect our freedoms by resisting attempts to make high-dose vitamin C illegal, and we need to learn the best ways to drink from this wonderful life-giving fountain.

You hold valuable information in your hands. This book is full of facts, evidence, studies, and a big dose of reality. Nothing here was intended to scare you, only to fully inform you. Together we can win the battle! But you will need your health and your strength to do so. You can start by optimizing your own vitamin C levels... here's how:

## *Optimizing Blood Levels of Vitamin C*

Vitamin C is the *Primal Panacea* — the primary defense in man's constant fight against toxins, pathogens, and oxidative stress. Because man must replace the vitamin C he once synthesized in abundance, this substance occupies an especially important position in the body's list of required nutrients.

Certainly humans have many other nutritional needs, but the body's intake requirements for most other micronutrients (vitamins, minerals, enzymes, and amino acids) and macronutrients (proteins, carbohydrates, fats) stay within more limited ranges.

Chapter 3 discussed the huge fluctuation in vitamin C production in C-synthesizing animals that occurs in response to their current toxic and pathogenic challenges. Man's need for vitamin C also varies greatly and in a range far above the government's RDA of 75 to 90 mg. The vitamin C starting point for healthy adults is approximately 6,000 mg and grows in proportion to their level of toxic exposure and the intensity of challenges to the immune system. It is a foregone conclusion that meeting this need solely through food intake is not possible.

Furthermore, the human digestive system is extremely inefficient at getting vitamin C into the bloodstream. This is yet more evidence of the importance of our lost ability to synthesize vitamin C. Studies show that as dose size increases, the percentage of vitamin C that gets into the blood dramatically decreases. One study found that around

19 mg of a 20 mg dose of water-soluble C made it into the bloodstream. As the dose sizes increased, however, that amount dropped precipitously.[1] Projections from the study's findings suggest that only 2,000 mg of a 12,000 mg dose will enter the bloodstream,[2] and delivering 3,000 mg of C into the bloodstream from a single ingested dose would be theoretically impossible.

This resistance to vitamin C assimilation from the digestive tract occurs because vitamin C (in all traditional tablets, capsules, liquids, and chewable forms) is absorbed by the body through a limited number of portals in the intestinal wall. Only one molecule of ascorbate can pass through a given portal at a time. So, at the point when all the portals are busy, any remaining unabsorbed vitamin C will pass on through to the colon and accumulate there. This is why the quantity of regular vitamin C the body can assimilate is so severely restricted.

Furthermore, this restriction explains the superiority of intravenous administration of vitamin C over traditional oral supplementation in the treatment of acute infectious diseases and severe toxin exposures. And on a practical note, bioavailability studies confirm improved absorption when daily vitamin C supplementation is broken into several smaller doses.

## The Monumental Breakthrough in High-Dose Vitamin C Supplementation

Frederick Klenner, MD, demonstrated the enormous therapeutic value of high-dose vitamin C in the treatment of an array of diseases and poisonings. When a patient's condition was critical, he often turned to massive doses given by intravenous infusion. He was so successful with this method that it quickly became the "gold standard" of vitamin C delivery.

Since Klenner's day, numerous variations of oral vitamin C supplement formulations (shape, size, additional ingredients, slight improvements in tableting processes, chewable, etc.) have entered the marketplace. But none of these significantly improved the bioavailability of oral vitamin C — that is, until vitamin C's marriage with liposome encapsulation science.

Liposomes were first discovered in the 1960s.[3] The science of liposome-enhanced bioavailability has enjoyed continued refinement during the last 50 years.[4] It rapidly became apparent that liposomes could envelop substances and enhance their delivery into the cells of the body. Because of its ability to dramatically increase the body's uptake of orally administered vitamin C, it has found a unique place in the realm of vitamin C supplementation. Liposome-encapsulated vitamin C has the convenience of an oral administration while offering a bioavailability technically superior even to C delivered by vein. In other words, an intravenous result delivered by mouth is now possible.

## What Are Liposomes?

When phospholipids (composed mainly of fatty acids) are placed in an aqueous solution under special conditions, their unique molecular structure forces them to form microscopic bubbles. These tiny spheres, called liposomes, have double-layered membranes almost identical to the bilayer membranes that surround most cells in the body. As liposomes are formed, they capture and enclose whatever was dissolved in the starting solution.

Because of their fatty acid composition, liposomes are not soluble in water and are not susceptible to breakdown in the stomach. Because of this composition — along with their infinitesimal size — liposomes can facilitate absorption of a large percentage of their encapsulated payloads before any significant enzymatic breakdown of the lipids takes place in the intestine.

As soon as they enter the small intestine, they slip through the intestinal wall without the need of the special molecular portals (receptor sites). Liposomes also penetrate cell walls in the same efficient manner. These and other properties make them ideal for carrying vitamin C (and many other water-soluble nutrients) into the blood and into cells.

## Bottom line:

### *Liposome-encapsulated vitamin C delivers intravenous impact in an oral form*

A peer-reviewed study demonstrated that liposome-encapsulated vitamin C was able to deliver roughly twice the maximum amount of vitamin C to the blood previously believed to be possible — even with spaced doses — of other more "traditional" forms of oral vitamin C.[5] My clinical experience with liposome-encapsulated vitamin C suggests that the clinical impact of liposome-encapsulated vitamin C may even exceed the clinical impact of intravenous vitamin C for some acute infections.

These findings do not negate the therapeutic importance of intravenous vitamin C. Clearly, when there is a clinical need to deliver a high dose of vitamin C quickly, as in a snakebite or barbiturate overdose, intravenous delivery is best. However, even in these situations, both routes of administration work synergistically in optimizing vitamin C's therapeutic benefits.

## *Determining Actual Vitamin C Need*

The human body has mechanisms for helping us determine our current need for vitamin C. Although far from perfect, one of these mechanisms — bowel tolerance — is a good starting point.

Often people who have used "megadoses" of traditional vitamin C to fight a cold or flu experience a watery diarrhea, called a C-flush. This phenomenon happens whenever a large amount of vitamin C is not absorbed in the small intestine. The unabsorbed C reaches the colon where it draws water into the bowels. A watery diarrhea naturally ensues, not as an adverse side effect, but simply because the intestines cannot handle the volume of water that the C draws into the large bowel.

The presence of a toxic or pathogenic challenge often increases bowel tolerance for ascorbate, most often in proportion to the severity of the challenge. In fact, Robert Cathcart, MD noted in his treatment of HIV/AIDS patients that bowel tolerance frequently rose to 75-100 grams per day, which is 20 to 50 times more than seen in healthy individuals.[6]

Another way to determine an optimum dose is simply by evaluation of bodily signals. When one doesn't "feel quite right," an increase in dose will usually be in order. If one reaches a sense of well-being and additional vitamin C does not produce any further improvement, the body's need has most likely been met.

For those with known C-deficiency diseases (like atherosclerosis, periodontal disease, cataracts, or osteoporosis) or continual toxic exposure (such as mercury-amalgam fillings, root canal-treated teeth, or toxic chemicals in the environment) upward adjustments in daily dose are also recommended.

## Practical Suggestions

Daily bowel tolerance dosing can be inconvenient and unpleasant, but a good strategy includes periodic utilization of this type of vitamin C supplementation to establish baseline need. A C-flush will cleanse the bowel and minimize its contribution to the body's toxin exposure as well. Once a month, or even once a week, take spaced doses of vitamin C powder dissolved in water until the onset of diarrhea. At this point a baseline dose can be determined, and the bowels will benefit from a healthy cleanse. Please note: Since the liposome formulation enjoys a nearly complete absorption, it will not cause a diarrheal flush.

When the baseline requirement is established, supplementation on subsequent days could include a combination of a liposomal formulation and sodium ascorbate powder or either type alone. Because liposome-encapsulated vitamin C is considerably more bioavailable than all other oral forms, especially as dose sizes increase, the following substitution schedule provides approximate values:

- 1,000 mg liposomal = 3,000 – 4,000 mg powder

- 2,000 mg liposomal = 8,000 – 10,000 mg powder

- 3,000 mg liposomal = 12,000 – 18,000 mg powder

The total daily dosage should be at least as much as determined by the last bowel tolerance result. Additional amounts often provide increased benefit.

Non-liposomal formulations of vitamin C abound. Without a lengthy discussion of each type, here are the main considerations. These forms are all water-soluble:

- Ascorbic acid powder is the least expensive form of vitamin C — because it is an acid, it is more likely to cause digestive stress

- Sodium ascorbate powder is inexpensive and easy to use — preferred over all other non-liposomal forms

- Ascorbyl palmitate is a fat-soluble form of vitamin C which gives a different absorption characteristic

- Bioflavonoids are good antioxidant nutrients — although they can help vitamin C improve the antioxidant capacity of the body, they are not necessary for this. A "natural vitamin C complex" is really just a marketing ploy that needlessly increases the price of vitamin C supplementation

- Ester C® is mainly composed of calcium ascorbate (which I do not recommend for other reasons) and may slightly improve absorption. The other components of Ester C® make it needlessly expensive

- Mineral forms: chromium ascorbate, magnesium ascorbate, manganese ascorbate, molybdenum ascorbate, potassium ascorbate, and zinc ascorbate present a problem because the associated minerals bring toxicities of their own to the table when used in the high dosages that you want to reach with your vitamin C supplementation. Avoid them except in lower doses.

Pills and capsules often contain non-nutritive fillers and ingredients that can add expense and adversely affect absorption. Also, liquid and chewable formulations may contain sugar — avoid them if possible.

In addition to direct supplementation with vitamin C, one can greatly improve its effectiveness by limiting the negative impact of toxins (*see Resource F*). Other nutrient supplementation can also be of substantial help (*see Resource G*).

## *Conclusion*

Supplementation of vitamin C is essential. It will protect people from dreaded pathogens, provide an inexpensive yet effective treatment for many diseases, and neutralize toxins of every kind. It can also provide an effective answer to some of the difficult challenges that currently threaten our nation. Good health and effective medicine do not have to bankrupt our system. People don't have to spend their last decades in line at the pharmacy picking up a handful of expensive maintenance prescriptions. The nursing home doesn't have to be the last stop before the grave. High-dose vitamin C, the **Primal Panacea**, can change these outcomes for a vast majority of people. Prove it for yourself — then share your discovery with others.

Special Resources

# For those who want more substantiation

# How vitamin C works

I fully appreciated vitamin C's ability to cure most infections, neutralize all toxins, and its effectiveness against many cancers long before I understood how it worked. And when supplemented correctly, I knew that it was probably the best way to forestall aging and prevent or slow most chronic degenerative diseases.

To be sure, the clinical responses to vitamin C therapy seemed nothing short of miraculous, especially to a traditionally-trained physician such as myself. Although I have no conflict with using any therapy that clearly benefits a patient and does no harm, I knew there was an underlying scientific mechanism to explain vitamin C's diverse abilities, and I had a driving curiosity to discover it.

It seemed logical to conclude there must be a final common pathway that allowed vitamin C to resolve or impede the impact of any infection or any toxin. This reasoning then posed the question:

- *What do all toxins and infections have in common?*

*The answer is as simple as it is elegant:*

- **All infections and all toxins cause their damage by increasing oxidative stress**

*No exceptions!* There is not a single infection (viral, bacterial, or other), or a single toxin, which does not generate substances known as "reactive oxygen species (ROS)."

Many ROS are free radicals, which are highly unstable molecules containing one or more unpaired electrons, causing them to always seek additional electrons. The addition of electrons "quenches" the free radical, causing it to become much more stable. Biochemical reactions nearly always seek to increase the chemical stability of the reacting molecules.

ROS can only do one thing (and they do it well), and that is to damage biological molecules by the process of *oxidation*. The same basic process that rusts away metal outside of the body breaks down biomolecules inside the body. Once a biomolecule is oxidized, its ability to do its job is compromised or eliminated completely, until it is chemically *reduced* (*the reverse of oxidation*) and thereby restored to its normal structure. So, the more oxidation (or "oxidative stress") is present in the tissues, the more abnormal that tissue will become over time.

So, what is oxidative stress? Let's start by understanding some basic terms.

> **Oxidation:** The process of a substance *losing* electrons
>
> **Reduction:** The process of a substance *gaining* electrons, or having them restored

All toxins are pro-oxidants, meaning they oxidize (or cause to be oxidized by ROS they generate) biomolecules, taking away enough of their electrons to impair or completely prevent their normal function.

All antioxidants reduce previously oxidized biomolecules, restoring electron content to the normal state, or they prevent normal biomolecules from becoming oxidized in the first place. When enough oxidized biomolecules are reduced back to their normal state, the tissue (or cell) involved can once again resume its normal functions.

It is also important to understand the difference between an *oxidized antioxidant* and a toxin. After all, when

vitamin C, or any other antioxidant, has donated its electrons, it is looking to take up electrons again to resume its
reduced, or active, state. So, what is the difference between a
toxin looking to take up electrons (oxidation) versus an oxidized antioxidant looking to take up electrons (oxidation)
in order to become a protective antioxidant again? Several
factors are involved:

1. A toxin strongly holds on to its electrons
   once it has oxidized something. In other
   words, once a toxin has taken the electrons
   away from a biomolecule (oxidation),
   it will **never** redonate the electrons to
   any other molecule seeking electrons. In
   other words, a toxin will never perform an
   antioxidant function, even if it has enough
   electrons to do so.

2. An antioxidant, such as vitamin C, is
   a classic **redox** (reduction-oxidation)
   molecule. This means that vitamin C
   is designed to take and give electrons
   repeatedly. When magnified millions of
   times, the vitamin C molecules actually
   promote electron **flow** through the cell
   by taking and giving electrons over and
   over again. A toxin, on the other hand, only
   **takes** and **keeps** the electrons it extracts
   from the molecules it oxidizes. By this
   mechanism, toxins **block** electron flow.

3. Toxins that have satisfied their hunger
   for electrons and are "relatively" inert,
   can exert additional "toxic" effects by
   **physically interfering** with the ability
   of normal biomolecules and normal
   cellular antioxidants to interact with
   each other. Most often this interference
   is simply a result of accumulation. If the
   toxin is not mobilized and excreted, it will

eventually accumulate and impair normal biomolecule function.

Vitamin C is an especially useful antioxidant since its simple chemical structure allows it access to nearly all parts of the body, including inside the cell as well as inside the cell's subcellular compartments.

Many toxins are ***directly*** pro-oxidant, meaning they oxidize biomolecules without any intermediate mechanisms. Vitamin C and other antioxidants can neutralize such toxins by directly donating their electrons, molecule for molecule, to those toxins. Such toxins are then "quenched," and no longer have the chemical ability to take electrons away from other molecules.

Other toxins are ***indirectly*** pro-oxidant, meaning they chemically interact with certain antioxidants, preventing them from doing their job and resulting in increased oxidative stress. Examples include heavy metals such as mercury and cadmium binding to sulfhydryl groups, as are found in many enzymes, amino acids, and antioxidants such as glutathione and N-acetylcysteine.

Regardless, whether directly or indirectly, all toxins cause excess oxidative stress, beyond what is produced in the course of normal metabolism. This can be couched in some basic laws of physiology:

- **Electrons are the fuel of life. The "combustion" of this fuel is simply the flow (exchange) of electrons by biomolecules**

- **All excess oxidative stress causes electron depletion and inhibits optimal electron flow**

- **All toxic effects are caused by excess oxidative stress**

That's it. There is no other way in which a toxin can be toxic beyond the impairment of electron supply and flow in the biomolecules of the affected tissues. And this is precisely why properly-dosed vitamin C, before the point of irreversible tissue damage, will neutralize the toxicity of *any* toxin exposure or poisoning encountered. It doesn't matter what chemical structure or molecular type the toxin is. Big, small, water-soluble, fat-soluble, ionic, neutral — it doesn't matter.

While all toxins have the same final common denominator of increased oxidative stress, it is the molecular structure of the toxin that determines its other known characteristics.

1. Water- or fat-solubility determines where the toxin will accumulate.

2. Molecular size determines access and ease of passage into different cells and tissue spaces.

3. The unique molecular structure, along with ionic charge or electrical neutrality, also determines where a toxin can go. These characteristics largely determine whether it tends to accumulate or whether it is more readily excreted and/or has access to endogenous chelators, such as glutathione transferases, or exogenous chelators that are administered.

4. More potent toxins can produce larger amounts of oxidative stress by generating ROS or free radicals that initiate oxidative *chain reactions*, rather than just producing increased ROS, molecule for molecule.

Therefore, any clinical poisoning or toxin exposure can be rapidly remedied by getting enough vitamin C (and other antioxidants as well) in the areas of toxin concentration as rapidly as possible. When this is achieved, health, at least in the short term, can always be restored.

Toxins that are difficult to reach and/or have already caused a great deal of damage when the vitamin C is first administered will be the most difficult to treat effectively. Also, when a toxin has an immediate and profound impact on biochemical pathways immediately critical to life (as with cyanide poisoning, for example), the patient may die before enough vitamin C can be administered. However, research shows that even with such profoundly toxic substances like cyanide, life can probably still be preserved if enough vitamin C and other antioxidants are present when the toxin is first encountered.

In the long term, after health has been acutely restored, other measures may need to be taken to optimize health. This would include any of a number of chelators or other measures known to support and increase the excretion of toxins. Furthermore, measures may need to be taken to lessen other new and/or ongoing toxin exposures, since all toxins have a cumulative effect in decreasing the overall antioxidant capacity of the body.

## Now, What About Infections?

In order to cure infections, an agent is needed to neutralize ongoing oxidative stress, repair oxidized molecules, and kill the pathogens, or at least render them more susceptible to eradication by a healthy immune system. Vitamin C does all of these things.

The effects of vitamin C on oxidation are noted above. Its effects in bolstering the immune system have been well documented in the scientific literature (*see Resource B*), including enhanced interferon production, enhanced natural killer cell activity, and stimulation of both T-lymphocyte and

B-lymphocyte production. However, it is what makes the pathogen proliferate that especially targets its demise.

Nearly all pathogens require large amounts of iron to thrive and multiply. Many effective antibiotics are actually iron chelators, removing readily accessible iron from the environment of the pathogens, slowing or stopping growth, and then allowing the immune system to kick in and finish the job.

Because of this absolute need for iron in order to thrive, infectious agents characteristically have relatively high concentrations of iron inside them. Furthermore, much of this iron is in an unbound, or reactive state. This presence of large amounts of reactive iron effectively places a **bullseye** on these microbes. Vitamin C helps load the arrows into the bow, as will be described below.

## Why Would Iron Facilitate Not Only the Growth of Pathogens But Also Their Death?

The answer is that iron is the ultimate double-edged sword. It is absolutely required for life, and, as it turns out, it is often also an absolute requirement for death (of cells). Just as iron is necessary for normal cell growth, it is also a critical component of programmed cell death.

Even the healthiest body or organism needs many cells to die on demand during the course of normal overall growth or just for the maintenance of a healthy state. Otherwise, a body would have no precise physical form or recognizable shape. A variation of the same mechanism that causes physiologically required cell death can also cause the death of a pathogen. It all depends upon the interrelationships among a few important factors.

A well-documented chemical reaction occurs whenever enough reactive iron and hydrogen peroxide get together inside the cell (or the pathogen). This is known as the **Fenton reaction**. This reaction involves the transfer of an electron from ferrous ion ($Fe^{2+}$) to hydrogen peroxide, generating a free radical known as the hydroxyl radical.

The hydroxyl radical will rapidly and irreversibly react with (oxidize) virtually *any* molecule in the body. The presence of the hydroxyl radical also facilitates the release of more reactive iron inside the cell which reacts with even more hydrogen peroxide — stimulating a self-sustaining oxidative chain reaction. That is why it is **the most toxic substance** known to science. The ability of hydrogen peroxide to kill bacteria has been shown to be directly dependent on the amount of hydroxyl radicals that are produced. Carbohydrates, RNA, DNA, lipids, and amino acids are all oxidized by the hydroxyl radical.

Finally, there exists no specific enzyme or enzymatic reaction that can neutralize the hydroxyl radical, meaning that the oxidative damage sustained by vital biomolecules is the *only* way to satisfy its hunger for electrons once it is produced.

All of this means that whenever the Fenton reaction is sufficiently activated by the presence of enough hydrogen peroxide and enough ferrous ions, cell (or pathogen) death will inevitably result. At least with regards to this Fenton reaction, the cell destined for programmed cell death and the rapidly dividing pathogen are very similar.

### How Does Vitamin C Fit into All of This?

The role of vitamin C in stimulating the Fenton reaction, also very well documented, occurs because the available unbound, or free, iron normally present inside the cell or pathogen is ferric ion ($Fe^{3+}$).

Ferric ion does not have an electron to donate to hydrogen peroxide, and no generation of hydroxyl radical occurs when only it and hydrogen peroxide are present. However, when vitamin C gets together with ferric ions, it readily converts (reduces) the $Fe^{3+}$ to $Fe^{2+}$ by the donation of an electron. The electron is then passed along to the hydrogen peroxide — producing the super-oxidizing hydroxyl radical. Note: it is still an antioxidant role (electron donation) by vitamin C that ultimately results in a very pro-oxidant effect. It is just a matter of location and concentration of the vitamin C, along with the presence of enough ferric ions and hydrogen peroxide.

It should also be mentioned that the ability of vitamin C to stimulate the Fenton reaction is the *singular* reason why there are so many studies in the literature claiming that vitamin C, in certain experimental situations, can "damage" biomolecules, cause genetic damage, or even promote the growth of cancer.

Tiny doses of vitamin C, in the presence of enough ferric ion and hydrogen peroxide, will *always* result in the production of the hydroxyl radical and result in a great deal of oxidative stress. However, large doses of vitamin C, thanks to the masterful design of Mother Nature, will *always* result in a net antioxidant, never pro-oxidant, effect in the tissues. Even when a small part of the vitamin C (milligrams) might be stimulating the Fenton reaction, the rest of the vitamin C (grams) "mops up" the oxidative stress generated very readily.

Even though excess oxidative stress is always undesirable and highly toxic, lesser amounts of it are absolutely necessary for the physiology of the cell to function normally. Non-lethal amounts of intracelluar oxidative stress often perform signaling functions: turning different enzymes and biochemical pathways on or off, as well as the reading of genes and the production of the molecules for which they are coded. As with much else in Nature, things are rarely just on or off, black or white. Shades of gray make biology what it is.

Because the role of vitamin C in the Fenton reaction is just the donation of an electron to a ferric ion, it should come as no surprise that anything else that is capable of donating an electron to a ferric ion in the presence of hydrogen peroxide will stimulate this reaction as well.

Another ROS known as superoxide, which contains an extra electron, can also convert ferric to ferrous ions by the donation of this electron and stimulate the Fenton reaction. This donation of an electron to ferric ion by superoxide, allowing the Fenton reaction to proceed, is known as the Haber-Weiss reaction.

Understanding the chemistry described above facilitates the understanding of how a number of **antioxidant enzymes** exert their influences in the cell. Three of the most important antioxidant enzymes in the body are superoxide dismutase (SOD), catalase, and glutathione peroxidase.

SOD converts superoxide to oxygen and hydrogen peroxide. This means that when enough SOD is present, the Fenton reaction will not be able to proceed directly by electron donation from superoxide, which helps to stabilize the cell.

In addition, the blood and nearly all cells contain an important antioxidant enzyme known as catalase. The role of catalase is to metabolize, or convert, hydrogen peroxide to water and oxygen. Catalase is exceptionally efficient in this task, with one molecule of enzyme capable of converting millions of hydrogen peroxide molecules per minute in the right medium.

Glutathione peroxidase functions by converting hydrogen peroxide to water when it is in the presence of reduced glutathione. Reduced glutathione, by virtue of its multiple functions and very high intracellular concentration, is the most important antioxidant *inside* the cell.

It can be seen, then, that maintaining normal levels of these three antioxidant enzymes plays a prominent role in suppressing the Fenton reaction inside the cell and keeping oxidative stress at minimal levels.

SOD helps by metabolizing superoxide and preventing it from directly feeding electrons into the Fenton reaction.

Both catalase and glutathione peroxidase work to keep hydrogen peroxide levels low, probably the most important factor in minimizing the production of Fenton-produced oxidative stress. An abundance of both the superoxide free radical and reactive iron, even in the presence of vitamin C, will produce very little oxidative stress if there are only trace amounts of hydrogen peroxide present.

To recap, nearly all pathogens contain large amounts of iron and a significant amount of this iron is in the unbound, reactive state. When vitamin C is administered to individuals with infections, the vitamin C enters the pathogens, converts the ferric ion to a ferrous ion, and the ferrous ion proceeds to break down the hydrogen peroxide present in the cell. Then, the resulting hydroxyl radicals literally oxidize the pathogen to death.

## What About Cancer?

Cancer cells, like pathogens, are also especially susceptible to the generation of hydroxyl radicals and oxidative stress to the point of cell death via the vitamin C-stimulated Fenton reaction. The reasons for the remarkable susceptibility of cancer to vitamin C therapy include the following:

1. Like pathogens, proliferating cancer cells require increased amounts of iron in order to multiply, and they generally have increased intracellular concentrations of iron.

2. Unlike normal cells, where most of the iron is stored in a bound, unreactive state, a substantial amount of the iron inside cancer cells is available in the cytoplasm in an unbound, reactive state.

3. Cancer cells often have low to undetectable levels of catalase, allowing hydrogen peroxide levels in the cytoplasm to increase.

4.  Cancer cells often have depressed levels of other antioxidant enzymes, including superoxide dismutase and glutathione peroxidase, causing the cells to already have increased levels of internal oxidative stress relative to normal cells, and making them more susceptible to induced cell death by further increasing those levels.

5.  The extracellular matrix surrounding cancer cells is highly dependent on vitamin C to maintain its integrity.

6.  While the cancer cells are being attacked, the immune system is being simultaneously stimulated and strengthened by the vitamin C.

7.  Similarly, while cancer cells are being attacked, normal cells (*without the high internal levels of reactive iron and hydrogen peroxide*) are being strengthened by accumulating vitamin C, bolstering their antioxidant defenses.

The typical cancer cell, then, has a high concentration of reactive iron in its cytoplasm. It also has an elevated level of oxidative stress even before vitamin C therapy is initiated. Most cancer cells, due to depressed levels of catalase, have increased levels of hydrogen peroxide in the cytoplasm. Overall, then, the typical cancer cell has all of the elements of the Fenton reaction in significant amounts, waiting to be triggered by the vitamin C-mediated reduction of ferric to ferrous ion. Subsequently, the cancer cell-killing hydroxyl radical is produced by the breakdown of hydrogen peroxide.

All of these characteristics are not shared by normal cells, which are being strengthened by the influx of vitamin C at the same time the cancer cells are being killed. Furthermore, the vitamin C has many different mechanisms of stimulating the immune system while the cancer cells are attacked and the normal cells improve their antioxidant capacity.

A separate but important way in which vitamin C impacts the treatment of cancer relates to the nature of the extracellular matrix, which is the substance that contains and surrounds cells in connective tissue.

Under normal circumstances, this matrix has a thick, gel-like quality. One important factor in the conversion of a normal cell to a malignant one relates to the conversion of the gel-like nature of this matrix to a loose and watery nature.

This change in the physical consistency of this extracellular matrix reliably occurs when vitamin C levels in this area of the tissues become significantly depleted. The collagen and connective tissue proteins are normally very elongated and substantially interconnected in the healthy state, when vitamin C levels are normal. When vitamin C is depleted, the elongated molecules break down into small segments, and many of the interconnections are lost. These changes cause the gel-like nature of the matrix to deteriorate to a watery state.

When a normal cell loses the physical restraint or resistance offered by the normally gel-like nature of the matrix, the cell often begins multiplying, and can eventually become malignant. When vitamin C is administered and normal levels are restored, there is a fairly rapid return to the gel-like state of this matrix, with a normal degree of physical support again being afforded the cells.

This restoration of a normal extracellular matrix by vitamin C is important in reverting malignant cells to their normal state, aside from the vitamin C-mediated killing of cancer cells by the mechanisms discussed above.

As a practical point, the lack of toxicity from vitamin C combined with its support of the immune system along with the bolstering of the antioxidant capacity of normal cells should be reason enough to include sizable doses of vitamin C as part of any cancer treatment protocol. Even if a traditional oncologist simply will not accept the ability of vitamin C to kill cancer cells, its benefits are still many.

Today there is increasing "concern" that vitamin C interferes in the treatment of cancer patients receiving traditional chemotherapy and is actually **contraindicated**! To the extent that nearly all standard chemotherapy drugs are highly toxic, it is absolutely correct that vitamin C will neutralize them as it would any other toxin or poison, if all are present in the same place at the same time. However, it is incredibly **easy** to completely avoid this potential problem by staggering the administrations of the chemotherapy and the vitamin C. Give the chemotherapy (if it must be done) and then follow it with the vitamin C a few hours later. The chemotherapy will be taken up by the cancer cells and do its damage, while the vitamin C administered later helps to repair the unintentionally damaged normal cells, which always occurs as well. Furthermore, the vitamin C that ends up going to the cancer cells will reliably augment the desired effects of the chemotherapy by triggering the Fenton reaction and helping to cause cancer cell death.

To recap, then, vitamin C by itself can serve as the perfect "chemotherapy" for very many cases of cancer. However, regardless of the therapeutic approach taken toward a given patient, vitamin C can **always** be expected to improve the long-term outcome. As well, the patient will also suffer from far less of the side effects normally experienced with traditional chemotherapy if vitamin C is included in the treatment protocol.

# 20 ways vitamin C boosts the immune system

In both Chapter Six and Resource A the power of vitamin C resulting from its incredible ability to donate electrons as an antioxidant is discussed. In fact, it is this very attribute of vitamin C that accounts for most of its potent antimicrobial and toxin-neutralizing qualities.

However, no other antioxidant can perform the many additional physiological and biological roles that vitamin C fills. To dismiss vitamin C as "nothing more" than an antioxidant greatly understates and misrepresents the range of vitamin C's positive effects on the body. Vitamin C is a strong stimulator and supporter of good immune function. Some of the ways that vitamin C promotes and boosts the immune system include the following:

1) Vitamin C enhances production of interferons.[1-6] Interferons are an important part of the body's immune system. The body produces them when the presence of pathogens — viruses, bacteria, or parasites — is detected. They facilitate the ability of cells to trigger protective cellular defenses against the detected attack.

2) Vitamin C enhances the function of phagocytes.[7-24] Phagocytes are a type of white blood cell that envelop pathogens and infection-related particles. Once the invaders are captured in this manner, they are enzymatically digested.

3)   Vitamin C selectively concentrates in
     white blood cells.[25-29] Some of the primary
     cells in the immune system concentrate
     vitamin C as much as 80 times higher
     than the level in plasma. This assures
     extra delivery of vitamin C to the sites
     of infection by the migration of these
     vitamin C-rich white blood cells.

4)   Vitamin C enhances the cell-mediated
     immune response.[30] There are 2 major
     ways that the body can respond to a
     pathogen: antibody-mediated immunity
     and cell-mediated immunity. Cell-
     mediated response refers to the activation
     of macrophages, natural killer cells, and
     antigen-specific T-lymphocytes that attack
     anything perceived as a foreign infectious
     agent.

5)   Vitamin C enhances cytokine production
     by white blood cells.[31] Cytokines are
     communication proteins released by
     certain white blood cells that transmit
     information to other cells, promoting the
     immune response.

6)   Vitamin C inhibits various forms of
     T-lymphocyte death.[32] T-lymphocytes are
     a type of white blood cell. They are an
     integral part of the cell-mediated immune
     defense system. Vitamin C helps to keep
     these important cells alive and viable.

7)   Vitamin C enhances nitric oxide production
     by phagocytes.[33,34] Phagocytes, as
     discussed in #2 above, are white blood
     cells that engulf invading microorganisms.
     Nitric oxide is produced in large amounts
     in these cells. It is one of the agents that
     will kill captured pathogens.

8)   Vitamin C enhances T-lymphocyte
     proliferation.[35-37] As mentioned in

#6 above, these cells are essential to cell-mediated immune responses, and vitamin C helps them to multiply in number.

9) Vitamin C enhances B-lymphocyte proliferation.[38] These white blood cells make antibodies as part of the antibody-mediated immune response. Antibodies are formed in reaction to the initial introduction of an invading pathogen or antigen. If and when the body detects a reintroduction of the same pathogen the body counters with a specific antibody attack.

10) Vitamin C inhibits neuraminidase production.[39] Some pathogenic viruses and bacteria create neuraminidase, an enzyme that keeps them from being trapped in mucus, one of the body's natural lines of defense. By inhibiting neuraminidase, vitamin C helps the body optimize this defensive mechanism.

11) Vitamin C enhances antibody production and complements their activity.[40-50] Good antibody function is important to combat both infections and toxins. The complement system is a complex group of proteins that interact to kill targeted cells and mediate other functions of the immune system.

12) Vitamin C enhances natural killer cell activity.[51] Natural killer cells are small lymphocytes that can directly attack cells, such as tumor cells, and kill them.

13) Vitamin C enhances prostaglandin formation.[52-54] Prostaglandins are hormone-like compounds that control a variety of physiologic processes, including the regulation of T-lymphocyte function.

14) Vitamin C enhances cyclic GMP levels in lymphocytes.[55,56] Cyclic GMP plays a central role in the regulation of different physiologic responses, including the modulation of immune responses. Cyclic GMP is important for normal cell proliferation (reproduction) and differentiation (specialization for specific purposes). Cyclic GMP also controls the action of many hormones, and it appears to mediate the relaxation of smooth muscle.

15) Vitamin C enhances localized generation of and/or interaction with hydrogen peroxide.[57-60] Vitamin C and hydrogen peroxide can kill microorganisms and can dissolve the protective capsules of some bacteria, such as pneumococci.[61]

16) Vitamin C detoxifies histamine.[62,63] This antihistamine effect of vitamin C is important in the support of local immune factors.

17) Vitamin C neutralizes oxidative stress.[64] Infections produce free radicals locally that further promote the infective process.

18) Vitamin C improves and enhances the immune response achieved with vaccination. [65-67]

19) Vitamin C enhances the mucolytic effect.[68] This property helps liquefy thick secretions, increasing immune access to infection.

20) Vitamin C may make bacterial membranes more permeable to some antibiotics.[69]

# The important metabolic roles of vitamin C

It is wrongly assumed by many that vitamin C is a trace nutrient (vitamin) and only required in tiny amounts sufficient to prevent scurvy. It is true that this C-deficiency disease spawned the chemical name [ascorbate] for vitamin C. Ascorbate literally means "against scurvy." And, were this its only function, the government's 90 mg RDA for vitamin C would be sufficient for most people on the planet. But, there's vastly more it can do.

Aside from its ability to prevent and cure scurvy, its ability to prevent and cure a great number of infectious diseases, and its power to neutralize nearly every toxin known to man (*see Resource H*), vitamin C is also a required component of many essential metabolic processes. A few of the more studied physiological functions are discussed below.

## *Collagen Synthesis*

Vitamin C is essential for the synthesis and maintenance of collagen, the most abundant protein in the human body. Collagen comprises about 25% to 35% of the total protein content in the body. Its strong, connective, elongated fibrils are found in skin, ligaments, tendons, cartilage, bone, blood vessels, the intestines, and the discs between spinal vertebrae. It is also found in the cornea and in muscle tissue. At least 19 molecules have been classified as types of collagen, but the most common, Type 1, accounts for about 90% of the body's total collagen content. Important facts relating vitamin C to collagen include the following:

157

- Vitamin C deficiency is an underdiagnosed contributor to degenerative disc disease in the elderly[1]
- Vitamin C helps protect the skin by promoting fibroblast proliferation, migration, and replication-associated skin injury repair[2]
- Formula containing vitamin C protects against skin wrinkles seen in premature aging[3]
- Increased vitamin C uptake by vascular smooth muscle cells increases both the synthesis and maturation of Type I collagen[4]
- Vitamin C induces an increase in Type I collagen deposits by normal human fibroblasts in a dose-dependent manner — an adequate supply contributes to the optimal density of collagen in the skin[5]
- High concentrations of vitamin C stimulate synthesis of Type IV collagen, which has important filtration characteristics in the kidney, the blood-brain barrier, and the arterial lining[6]

## Basement Membrane Synthesis

Basement membrane is a thin, sticky layer that supports epithelial cell layers — tissues that line the surfaces and cavities throughout the body (e.g. the lining of the stomach and the lining of blood vessels). It binds the glomerular capillaries in the kidneys to the Bowman's capsule which is necessary for blood filtration. It also attaches the pulmonary capillaries in the lungs to the lung alveoli. In addition, basement membrane functions as a restrictive barrier to prevent cancer cells from passing deeper into tissues. Vitamin C is related to the basement membrane in the following ways:

- Vitamin C maintains the gel-like state of the basement membrane, helping to suppress tumor invasion through the basement membrane[7]
- Vitamin C deficiency reduces the expression of basement membrane components (Type IV collagen, laminin, elastin) in blood vessels[8]
- Vitamin C accelerates the deposition of other important basement membrane proteins in the junction between the dermis and epidermis[9]

## Facilitates Wound Healing

As skin wounds heal, dermal and epidermal cells must replicate to close the wound. This process consumes a great amount of vitamin C. Vitamin C is important in the following ways:

- Vitamin C treatment results in better organization of basal keratinocytes, an increase in fibroblast number and a faster formation of the dermal-epidermal junction[9]
- Vitamin C regulates keratinocyte viability, epidermal barrier, and basement membrane *in vitro*, and it reduces wound contraction after grafting of cultured skin substitutes[10]
- Formulations with vitamin C significantly reduce bed sores (pressure ulcers) of long-term nursing home residents[11]

## Carnitine Synthesis

Carnitine is an amino acid that is essential for the transport of fatty acids into mitochondria for the production of ATP via the citric acid cycle (Krebs cycle). This process provides the major source of cellular energy. Vitamin C is an essential cofactor for the synthesis of carnitine, and high-dose vitamin C helps optimize this synthesis.[12,13]

## Neurotransmitter Synthesis

Neurotransmitters are biomolecules that facilitate the electrical flow between neurons and nerve cells in the body and in the brain. The body's ability to respond to the environment as well as the brain's ability to think and to remember is dependent on these essential substances. Vitamin C is also directly involved in the synthesis of neurotransmitters.[14]

## Promotes Calcium Incorporation into Bone Tissue

The formation and maintenance of quality, high-density bone material requires vitamin C. Vitamin C promotes assimilation of calcium into the bone, protects against leaching of calcium out of the bones (resorption), and fights the oxidative stress that works against assimilation and for resorption.[15,16] Additional relationships between vitamin C and bone metabolism include the following:

- Vitamin C stimulates the formation of the cells that incorporate calcium into bone tissue (osteoblasts)[17,18]
- Vitamin C inhibits the development of cells that dissolve calcium out of bone tissues (osteoclasts)[17,18]
- As a powerful antioxidant, vitamin C fights oxidative stress in bone tissues[19]
- Collagen cross-linking, required to form the dense matrix for optimal bone strength, requires vitamin C[20,21]
- Deficiency of vitamin C can result in bone fragility[22]
- Vitamin C supplementation helps to prevent bone loss[23-28]

- Supplementation with vitamin C provides a dose-dependent protection against bone fractures in the elderly — the higher the dose, the fewer the fractures[29]
- Elderly patients sustaining hip fractures typically have low vitamin C blood levels[30]

## Natural Antihistamine

Histamines are biomolecules that trigger allergic responses in the body. Although some of that response is necessary and helpful as a mediator of inflammation against antigens, in many individuals the response can be protracted. This results in a more chronic inflammatory response that can produce unwanted symptoms (like itchy eyes and a stuffy nose), as well as promote significant chronic diseases such as atherosclerosis. Vitamin C not only helps eliminate or neutralize the offending allergens and toxins, it also neutralizes the toxic effects of the histamine itself — functioning as a natural antihistamine.[31-34]

## Plays Many Roles in Immune System Function and Maintenance

These functions of vitamin C are so important that a separate listing has been provided. Here is a list. Refer to Resource B for a broad explanation.

### Vitamin C enhances:
- Production of interferons
- Function of phagocytes
- Cytokine production by white blood cells
- Cell-mediated immune response
- Nitric oxide production by phagocytes
- T-lymphocyte proliferation
- B-lymphocyte proliferation
- Antibody production and complement activity

- Natural killer cell activity
- Prostaglandin formation
- Cyclic GMP levels in lymphocytes
- Localized generation of, and/or interaction with, hydrogen peroxide
- Mucolytic effect
- Nonspecific vaccination effect

***Vitamin C inhibits:***
- Various forms of T-lymphocyte death
- Neuraminidase production

***Vitamin C also:***
- Selectively concentrates in white blood cells
- Detoxifies histamine
- Neutralizes oxidative stress
- May make bacterial membranes more permeable to some antibiotics

# Vitamin C and its relationship to heart disease risk factors

This resource provides a starting place for those interested in studying the relationship between heart health and vitamin C. By no means is it exhaustive in scope. A handful of the major coronary heart disease risk factors have been selected simply to provide an exemplary exposure to the vast substantiation available. A much more complete treatment of this topic is available in my book, *Stop America's #1 Killer!* (available directly from the publisher at www.MedFoxPub. com. or Amazon.com). It discusses nearly 30 risk factors and offers practical suggestions for the treatment and prevention of arterial blockages.

In this Resource, a short discussion and a list of published studies showing the role that vitamin C plays in each of seven major risk factors is provided. These factors are: High blood pressure, cholesterol and triglyceride levels, arterial inflammation, lipoprotein(a) levels, diabetes, smoking, and fibrinogen levels.

## High Blood Pressure

High blood pressure does not act alone in contributing to arterial narrowings and blockages. Studies show that high blood pressure requires an accompanying lack of arterial vitamin C to initiate these damaging affects. Sufficient vitamin C must be taken on a regular basis to keep the collagen content in all three layers of the blood vessel at a level that will maintain arterial integrity.[1-3] It is the progressive lack of wall integrity that prompts the body's compensatory response of stabilizing the arterial structure by bulking up with atherosclerotic plaques. Many studies help to demonstrate these conclusions. Here are a few:

- Combined antioxidant supplementation, including vitamin C, reduces blood pressure[4]
- Vitamin C is effective as a monotherapy in lowering the blood pressure of hypertensive patients[5]
- Higher blood levels of vitamin C relate to lower blood pressure in humans[6-9]
- Healed wounds in C-deficient animals have "greatly inferior tensile strength" compared to those with adequate vitamin C[10]
- Normally formed collagen breaks down upon withdrawal of vitamin C[11]
- Vitamin C is essential for normal tissue healing and maintenance of previously formed scar tissue[12]
- Scar tissue is more sensitive than normal connective tissue to vitamin C deficiency[13]
- Vitamin C deficiency plays an integral role in the actual causation and sustaining of high blood pressure[14-16]

## Cholesterol and Triglyceride Levels

One of cholesterol's many functions in the body is to neutralize or inactivate toxins. As a result, cholesterol levels are routinely elevated in conditions of increased toxin exposure.[17,18] Unfortunately, this important compensatory mechanism, left unchecked, can cause its own significant harm by accelerating atherosclerosis as it infiltrates arterial walls.

A triglyceride, like cholesterol, is another lipid (fat or fat-like substance) that has been linked to heart disease. An elevated level of triglycerides in the blood is an independent risk factor tied to a greater chance of death by heart attack.[19]

Vitamin C greatly limits and can even prevent the negative impact of cholesterol and triglycerides on the development of atherosclerosis. Many studies are consistent with this finding. Here are a few:

- Cholesterol neutralizes a large number of different bacterial toxins capable of causing direct cellular damage[20,21]
- Elevated serum cholesterols are seen as a marker of, if not a direct response to, a variety of toxic exposures[22]
- Cell membrane-bound cholesterol in the arterial walls binds bacterial toxins, becoming a focus of reactive immune activity, and promoting atherosclerotic damage[23]
- Increased toxic pesticide exposures correlate with increased cholesterol levels[24]
- Striking elevation of cholesterol is seen in animals exposed to lead[25]
- Aflatoxin exposure increases cholesterol levels in rabbits — vitamin C administration significantly lowers those levels and alleviates the harmful effects of exposure[26]
- Vitamin C deficiency results in the development of atherosclerosis — under this deficiency, cholesterol and triglycerides accumulate in plaques, even without adding cholesterol to the diet[27,28]
- Injected vitamin C demonstrates a protective effect against the development of atherosclerosis in guinea pigs fed increased amounts of cholesterol[28]

- Vitamin C administration reduces the incidence and severity of atherosclerosis in rabbits fed a diet high in cholesterol and hydrogenated fat[29]
- Some form of injury to a blood vessel is needed to initiate cholesterol deposition in the vessel — this injury is accompanied by a localized deficiency of vitamin C[30,31]
- Presence of vitamin C limits cholesterol penetration into the blood vessel and increases release of cholesterol already in the vessel[32]
- Vitamin C supplementation lessens intimal thickening and lipid infiltration in rabbits fed a cholesterol-rich diet[33]
- High doses of cholesterol exert toxic effects and rapidly metabolize vitamin C, just like any other toxin or toxic effect[34-36]
- Vitamin C deficiency leads to increased blood levels of cholesterol[37-39]
- High levels of vitamin C lower the cholesterol concentration in both the serum and the liver of guinea pigs[40]
- Vitamin C prevents the cholesterol level in the blood from increasing after cholesterol feeding in lab animals[41,42]
- Low levels of vitamin C reduce the rate of metabolic transformation of cholesterol into bile acids leading to increased levels of cholesterol[43,44]
- Daily vitamin C supplementation decreases cholesterol levels in humans[45,46]
- Vitamin C lowers the levels of cholesterol and triglycerides in rabbits and rats with high cholesterol levels and enhances the activity of LPL (lipoprotein lipase), the enzyme that helps clear fats from the blood[47]

- Daily supplementation with 2 to 3 grams of vitamin C in 50 of 60 patients with increased cholesterol levels and/or heart disease increased the average LPL activity by 100% and decreased the average triglyceride level by 50% to 70%[47]
- Two-gram daily doses of vitamin C decreased both the triglyceride and cholesterol levels,[48] while doses of 500 mg were found ineffective[49]
- As vitamin C blood levels increase, triglyceride levels drop and HDL cholesterol increases[50-52]

Polyunsaturated lecithin, or polyunsaturated phosphatidylcholine (PPC), is a term referring to a substance that directly impacts the cholesterol metabolism in the arterial wall.

The positive anti-atherosclerotic interactions between vitamin C therapy and lecithin therapy are significant. Vitamin C is known to help maintain the normal physical characteristics of the ground substance and basement membrane areas, making them substantially less receptive to the deposition of cholesterol from the blood. The following effects of lecithin and PPC, along with the many positive effects of vitamin C, provide further reason to supplement with a liposome-encapsulated product when possible — especially for those who need heart-protective help.

- Administration of a soybean-derived PPC was able to protect cholesterol-fed rabbits from the development of atherosclerosis[53]
- A soy lecithin-rich diet in monkeys and hamsters reduced total plasma cholesterol without reducing the HDL-bound, or "good" cholesterol; the early stages of atherosclerosis were significantly reduced in the hamsters as well[54]

- Soy lecithin lowers cholesterol in rabbits and rats; human endothelial cells incubated with soy lecithin significantly expel internal cholesterol[55]
- Soy lecithin-rich diets stimulate the liver uptake of HDL-cholesterol in rats[56]
- Soy lecithin-rich diets significantly increase the amounts of cholesterol excreted into the bile via the liver in rabbits[57]
- Vitamin C and lecithin synergistically prevent arterial lesions in cholesterol-fed rabbits — given alone each is helpful but together they provide more than just the sum of their individual effects[58]

## Arterial Inflammation

Inflammation, by multiple mechanisms, is a significant risk factor for atherosclerotic heart disease. One mechanism involves its tendency to induce vasoconstriction in blood vessels. This results in a significant narrowing of the caliber of those vessels. Research shows that this inflammation-induced vasoconstriction can be corrected by injecting vitamin C directly into the artery.[59]

A vitamin C deficiency, on the other hand, stimulates the inflammation process with the body's need for more vitamin C in depleted areas. This compensatory response can succeed in bringing vitamin C into an inflamed area. However, in a continuing state of vitamin C deficiency, it brings other factors into play that also stimulate development of atherosclerotic plaques. In addition, vitamin C deficiency definitely leaves the door open for other inducers of inflammation, such as bacterial and viral infections, as well as the toxins and autoimmune reactions they often produce.

Here are some studies that demonstrate these aspects of vitamin C:

- Human arteries are commonly depleted of vitamin C, even in individuals who are "apparently well-nourished" — localized depletions of vitamin C often exist in the segments of arteries subjected to greater mechanical stress[60]
- Inflammation is thought to be a major player in the development, progression, and eventual destabilization of atherosclerotic lesions, ultimately leading to the complete obstruction of an artery[61-63]
- Plaques prone to complications — such as sudden complete obstruction — contain large numbers of inflammatory cells, while stable plaques that have a lesser complication rate have less evidence of inflammation[64-66]
- Low vitamin C levels are most likely related both to the presence of inflammation and the severity of the vascular disease[67]
- Chronic inflammation in atherosclerosis, with an increased risk of heart attack from the total blockage of a heart artery, is related to chronic periodontal (gum and adjacent bone) disease[68-70]
- The DNA specific for multiple periodontal microbes/pathogens is detected in atherosclerotic plaques[71]
- Periodontal disease is associated with the development of carotid artery atherosclerosis[72]
- Localized vitamin C deficiency in areas of developing atherosclerosis significantly enhances the ability for microbes to continue to infect or colonize there[73]
- Infection is implicated as a primary reason for chronic inflammation of the arterial wall[74]

- Various infections, including streptococcal, tend to stimulate cell proliferation in the intima and inner medial layers of the blood vessel, much like the "traditional" form of atherosclerosis[75,76]

- Infections can further contribute to the development of atherosclerosis by stimulating autoimmune reactions against components of the blood vessel wall[77-79]

- Autoimmune antibodies attack endothelial cells in culture[80] and have been correlated with atherosclerotic disease in the carotid artery[81]

- Patients known to have atherosclerosis have also demonstrated elevated levels of autoimmune antibodies[82]

- Autoimmune disease increases the prevalence of atherosclerosis[83-86]

- Vitamin C is effective in treating autoimmune disease[87]

- Viral infections are specifically implicated in the development of atherosclerosis[88-94]

- Higher viral loads in patients infected with human immunodeficiency virus (HIV) are associated with poorer endothelial function, a condition thought to play an important role in the evolution of atherosclerosis[95]

- Herpesviruses are thought to act as blood-clotting activators, playing a role in provoking the total arterial blockages often seen in the late stages of atherosclerosis[96]

- High blood levels of C-reactive protein are associated with greater degrees of inflammation and greater risk of atherosclerosis[97-100]

- C-reactive protein is frequently found deposited in atherosclerotic lesions[100]

## *Lipoprotein(a) Levels*

Fat-protein complexes that transport fat in the blood are called lipoproteins. Examples of these complexes are high-density (HDL) and low-density lipoproteins (LDL) that are known for their cholesterol transport functions. HDL transports cholesterol to the liver for metabolism and excretion, while LDL transports cholesterol to non-liver tissues and into the arterial walls. Because of these transport character-istics, HDL-bound cholesterol is known as the "good" cho-lesterol and LDL-bound cholesterol is known as the "bad" cholesterol.

HDL is considered a good lipoprotein since a high blood level of it means there is a greater capacity for trans-porting more cholesterol out of the arterial walls to the liver for excretion into the intestine via the bile. Just the opposite is considered to be the case for LDL, which is known to help bind cholesterol and bring it into the arterial wall.

Another of these fat-protein complexes is known as lipoprotein(a), or Lp(a). Lp(a) is adept in promoting ath-erosclerosis and has emerged as an independent coronary artery disease (atherosclerosis) risk factor. When high blood levels of Lp(a) are found with elevated LDL cholesterol, depressed levels of HDL cholesterol, and hypertension, the combination can be particularly aggressive in the devel-opment of arterial blockages.[101] Unstable angina patients with elevated Lp(a) are more likely to proceed to a signif-icant cardiac complication, such as blockage of the artery and heart attack.[102] Additional Lp(a)-related information includes the following:

- Bodily production of Lp(a) is believed to be a compensatory mechanism to counteract vitamin C deficiency[103]
- Lp(a) is only found in non-C-synthesizing animals[103]

- Prolonged elevations of Lp(a) result in excessive deposition in the arterial wall, promoting the development of atherosclerosis[104]
- Vitamin C deficiency increases plasma concentrations of Lp(a) and fibrinogen[105]
- Lp(a) deposits in arterial walls correlate with the extent of atherosclerotic lesion development in the coronary arteries and the aorta[106]
- Lp(a) accumulation is significant in the development of atherosclerosis in coronary artery bypass vein grafts[107]
- A regimen of vitamin C and lysine dramatically reduced anginal chest pains in 3 case studies[108-110]
- Vitamin C restores impaired blood flow throughout the small blood vessels (microcirculation) of the heart typically seen in smokers[111]
- Human atherosclerotic lesions are primarily composed of Lp(a)[112]
- Administration of vitamin C, lysine and proline, along with niacin, guar gum and the ayurvedic herb gum guggulu for 19 months, significantly lowered Lp(a) levels, reducing a 75% narrowing of the right coronary artery to 40% and resolving other 50% narrowings in a cardiac patient case study[113]

## Diabetes

Diabetes mellitus is a chronic disease in which the metabolism of carbohydrate, protein, and fat is impaired due to the inadequate production of insulin or due to resistance of the target tissues to the effects of insulin. It appears to exert much, if not most, of its negative impact on the body by virtue of the associated chronic deficiency of vitamin C found in both the tissues and the blood. Very commonly, hypertension and lipid disorders (such as elevated Lp(a) and elevated cholesterol) coexist with diabetes.

The local deficit of vitamin C in the blood vessel wall induced by diabetes can easily initiate the atherosclerotic process. After this damage to the blood vessel wall is initiated, other risk factors such as inflammation and elevated blood fats like cholesterol and Lp(a) can more easily make their contributions to plaque development.

Finally, the unique interrelationship between insulin and vitamin C also offers strong evidence that the chronic diabetic state is both the result of vitamin C deficiency and a very strong contributor to a continuing state of significant vitamin C deficiency. Consider the following findings:

- Diabetes is a well-established risk factor for atherosclerosis and coronary heart disease[114,115]
- Daily vitamin C supplementation in diabetic patients results in striking cholesterol drops, ranging from 40 mg to 100 mg per 100 ml of blood in a majority of the patients[116]
- Diabetes is marked by high levels of oxidative stress from increased free radical production and/or reduced antioxidant defenses[117,118]
- Complications of diabetes spring from its increased oxidative stress[119-121]
- Diabetics have reduced plasma levels of vitamin C[122-126]
- Elevated glucose levels (hyperglycemia) seen in diabetes may directly induce a state of latent scurvy, or advanced vitamin C deficiency[127]
- Glucose competes with vitamin C for uptake into the cell and mitochondria[128-132]

- Insulin promotes the cellular uptake of vitamin C as well as the cellular uptake of glucose[133]
- Injection of insulin produces a fall in the plasma levels of vitamin C and a rise in the white blood cell and platelet content of vitamin C[134]
- Hyperglycemia works to decrease the ability of the natural filters in the kidney to reabsorb vitamin C, resulting in more vitamin C being excreted in the urine and less vitamin C remaining in the blood[135]
- High glucose levels inhibit some important functions of vitamin C[136]
- Hyperglycemia is also especially effective in depleting the vitamin C content in monocytes — a primary part of immune response[137]
- Platelets, the sticky elements in the blood that aggregate to initiate blood clot formation, have decreased levels of vitamin C in diabetic patients[138]
- Greater amounts of vitamin C in platelets directly lessen their tendency to aggregate, or initiate the focus for a blood clot[139]
- Blood clotting is an integral part of the small vessel disease (angiopathy) seen in diabetics, and this anti-platelet sticking effect of vitamin C is typically less in evidence in the diabetic[140]
- Average vitamin C levels in the blood are "significantly lower" in persons with newly diagnosed diabetes than in nondiabetics[141]
- Vitamin C administration has a powerful protective effect against abnormal blood clotting[142]
- Vitamin C also appears to play an essential role in regulating the release of insulin

from the cells that produce it in the
pancreas[143]
- Diabetic patients show clinical
  improvement when an infusion of
  vitamin C is combined with insulin
  injections[144]
- Individuals with diabetes are also much
  more likely to have advanced periodontal
  disease than nondiabetics[145,146]

## Smoking

Smoking is another well-established, independent,
and major risk factor for the development of atherosclerosis and coronary heart disease.[147,149] Many, if not most,
of the mechanisms in which smoking causes atherosclerosis
appear to at least utilize vitamin C deficiency as a cofactor.
Consider the following points:

- Smoking lowers the blood level of
  vitamin C, and adding nicotine to samples
  of whole human blood significantly lowers
  the vitamin C content of the blood[149]
- Vitamin C blood levels in smokers are
  markedly reduced[150-152]
- Even after adjusting for age, gender,
  vitamin C intake, and multivitamin intake,
  exposure to tobacco in the immediate
  environment remained "significantly
  associated" with lower blood levels of
  vitamin C in children chronically exposed
  to tobacco smoke[153]
- Environmental tobacco smoke, even with
  "minimal" exposure, produces a "highly
  significant" reduction of plasma ascorbate
  levels[154]
- Cigarette smokers have average blood
  levels of vitamin C that are inversely

  proportional to the amount of tobacco
  smoked[155,156]

- A single puff of smoke contains 1,015
  different pro-oxidants[157]

- A severe form of vascular disease known
  as Buerger's disease is always associated
  with smoking, and it is characterized by
  such rapidly progressive narrowings and
  blockages of the arteries that gangrene
  often occurs when the blood supply
  becomes compromised enough, resulting
  in loss of fingers or toes[158]

- Periodontal disease (characterized
  by focal vitamin C deficiency) is much
  more common in smokers than in
  nonsmokers[159]

- A strong correlation exists between
  lower whole blood vitamin C levels
  and increasing severity of periodontal
  disease[160]

- Administration of vitamin C to children
  with significant gum disease clearly
  improves the condition[161]

- Typical cigarette-induced reductions
  in microcirculatory blood flow are
  greatly reduced with vitamin C
  supplementation — these blood flow
  reductions can result in, or help to cause,
  anginal chest pain and heart attack just
  like the blockages in the much larger
  arteries[162]

- Vitamin C protects against some
  cardiovascular and microvascular changes
  seen after cigarette smoke inhalation[163]

- Cigarette smoking promotes
  atherosclerosis by causing white blood
  cells to clump together and stick to the

blood vessel walls[164,165] — once they
adhere, acute and chronic damage can be
inflicted on the blood vessel wall[166,167]

- Vitamin C pretreatment "almost entirely
  prevented" smoke-exposure-induced
  clumping of white blood cells and a
  subsequent tendency to adhere to blood
  vessel walls in laboratory animals[168]

## Fibrinogen Levels

Fibrinogen is a pivotal protein involved in the clotting
mechanism in the blood plasma. It also factors directly into
how viscous ("thick") the blood is. Fibrinogen can play
a role in how readily the platelets in the blood will stick
together and promote the initiation of blood clots. Fibrin,
an important component in the blood clot, results from the
direct conversion of fibrinogen when the clotting mechanism in the blood has been initiated.

Fibrinogen appears to be a risk factor that involves a
vitamin C deficiency in exerting its effects as a heart disease
risk factor. At the very least, there is a clear correlation
between elevated fibrinogen levels and decreased vitamin C
levels. It is also very possible that the vitamin C deficiency
itself directly results in the elevation of fibrinogen levels in
the body.

An elevated fibrinogen level in the blood can be
expected to increase both the size of atherosclerotic plaques
as well as the likelihood of sudden complete blockages by
acutely formed blood clots on top of developing plaques.
Fibrinogen facts include the following:

- An increased level of fibrinogen in the
  blood is an independent risk factor for
  cardiovascular disease[169-173]

- Higher fibrinogen levels are tied to lower levels of vitamin C[174]

- Blood fibrinogen levels were up and blood vitamin C levels were down in stroke patients[175]

- Vitamin C supplementation (1,000 mg) substantially increases the ability to dissolve blood clots in healthy individuals as well as in those with coronary heart disease — this effect persists only as long as the increase of vitamin C in the blood is maintained[176]

- Vitamin C supplementation (1,000 mg) helps prevent excessive fibrinolysis (blood clot breakdown) in patients with chronic nephritis, showing that vitamin C is important in maintaining the balance between fibrin formation and fibrin breakdown[177]

# Kidney stone formation risk factors

Concern about the development of kidney stones is often a reason that high-dose vitamin C is discouraged or denied. Under certain conditions, vitamin C — and a large list of many other factors — can contribute to an increase in oxalate concentration in the urine. Because calcium oxalate comprises many kidney stones, some may conclude that vitamin C causes kidney stones, since it can increase urinary oxalate. This myth is debunked in Chapter 7. Although research presented in that chapter shows that a high intake of vitamin C actually *lowers* the incidence of kidney stones, those with preexisting kidney disease (renal insufficiency or failure) should seek the advice of a physician before undertaking a high-dose vitamin C supplementation program.

Many factors are involved in the precipitation of calcium oxalate out of the urine, leading to stone formation. Increased vitamin C supplementation is but one of those factors. It is important to realize that a given risk factor can only produce a given medical condition when other surrounding circumstances favor the development of that condition as well. These risk factors, with appropriate references, include the following:

1) Increased oxalate in the urine[1,2]
2) Presence and high concentration of other dissolved substances (solutes) in the urine[3,4]

3) Presence of heavy metal chelation agents, such as DMPS, DMSA, and EDTA, which have their own independent kidney toxicities, due to increased urinary solute load and toxin damage to the kidneys[4]

4) Increased calcium in the urine[5-8]

5) Low magnesium levels in the urine[9]

6) Low citrate in the urine[10-12]

7) Low potassium in the urine[6]

8) Increased cystine in the urine[13]

9) Increased phosphorus in the urine[14]

10) Increased uric acid in the urine[15,16]

11) Increased lipids in the urine[17,18]

12) Increased cholesterol in the urine[17,18]

13) Increased age, with age-associated decrease in the flow rate of fluid filtered through the kidneys[19]

14) Intake of hard water[20]

15) Overall state of hydration[21,22]

16) Decreased daily volume of urine flow and formation[23,24]

17) Urinary pH[6,25-28]

18) Low dietary calcium[29]

19) Supplemental calcium[29,30]

20) Vitamin D supplementation[31-34]

21) Low intake of magnesium and vitamins[35]

22) Preexisting calcium deposits throughout the body, especially in the vascular system

23) Preexisting kidney insufficiency or failure, including being on hemodialysis[36-38]

24) Any injury to the cells lining those parts of the urinary system susceptible to stone formation[39]

25) Intake of oxalate stone-generating or oxalate-containing foods[1,40,41]

    a. Fruits: rhubarb, blackberries, blueberries, raspberries, strawberries, currants, kiwifruit, concord grapes, figs, tangerines, lemon peel, lime peel, plums

  b. Vegetables: green beans, beetroot, spinach, escarole, okra, parsley, pokeweed, sweet potatoes, swiss chard, beet greens, collards, leeks

  c. Meats: liver

  d. Grains: wheat bran, wheat germ, millet, grits, quinoa

  e. Nuts: peanuts, pecans, almonds, cashews, soybeans

  f. Miscellaneous: chocolate, pepper

26) Intake of oxalate stone-generating or oxalate-containing beverages[42,43] (black tea, cocoa, coffee)

27) Intake of oxalate stone-generating or oxalate-containing supplements and medicines[44-55]

28) Intake of oxalate stone-generating toxins[1,56,57]

29) Receiving all nutrition via intravenous infusion[58,59]

30) Deficiency of pyridoxine (vitamin B6)[60-65]

31) Deficiency of thiamine (vitamin B1)[64,66]

32) Having had intestinal bypass or resection surgery, or small bowel malabsorption from any cause[67-70]

33) Urinary tract infection or presence of bacteria[71-76]

34) Presence of increased oxidative stress in the urinary tract[77,78]

35) Primary hyperoxaluria (excessive excretion of oxalate in the urine), a hereditary disorder[79]

36) Hyperparathyroidism[80,81]

37) Urinary stasis (stoppage or lessening of normal urinary flow) or incomplete voiding[82,83]

38) Obstructive urinary disease[76]

39) Polycystic kidney disease[84,85]
40) Cirrhosis[1]
41) Diabetes[1]
42) Congestive heart failure[1]
43) Crohn's disease[86-88]
44) Cystic fibrosis[89-90]
45) Renal tubular acidosis (this is a disease marked by an inability of the kidneys to remove excess acid from the blood into the urine resulting in overly acidic blood)[1]
46) Sarcoidosis (a chronic inflammation of unknown origin that results in the formation of lumps [granulomas] in various organs of the body)[91,92]
47) Klinefelter's syndrome[1]
48) Parasitic diseases including amebiasis, schistosomiasis, giardiasis, and ascariasis[1]
49) Antibiotic therapy[93]
50) Increased fluoride intake[94]
51) Prolonged bedrest[95]
52) Kidney transplantation[96]
53) Hypertension[97,98]
54) Increased alcohol intake[99]
55) Increased glucose intake[100,101]
56) Pregnancy[102,103]
57) Methoxyflurane anesthesia[104-106]
58) Ketogenic diet (a high-fat, high-protein, low-carbohydrate diet)[107]
59) Space travel[108-109]
60) Increased vitamin C supplementation[110-112]
61) Calcium ascorbate as the type of supplemental vitamin C[113,114]

# Minimizing toxin impact

Two basic aspects of toxin exposure must be addressed:

1) Daily exposure to new toxins

2) Accumulation and storage of new toxins in bodily tissues rather than neutralization and excretion

A heavy metal such as mercury is a good example of a toxin that tends to exert its maximum toxicity after it has significantly accumulated in target tissues after extended chronic exposure. Other toxins, like alcohol, are readily excreted after their initial exposure and long-term accumulations are not an issue.

Whether an individual should undergo a mild, moderate, or aggressive program of detoxification is a decision that should be made in concert with a healthcare practitioner. The practitioner should be familiar with the wide array of interventions available for mobilizing and excreting toxins.

Although a good program of supplementation will generally stimulate at least a mild degree of detoxification, the need for deeper detoxification should be determined scientifically. Clinical status, standard laboratory tests, and special testing for the degrees of toxin accumulations all need to be a part of this decision. Sometimes an individual is suffering from a medical condition that is not likely to show substantial improvement until a major portion of accumulated toxins have been mobilized and excreted.

## *Poor Dental Health: A Major Source of Toxin Exposure*

With few exceptions, individuals who are unable to optimize their antioxidant capacity with quality supplementation are dealing with a significant amount of dental toxicity. Dental toxicity is often both infectious and toxic in nature, representing a "double whammy" in consuming the body's stored antioxidant supplies. Also, since the infections and toxins are generated "within" the body, 100% of all such toxins are assimilated by inhalation, swallowing, mucous membrane absorption, or direct release into the bloodstream. Toxins external to the body are never this effectively absorbed and assimilated.

This is why the root canal procedure is the most important single factor in the causation of chronic degenerative diseases, especially cancer and coronary heart disease. The enormous toxicity secreted directly into the bloodstream always keeps the antioxidant levels in the tissues knocked down, allowing any of a number of diseases to take hold and progress.

Addressing dental toxicity, then, should be the first, or at least a very early part of one's program targeted at optimizing antioxidant capacity. This involves the following:

1) Finding a supportive dentist who will work with you

2) Properly extracting all root canals

3) Properly extracting all infected or abscessed teeth

4) Proper cleaning/revision of jawbone cavitations

5) Properly addressing periodontal disease (a cup of warm water with a few capfuls of 3% hydrogen peroxide administered with a water irrigation device will resolve many cases of this disease, even when advanced with gum recession and bone resorption)

6) Replacement of mercury amalgam fillings with biocompatible replacement materials

7) Using biocompatible replacement materials for crowns and other dental appliances

8) Probable removal of dental implants, depending upon how well the patient improves clinically with the other dental/supplementation interventions

Items 1 through 3 are the most important factors to address. Allowing root canal-treated teeth, as well as any other infected teeth, to remain unextracted will severely compromise your path to recovery or your attempts to maintain good health.

For those who want more details, the enormous toxicity of the root canal-treated tooth is the subject of another book, *The Roots of Disease,* that I coauthored with Dr. Robert Kulacz.

## *Poor Digestion: A Huge Source of Toxins*

Another common source of substantial daily toxin exposure comes from a poorly functioning gastrointestinal tract. Proper digestion is of paramount importance. Many toxins of the same variety and toxicity level as can be seen in root canal-treated teeth are generated in substantial quantity in the sluggish, constipated gut.

Daily bowel movements, preferably at least twice daily, are your best evidence that your bowel function is normal or near-normal. A short list of important recommendations to help normal bowel function include the following (this issue is addressed in greater depth in my book, *Optimal Nutrition for Optimal Health*):

1) Combine your foods properly (*extremely important*)

2) Minimize high glycemic index foods (*choose complex carbohydrates rather than simple carbohydrate foods*)

3) Chew thoroughly!!! (*a simple but extremely important factor in achieving normal digestion*)

4) Minimize water and liquids with meals (*dilutes digestive enzymes*)

5) Take a broad-spectrum digestive enzyme supplement with or before meals

6) Eat smaller amounts more frequently rather than having one or 2 large meals daily

7) Minimize dairy in general, and do not consume pasteurized milk as a beverage (*too much calcium, impairs digestion*)

8) Try to limit meat protein to between 2 to 4 ounces at a time (*difficult to completely digest larger amounts*)

9) Minimize seafood (*mercury exposure*)

10) Choose organic foods when possible

## *Minimizing Reactive Iron*

This very important key to achieving optimal anti-oxidant capacity needs to be addressed separately. Free, or reactive, iron levels in the body must be minimized. Such iron is a powerful oxidative catalyst, and it is probably the primary factor in promoting excess oxidative stress wherever it has excessively accumulated in the body.

Ferritin levels are currently the best test to check for excess iron stores, corresponding to excess levels of free iron in the body. Currently, some laboratories consider ferritin levels as high as 400 ng/ml to be normal. This level is **never** normal. Every effort should be made to bring ferritin levels down to 15 to 25 ng/ml, or less. As long as the hemoglobin level is normal, the body has enough iron in it. When a borderline anemia is finally being approached, measures to facilitate iron excretion can be withheld. The best ways to lower the body's stores of iron are:

1) Phlebotomy. Giving up to 6 units of blood annually is a good goal, and this will drop ferritin levels significantly.

2) Sweating excessively (*aerobic athletes can achieve this, but it is more readily accomplished with a far infrared sauna*); magnesium and other electrolytes can be wasted as well, and should be monitored and supplemented

3) Inositol hexaphosphate (IP6, phytic acid). Doses between 2 and 3 grams should be taken daily, but on an empty stomach; it will bind iron and calcium in food if taken with meals (best to take in the middle of the night when arising to go to the bathroom, or first thing in the morning by itself)

4) Prescription iron chelation; this should be done only if difficulty is encountered in stabilizing an acute clinical situation that is likely being exacerbated by, or primarily due to, excess iron (*such as progressive coronary artery disease, with clear progression of arterial narrowings on serial angiography that are not responding adequately to other measures*)

# Balancing high-dose vitamin C with other supplements

Although vitamin C is perhaps the premier supplement, additional supplementation with a range of other nutrients often deficient in the daily diet is very beneficial. This is not a "one size fits all" matter, however. What is optimal for any given person depends on multiple factors. These factors include new daily toxin exposure, types and levels of toxins already accumulated, and pre-existing diseases.

Also, largely due to these three factors, different individuals will have variable requirements for the different vitamins and minerals. Some conditions will consume or deplete some nutrients more than others. The following supplements are important, but the dose ranges are only very approximate. They are best adjusted over time in concert with a knowledgeable healthcare practitioner monitoring you and your test results on a regular basis.

- L-lysine: 3,000 to 6,000 mg daily (*especially when trying to slow or even reverse coronary artery disease*)

- Magnesium chelate (*glycinate or other*): 200 to 1,000 mg daily (essential to maintaining normal calcium metabolism and mobilizing abnormal calcium depositions)

- Vitamin K2: 1 to 3 mg daily (*critical for calcium balance as with magnesium*)

- Vitamin D3 (*cholecalciferol*): 5,000 to 10,000 IU daily (*adjust up or down depending on blood levels, generally aiming for 60 to 80 ng/cc*)

- Vitamin E (*mixed tocopherols and tocotrienols*): 200 to 1,000 IU daily

- Beta Carotene (*vitamin A source*): 25,000 IU daily

- Vitamin B complex: 1 daily or a portion of a vegetable/fruit powder blend (*individual B vitamins can be supplemented in greater amounts depending upon needs*)

- Multimineral: 1 daily or a portion of a vegetable/fruit powder blend (*individual minerals can be supplemented in greater amounts depending upon needs; AVOID copper and iron, unless a clear deficiency has been identified*)

- Omega-3 krill oil: 300 to 600 mg daily

- Digestive enzymes: before or with meals

- Any of a wide variety of quality antioxidants and other supplements including, but not limited to:
  — N-acetylcysteine
  — coenzyme Q10
  — alpha lipoic acid
  — silymarin
  — resveratrol
  — L-arginine
  — amino acids
  — MSM
  — nattokinase
  — polyphenols
  — superoxide dismutase
  — catalase
  — rutin
  — quercetin
  — whey protein powder
  — wheat germ
  — lecithin

Finally, in concert with a healthcare practitioner who is working with you, periodic assessment with coronary artery calcium testing should be performed, initially at 6-month to one-year intervals. If your total "program" results in progressively increasing coronary artery calcium scores, more evaluation needs to be done and a better program should be instituted. On the other hand, a progressively declining score is an excellent indicator that you are treating your entire body well, in addition to your coronary arteries.

# Published studies supporting the use of vitamin C in the treatment of infectious diseases and toxin exposures

This is not an exhaustive resource. Time and space do not permit such a treatment; furthermore, new studies are published daily. Hopefully, the information provided in this resource will stimulate a greater appreciation of what researchers have already solidly established.

The vast majority of studies cited are indexed on the government's *PubMed* website. For those who want to "see" the abstracts of the actual studies, here are some basic instructions:

1. Go to the *PubMed* site at
   **http://www.ncbi.nlm.nih.gov/pubmed**

2. Type the last name of the first author listed in the reference followed by the year, volume, number, and first page of that reference (*e.g., the underlined items with simple spaces separating those items, as in the sample citation listed below*)

   Riordan NH, Riordan HD, Jackson JA: Intravenous ascorbate as a tumor cytotoxic chemo-therapeutic agent. *Med Hypoth*, 1995; 44(3):207-213.

   You will type: Riordan 1995 44(3) 207

3. Click the "Search" button

In most cases, the search will retrieve an abstract of the study. In some cases the whole study may be available at no charge. For the remaining studies, a copy of the entire study can often be obtained for a fee.

Remember that all studies should be evaluated critically. The goal of this book is to promote honest, science-based research on the medical uses of "high-dose" vitamin C. The work of such pioneers as Dr. Klenner, Linus Pauling, Dr. Cathcart, Dr. Riordan, and others provides sufficient basis and direction for the continued investigation on the applications of vitamin C, the *Primal Panacea*.

Therefore, particular caution should be exercised regarding the definition of "high-dose." These definitions vary widely! Those who have swallowed the 90 mg RDA mantra consider 500 mg to be "high-dose," while the pioneers listed above define a daily "high-dose" in the 10,000 to 150,000 mg (or more) range. It is essential for readers and future researchers to acknowledge that obtaining the types of results reported by Dr. Klenner — and those who followed him — requires the use of "Klenner-sized" doses. Time after time, studies have shown that successful clinical responses to vitamin C are extremely dose-dependent. Klenner himself repeatedly emphasized this important fact.

*Very few* of the studies cited in the following pages employed true "high-dose" vitamin C. Even with that great handicap, positive results have still been achieved with doses considerably below optimum. Much better outcomes await those who are willing to break though this low-dosage "barrier." Cures and good health at low cost are ahead. There is absolutely no valid reason to be timid. Let's move forward!

## Aflatoxin Poisoning

**Description:** Aflatoxins are a family of poisons produced by several fungal species (molds) of the *Aspergillus* variety. These toxins are among the most carcinogenic substances known to man. Continued exposure significantly increases the risk of hepatocellular carcinoma (liver cancer), which is the third most common cause of cancer deaths worldwide.[1] The typical sources for aflatoxin are found in decaying vegetation, nuts, spices, and grains. Examples include: contaminated millet, rice, wheat, peanuts, soybeans, sunflower seeds, chili peppers, black pepper, ginger, almonds, pistachio, walnuts, coconuts, and brazil nuts.[2]

**Traditional Approach:** No specific treatment for aflatoxin poisoning prior to diagnosis of hepatocellular carcinoma is listed in *Cecil Medicine*.

**Studies Show:**

- Vitamin C protects guinea pigs from acute aflatoxin poisoning[3]

- Negative effects of aflatoxin on the rabbit reproductive system are greatly reduced with vitamin C[4]

- Vitamin C affords significant protection against aflatoxin-induced rupture of red blood cells *in vitro*[5]

- Aflatoxin-induced chromosomal abnormalities in bone marrow cells of mice are decreased by vitamin C[6]

- Vitamin C lessens aflatoxin-induced mutations in some bacteria[7,8]

## AIDS/HIV

**Description:** Acquired Immunodeficiency Syndrome (AIDS) results from advanced Human Immunodeficiency Virus (HIV) infection. This virus attacks the immune system, profoundly depleting T-lymphocytes (cell-mediated immunity). These lymphocytes initiate and control many necessary immune responses, and the ability of HIV to destroy CD4+ lymphocytes reduces/eliminates the body's ability to defend against a host of opportunistic pathogens.[1]

**Traditional Approach:** Treatment of HIV and AIDS is divided into three major areas: (1) anti-retrovirus therapies, (2) treatment/prevention of opportunistic infections, and (3) treatment of HIV-related complications. The goal is simply to slow the progression of the disease with the least disruption to the patient's lifestyle.[2]

**Studies Show:**

- AIDS and HIV infection are preventable and reversible with aggressive vitamin C therapy continued for a long enough time[3]

- Clinical improvement is proportional to vitamin C dosage size — a patient can be put into remission if enough vitamin C is administered[4]

- AIDS patients who die of nervous system toxicity are found to have significantly reduced vitamin C levels in the most-effected areas of brain[5]

- Even small doses of oral vitamin C to HIV-infected patients lessen evidence of oxidative stress and result in a reduction in actual viral load[6,7]

- CD4 depletion can be slowed, stopped, and even reversed for several years when vitamin C is optimally dosed[8]

## AIDS/HIV (cont.)

- Vitamin C inhibits the ability of HIV to replicate in chronically infected T-lymphocytes with a mechanism not characteristic of antioxidants in general[9]

- Vitamin C concentrations not directly toxic to HIV-infected cells are still able to inhibit virus reproduction inside the cells[10]

- Supplementation with vitamin C and N-acetyl cysteine for 6 days in HIV-infected patients increases CD4 T-lymphocyte count, increases glutathione levels in those cells, and decreases plasma levels of HIV-related RNA[11]

- High intakes of vitamin C, niacin, and vitamin B1 by HIV-infected patients slows progression to AIDS after adjustment for confounding variables[12]

- HIV-infected patients have lower plasma concentrations of vitamin C than found in non-HIV controls[13]

- AIDS patients with myelopathy "respond well" to vitamin C therapy[14,15]

- "Supranutritional" dosing of vitamin C and vitamin E protects against AZT-mediated oxidative muscle damage in both AIDS patients and in mice[16]

## Alcohol (Ethanol) Poisoning

**Description:** The major toxicity associated with ethanol consumption springs from the breakdown of alcohol into acetaldehyde. At a certain point, acetaldehyde becomes lethal. Vitamin C not only reduces the production of acetaldehyde, but it also appears to reduce the loss of perception and motor skills that can accompany acute ethanol consumption.

**Studies Show:**

- Vitamin C lessens body movement abnormalities produced by the administration of methanol (another alcohol) in mice[1]

- Motor coordination and color discrimination are significantly better in men supplementing vitamin C for 2 weeks prior to alcohol consumption in a placebo-controlled study — alcohol elimination from the blood is also improved by vitamin C[2]

- A vitamin C dose (equivalent to 4,400 mg dose for a 150-pound person) produces no clear improvement in motor coordination in alcohol-intoxicated lab animals; while high-dose vitamin C (equivalent to 35,000 mg for a 150-pound person) completely prevented motor coordination loss[3]

- 40 grams of intravenous vitamin C along with vitamin B1 can neutralize the intoxication effects of alcohol[4]

- Vitamin C reduces abnormal elevations of oxidative stress in patients with chronic alcoholic liver disease[5]

- Alcoholics have much lower blood levels of antioxidant enzymes and antioxidants, including vitamin C[6]

## Alcohol (Ethanol) Poisoning (cont.)

- Alcoholics both metabolize and eliminate vitamin C more quickly, indicating a much greater need for supplementation[7]

- Vitamin C blood levels are reduced by 12-15% from "moderate" alcohol consumption[8]

- Supplementation with only 1,000 mg of vitamin C daily for 3 days prior to acute alcohol consumption decreases the associated acetaldehyde-mediated poisoning[9]

- There is a direct correlation between levels of vitamin C in white blood cells and the rate of ethanol clearance from the blood[10]

- Vitamin C given 90 minutes before an otherwise fatal injection of acetaldehyde significantly reduces mortality in mice[11,12]

- Vitamin C, along with glucose and cysteine, blocks otherwise lethal doses of acetaldehyde given to mice[13]

- Pretreatment with vitamin C lessens alcohol-induced oxidative stress and blocks the otherwise-expected DNA damage[14]

- High-dose vitamin C (equivalent to 140 grams for a 150-pound person) clearly reduces alcohol-induced poisoning in rats[15]

- Guinea pigs receiving a 5-week pre-treatment with large amounts of vitamin C are able to metabolize ingested alcohol much more quickly then those receiving minimal amounts[16]

- Administration of "large amounts" of vitamin C accelerates the metabolism of both ethanol and acetaldehyde, while reducing some of their adverse health effects[17]

## Alcohol (Ethanol) Poisoning (cont.)

- The alcohol-induced increase in blood fats is significantly reduced with supplemental vitamin C in guinea pigs[18]

- The same ethanol dose that caused SGOT (a liver enzyme) levels to increase 12-fold in animals with vitamin C levels below 16 mg/100 g of liver weight was given to animals with C levels above this threshold — researchers reported a 60% reduction in SGOT[19]

- A thorough review of the literature demonstrates that adequately-dosed vitamin C is the best way to detoxify alcohol, prevent future alcohol-induced damage, and repair past alcohol-induced damage[20]

## Aluminum Poisoning

**Description:** Aluminum in the blood causes oxidative damage through lipid peroxidation (LPO), which can then result in damage to cell membranes and cellular DNA. Aluminum toxicity can damage the central nervous system, and it can greatly impair speech, cognitive abilities, memory, and muscle coordination. As it accumulates in bones, it inhibits the incorporation of calcium. High aluminum exposure increases the risk for lung and bladder cancer.[1]

**Traditional Approach:** Removal of aluminum from the blood can be accomplished through hemodialysis and hemofiltration. Deferoxamine is used to chelate aluminum from blood and tissues when serum levels exceed 100 µg/L.[1]

**Studies Show:**

- An antioxidant treatment protocol including vitamin C largely blocks the ability of aluminum to increase LPO activity[2]

- Vitamin C prevents aluminum-induced LPO damage *in vitro*[3]

- Vitamin C supplementation in rabbits enhanced excretion (chelation) of aluminum accumulated in bone tissues [4]

- Vitamin C prevents some aluminum-induced LPO breakage of chromosomes in bone marrow cells of mice[5,6]

## Alzheimer's / Dementia

**Description:** Dementia is defined as a cognitive disorder
that interferes with daily functioning and results in
a loss of independence. Its incidence increases with
age.[1] It is generally accepted that oxidative stress from
reactive oxygen species (ROS) is largely responsible
for the genesis and progression of dementia diseases.[2]

**Traditional Approach:** There are no established preventative therapies. There are two classes of drugs
are approved and used in treatment: cholinesterase
inhibitors and memantine.[3]

**Studies Show:**

- Animal studies validate an important role for
  vitamin C in preventing and reducing excess
  oxidative stress in models of neurodegenerative
  diseases[4-6]

- A combination of vitamin C, vitamin E, and non-
  steroidal anti-inflammatory drugs slows the
  cognitive decline of Alzheimer's disease[7]

- A randomized, double-blind, placebo-controlled
  study concludes that Alzheimer's patients who
  received an antioxidant formula, including
  vitamin C, demonstrate significantly improved
  cognitive scores[8]

## Amphetamine Poisoning

**Description:** Seizures, tachycardia, hyperthermia, hallucinations, stroke, hypertension, and death can result from acute amphetamine overdose. Toxic exposure to amphetamine causes neuronal cell damage and even destruction, as well as heart damage.[1]

**Traditional Approach:** Treatment can include sedation, ice pack therapy for hyperthermia, and use of drugs like benzodiazepines and haloperidol.[1]

**Studies Show:**

- A 17 year-old male suffered an Ecstasy overdose, entered the hospital after a grand mal seizure, and awoke from a comatose state, talking within 50 minutes after starting intravenous vitamin C[2]

- Pretreatment with vitamin C lessens the neurotoxic effects of methamphetamine in laboratory animals[3,4]

- Vitamin C pretreatment along with other antioxidants lessens the long-lasting depletions of dopamine in the brains of rats given methamphetamine[5]

- The anti-amphetamine effects of haloperidol are substantially enhanced by vitamin C administration[6]

- Vitamin C lessens the behavioral abnormalities associated with amphetamine administration in rats[7]

## Arsenic Poisoning

**Description:** Arsenic poisoning commonly results from chronic exposure to the trivalent form of this element (arsenite). Signs and symptoms include weakness, malaise, discoloration of the tongue and inside the mouth, lung disease, neuropathy, liver toxicity, and brittle nails.[1]

**Traditional Approach:** Chelation with the drug, 2,3-dimercapto-1-propanesulfonate [DMPS] (not FDA-approved), when blood levels are above 50 µg/L.[2]

**Studies Show:**

- In the 1940s doctors treated syphilis with arsenic; vitamin C was found to be the "safest way" to protect patients from the toxic effects of the medicine[3]

- Vitamin C protects lab animals from the toxic effects of sodium arsenite on ovarian and brain functions[4]

- Vitamin C enhances the effectiveness of arsenic trioxide in killing cancer cells seen in leukemia and multiple myeloma[5-7]

## Arthritis

**Description:** Arthritis diseases (polyarthritis, osteoarthritis, and rheumatoid arthritis) all result in a degeneration of joint tissues. Oxidative stress has been blamed for cartilage senescence, chondrocyte telomere instability, and a lessening of chondrocyte function in arthritis.[1] A compromised antioxidant defense system is also tied to the development of arthritis.[2]

**Traditional Approach:** *Cecil Medicine* has no listing for osteoarthritis. The treatment for rheumatoid arthritis attempts to put the disease into remission and manage pain. It includes the use of non-steroidal anti-inflammatory drugs (NSAIDs), corticosteroids, and disease-modifying antirheumatic drugs (DMARDs).[3] Treatment for polyarthritis includes the use of NSAIDs, corticosteroids, sulfasalazine and methotrexate.[4]

**Studies Show:**

- Osteoarthritis patients have significantly lower vitamin C stores than normal[5]

- Scurvy victims exhibit arthritis symptoms[6,7]

- Lower levels of vitamin C and GSH (an intracellular antioxidant) are seen in the synovial fluid of arthritic joints and are tied to damage of cartilage tissue[8]

- A lower intake of vitamin C is associated with development of polyarthritis[9,10]

- A greater vitamin C intake reduces the bone marrow lesions that help cause knee osteoarthritis[11]

- High-dose vitamin C administration reduces extremity arthritis and its associated inflammatory edema, as well as the infiltration of the inflammatory cells into the synovial tissue in arthritic rats[12]

## Barbiturate Overdose

**Description:** Barbiturates are used as anticonvulsants, tranquilizers, and sedatives. Phenobarbital is the most commonly known of these drugs, and it remains the most common drug used to treat seizure disorders throughout the world. Symptoms of a barbiturate overdose range from sluggishness to a life-threatening coma.[1]

**Traditional Approach:** After intubation (insertion of a breathing tube) and beginning intravenous fluid therapy, the patient is often given drugs to boost their blood pressure like norepinephrine or dopamine. Activated charcoal may then be given in hopes of absorbing any of the barbiturate that remains in the gastrointestinal tract.[2]

### Studies Show:

- A comatose patient who had overdosed on barbiturates, with a blood pressure of 60/0, promptly awakened and completely recovered with 125,000 mg of vitamin C administered over a 12-hour period[3]

- Fifteen cases of severe barbiturate overdose completely resolved within hours with the combination of intravenous and oral vitamin C administration totaling 100,000 mg or more[3]

- Injection of high-dose vitamin C reverses the low blood pressure, the respiratory failure, and the central nervous system depression seen with barbiturate overdose in dogs and mice[4]

# Benzanthrone Poisoning

**Description:** Benzanthrone is an aromatic hydrocarbon derivative used as a solvent in the industrial manufacture of dyes, and in fireworks.[1] Exposure over a period of time can produce severe skin irritation, a loss of appetite, fatigue, and weakness. It can also impair liver function and cause gastritis.[1] Ingestion of this toxic substance can cause burns in the esophagus and G.I. tract.[2]

**Traditional Approach:** Treatment of external exposure involves removal from the source, along with topical creams. For ingestion, stomach pumping or irrigation-followed by doses of activated charcoal is employed in an attempt to block further absorption of any remaining benzanthrone.[2]

**Studies Show:**

- Exposure to benzanthrone consumes vitamin C and glutathione[3]

- Vitamin C in a dose equivalent to 1,750 mg for a 150-pound person lowers benzanthrone-induced death by 40% in laboratory animals[4]

- Small doses of vitamin C produce significant improvement in the appearance and the biochemical changes seen in the liver, testis, kidney, and bladder of animals exposed to benzanthrone[5]

- Oral and topical vitamin C treatments provide substantial protection against benzanthrone-induced toxic effects on skin and liver[6]

- Pretreatment with vitamin C increases excretion and greatly reduces organ retention of benzanthrone[7,8]

## Benzene Poisoning

**Description:** Benzene is a clear, liquid, aromatic hydro-carbon commonly used as a solvent. Exposure can occur through contact with the skin, breathing the vapors, or ingestion. Symptoms of poisoning include: blurred vision, irritated nose/throat, loss of appetite, nausea, vomiting, irregular or rapid heartbeat, rapid/shallow breathing, dizziness, drowsiness, nervousness, convulsions, headache, staggering, unconsciousness, and weakness.[1]

**Traditional Approach:** "There is no antidote for acute benzene poisoning."[2] Those exposed should be immediately removed from the source and cardiopulmonary status must be monitored and treated. Stomach pumping is indicated if significant quantities have been ingested.[2]

**Studies Show:**

- Severe benzene poisoning resulted in "symptoms like those of scurvy," and high-dose vitamin C administration forced excretion of benzene in the urine[3]

- A benzene-induced scurvy-like state was successfully treated with high-dose vitamin C[4]

- Vitamin C supplementation is recommended to prevent benzene poisoning[5]

- Vitamin C in a dose-dependent fashion provides protection in animal cell preparations from the toxic effects of bromobenzene[6]

- Increased vitamin C lessened symptoms and lowered mortality rate by 57% in guinea pigs[7]

# Brucellosis

**Description:** Brucellae are animal-borne bacteria that can infect humans, typically through contact or ingestion of contaminated milk products. Symptoms of the disease include joint pain, enlargement of the spleen and/or liver, and swollen lymph nodes. Severe cases may cause damage to the heart and can result in death.[1]

**Traditional Approach:** If detected early and treated with an extended protocol of antibiotics, the infection is sometimes curable. Relapses can occur throughout a patient's life, even when treated aggressively early in the course of the infection. Chronic brucellosis is considered to be incurable.[1]

**Studies Show:**

- Significantly lower vitamin C levels are found in chronic brucellosis patients[2]

- Vitamin C supplementation for 15 days restores specific parameters of monocyte immune function needed for combating brucellosis[2]

- In a brucellosis case study with a 35 year-old woman suffering with symptoms for 15 years, 15 months of vitamin C supplementation at 3,000 mg per day eradicated her recurring symptoms[3]

- Daily vitamin C supplementation at 3,000 mg eliminated chronic symptoms and enabled a 6-year brucellosis sufferer to return to work and to regain the 70 pounds he lost because of the disease[3]

- 11 of 12 brucellosis cases show dramatic improvement with daily vitamin C supplementation at 3,000 to 4,000 mg — the non-responder was the only patient refusing an occasional intravenous injection of C to bolster the oral C dosing[3]

## Cadmium Poisoning

**Description:** Flu-like symptoms can result from an acute exposure to cadmium vapor. Tracheobronchitis, pneumonitis, and pulmonary edema result from more serious exposure. Inhalation can damage the respiratory tract and cause kidney failure. Ingestion can cause immediate damage to the liver and the kidneys. Chronic exposure has been linked to calcium loss in the bones.[1]

**Traditional Approach:** "The clinical picture of chronic cadmium poisoning is one of irreversible renal toxicity... Treatment of the toxic effects of cadmium is symptomatic and supportive. There is no accepted way to reduce the body burden of cadmium."[2] [*Translation: There is no effective treatment.*]

**Studies Show:**

- High-dose vitamin C provided substantially better protection against cadmium poisoning than low-dose vitamin C in guinea pig studies[3-5]

- Vitamin C inhibits the accumulation of cadmium in the brain, heart, and testes of test animals[6]

- 93% of lab animals pretreated with vitamin C survived a dose of cadmium that was fatal for all the non-treated animals[7]

- Vitamin C provides significant protection against the chromosomal damage induced by cadmium chloride exposure in cultured mouse cells[8]

- Vitamin C added to animal feed lowers cadmium accumulation in the kidney and liver by up to 40%[9,10]

# Cancer

**Description:** Cancer is a class of diseases in which a group of cells displays uncontrolled growth, invading and sometimes destroying adjacent tissues. In its advanced stages it frequently metastasizes or spreads to other locations in the body via lymph or blood. These three malignant properties of cancers differentiate them from benign tumors, which do not rapidly proliferate, invade or metastasize.[1]

**Traditional Approach:** Often a combination of one or more of the following is used: surgery, radiation, and chemotherapy. The theory behind radiation and chemotherapy is that the more rapidly growing cancer cells are less able to defend themselves from toxic assault than the normal cells. Radiation and nearly all chemotherapy drugs are themselves carcinogenic (cancer-causing), since they increase oxidative stress in all the cells treated, not just the cancer cells.[2]

**Studies Show:**

- Case studies demonstrate success in treating and even completely resolving various cancers with high-dose vitamin C[3-12]

- In advanced cancer patients, high-dose vitamin C therapy compared to conventional therapy at one facility over a 3-year period shows:[13]
    - 75% better breast cancer survivor rate
    - 867% better lung cancer survivor rate
    - 107% better colorectal cancer survivor rate
    - When breast cancer patients made this facility as their first treatment option, the 3-year survival rate improved by 134%

- High-dose vitamin C enhances the effectiveness of traditional chemotherapies[14-16]

## Cancer (cont.)

- Vitamin C has its own cancer cell-killing ability, and it also significantly improves the cell-killing ability of doxorubicin — even when the vitamin C is given at a non-cytotoxic dosage, it still improves the cell-killing ability of doxorubicin[17]

## Carbon Tetrachloride Poisoning

**Description:** Although once used as a common cleaning solvent, its toxic properties have limited its current use. Chronic exposure to carbon tetrachloride can result in kidney damage and cancer. Acute exposure to high concentrations of the liquid or vapor can damage the central nervous system, as well as the liver and kidneys. Prolonged exposure can result in coma and even death.[1]

**Traditional Approach:** No accepted antidote for this poisoning exists. Two experimental treatments are sometimes used: Hyperbaric oxygen and/or N-acetyl-cysteine[2] [*a precursor of glutathione, a powerful intra-cellular antioxidant that is recharged by vitamin C*]

**Studies Show:**

- Repeated doses of vitamins C and E reduce toxic effects of carbon tetrachloride on the liver in rats[3,4]

- Vitamin C can prevent carbon tetrachloride from causing liver damage in rats[5]

- The intravenous injection of vitamin C into mice prior to the administration of an LD10 (lethal dose for 10% of the test group) of carbon tetrachloride completely prevents any deaths and minimizes the tissue damage normally expected[6]

- Vitamin C prevents carbon tetrachloride-induced gonadal damage in rats[7]

# Cholesterol (High Levels of LDL)

**Description:** Cholesterol is manufactured by the body, and it is also supplied via dietary intake. It is necessary for the neutralization of several different toxins and it is a natural anti-inflammatory agent. Unlike cholesterol linked with high-density lipoprotein (HDL, "the good cholesterol") that is transported to the liver for excretion, the cholesterol linked with low-density lipoprotein (LDL, "the bad cholesterol") is transported into arterial walls during times of a focal vitamin C deficiency in the coronary arteries, facilitating plaque formation.

**Traditional Approach:** Statin drugs are used as "first-line therapy for lowering LDL cholesterol in patients with diabetes" as well as for other patients with high levels of LDL cholesterol.[1] [*A meta-analysis of statin studies published in 2011 found that the evidence for cost-effective primary prevention with statins is not clear-cut. The authors cautioned against prescribing these drugs for primary prevention among people with low cardiovascular risk.*[2]]

**Studies Show:**

- Serum cholesterol levels increase with a vitamin C deficiency[3-9]

- Excessive cholesterol depletes vitamin C[10-16]

- Vitamin supplementation lowers serum cholesterol[18]

- High-dose vitamin C stimulates cholesterol transformation into bile[19]

- Vitamin C protects arteries from plaque buildup even in the presence of high serum cholesterol[20,21]

# Chromium Poisoning

**Description:** Several forms of chromium exist but the most toxic form is chromium VI (hexavalent chromium). Topical exposure to this metal can cause serious dermititis. Inhaling chromium can cause breathing disorders (like asthma attacks) and even lung cancer. Ingesting chromium VI can cause stomach upset, ulcers, convulsions, kidney damage, liver damage, and even death.[1]

**Traditional Approach:** "Treatment of chromium poisoning is symptomatic and supportive.[2] [*Translation: There is no effective treatment.*]

**Studies Show:**

- Vitamin C is an effective antidote for chromium poisoning in lab animals from both internal and external exposures[3]

- Topical vitamin C shortens healing time for chromium-induced skin ulcers in guinea pigs[4]

- Vitamin C-impregnated filters protect against the toxicity of inhaling chromic acid mist[5]

- Vitamin C is considered a "true antidote" for hexavalent chromium poisoning[6]

- Chromate-induced kidney toxicity is greatly lessened by vitamin C[7]

- Vitamin C offers definite protection against both the toxic and mutation-causing effects of chromium in guinea pigs[8]

- Vitamin C is effective at removing (chelating) chromium from the tissues of laboratory animals[9]

## Common Cold

**Description:** Also called an upper respiratory infection, the common cold is caused by a virus that is passed from human to human. Irritation and swelling of the nasal passages and sinuses, scratchy throat, and cough are the associated symptoms. Although the cold is considered to be incurable, it is self-limiting, meaning it eventually runs its course. Secondary infection is common, and this can be serious to life-threatening in the very young and the elderly.[1]

**Traditional Approach:** "Given the self-limited nature of colds, any treatment should be completely safe... Because the subjective symptoms of a cold disappear in seven days without intervention, a variety of actually ineffective treatments, such as vitamin C and zinc gluconate lozenges, have been reported to be effective as a result of inadequate 'blinding' of placebo recipients. Herbal remedies are widely used, but evidence does not indicate any benefit."[1]

**Studies Show:**

- Vitamin C shortens the duration of the common cold[2]

- The common cold requires much more vitamin C than previously suggested — a mild cold requires 30,000 to 60,000 mg; a severe cold requires 60,000 to 100,000 mg[3]

- Early loading of vitamin C at the first sign of symptoms reduces cold and flu symptoms by 85%[4]

- Vitamin C lessens the severity and duration of the common cold[5,6]

- Vitamin C alleviates cold-like symptoms, delays the onset of disease, and decreases chances of death from infection[7]

# Diphtheria

**Description:** The *Corynebacterium diphtheriae* organism primarily infects the respiratory tract, resulting in inflammation of the tonsils, throat, and larynx. Exotoxins produced by this infection can sometimes damage the heart and the nervous system. The disease is highly contagious and between 5% to 10% of cases in the U.S. are fatal.[1]

**Traditional Approach:** Patients are quickly quarantined and treated with large doses of an antitoxin obtained from horses. Because production by U.S. manufacturers has stopped, no licensed product is available here. Antibiotics are also prescribed to combat the infection and to limit the continued production of exotoxin. For all these reasons, the emphasis in this disease has been prevention through the use of vaccination.[1]

**Studies Show:**

- Lethal doses of diphtheria toxins were no longer lethal in guinea pigs when premixed with vitamin C — the toxin doses without added vitamin C killed the guinea pigs in 4 to 8 days[2]
- Vitamin C increases resistance to diphtheria toxin in guinea pigs[3]
- Vitamin C inactivates diphtheria toxin in the test tube and protects guinea pigs from a lethal dose of diphtheria toxin[4]
- Scurvy-stricken guinea pigs infected with diphtheria show twice the mortality rate as non-scurvy animals[5]
- Small intramuscular injections of vitamin C saved 50% of pigeons injected with fatal doses of diphtheria toxin[6]

## Diphtheria (cont.)

- Small (1,000 to 2,000 mg) oral doses of vitamin C
  have little effect on diphtheria but large,
  frequent doses via intramuscular or intravenous
  administration are able to routinely cure the
  infection[7]

- Three children with nasal diphtheria; all received
  antitoxin injections — 1 also received 10,000 mg
  of vitamin C via injection every 8 hours for 3 doses
  and then every 12 hours for 2 more doses followed
  by oral dosing; the patient receiving the vitamin C
  was the lone survivor[8]

## Distemper (Cat & Dog)

**Description:** Although different viral strains are responsible for feline and canine distemper, the symptoms are very similar. Infection is accompanied by "runny nose, vomiting and diarrhea, dehydration, excessive salivation, coughing and/or labored breathing, loss of appetite, and weight loss. When and if the neurological symptoms develop, incontinence may ensue."[1]

**Traditional Approach:** Most often the treatment is simply to make the animal more comfortable. Unless the immune status of the animal is especially strong, the disease is often fatal, especially in very young or older animals. Although most dogs are vaccinated for distemper, there is still a high prevalence of the disease in the U.S.[1]

**Studies Show:**

- Twelve pets (cats/dogs) were treated with 1,000 to 2,000 mg of intravenous vitamin C per day for 3 days — all 12 recovered, even 2 that were given no hope of recovery by other veterinarians[2]

- Many dogs suffering with distemper were cured with multigram injections of vitamin C every 2 hours[3]

- The treatment of distemper in 67 dogs with vitamin C produced excellent results[4]

# Dysentery, Amebic

**Description:** An ameba, *Entamoeba histolytica*, causes this protozoan infection that often results in intestinal cramps, bloody diarrhea, abdominal soreness, painful straining during bowel movements, and fever. The intestinal wall can develop lesions that sometimes perforate the colon, often resulting in a fatal outcome. The infection is transferred by the ingestion of untreated drinking water or of contaminated foods.[1]

**Traditional Approach:** Prevention is important. Infections are treated with an array of antimicrobial drugs.[1]

**Studies Show:**

- Guinea pigs fed a vitamin C-deficient diet are especially susceptible to ameba infection, even when the microbe count in the inoculating dose is decidedly small[2]

- Vitamin C-deficient guinea pigs more easily contracted amebic infections, had more severe clinical courses, and all died — vitamin C supplementation in animals on the same diet resulted in more resistance to severe infection, and a significant number survived[3]

- 106 ameba-infected patients receiving only 150 mg of vitamin C daily experienced milder symptoms[4]

- Ameba-infected patients treated with 500 mg of vitamin C daily had shorter illness durations and quicker resolution of symptoms than patients not given vitamin C[5]

## Dysentery, Bacillary (Shigellosis)

**Description:** Bacillary dysentery is caused by four pathogenic species of *Shigella* bacteria. Infection causes a severe irritation of the colon that can result in diarrhea, bloody stools, abdominal cramping, and fever. This extremely contagious infection can occur with the ingestion of as few as 10 to 100 organisms in contrast to other gut pathogens that require the presence of 1,000 to 10,000 organisms to initiate infection. *Shigella* bacteria are becoming increasingly antibiotic-resistant, and the infection can still be passed by recovering individuals for up to six weeks after all symptoms have subsided.[1]

**Traditional Approach:** Maintaining good hydration, with water and electrolyte replacement, is necessary. Most cases resolve within 4 to 8 days. In severe infections symptoms can last for up to six weeks, even when antibiotics are prescribed.[2]

**Studies Show:**

- Patients given 500 to 1,000 mg of vitamin C by intramuscular injection were readily cured of dysentery — children having "10 to 15 bloody stools per day" would clear up in 48 hours[3]

- Adrenal levels of vitamin C were 60% lower in monkeys in the wild that died of naturally-acquired dysentery, indicating significant vitamin C consumption by the infection[4]

- Vitamin C administration provided 100% protection from dysentery infection in animals injected with the *Shigella* bacteria[5]

- Non-vitamin C-producing monkeys can develop severe scurvy after being exposed to *Shigella*[5]

## Encephalitis

**Description:** Encephalitis is an inflammation of the brain that causes dangerous swelling, often occurring as a complication of a viral infection. Viruses that can cause encephalitis include: herpes simplex, measles, mumps, chickenpox, and West Nile virus. An allergic reaction to a vaccination, autoimmune diseases, and certain bacterial infections can also cause encephalitis. Symptoms include extremely high fever, headache, confusion, drowsiness, stiff neck and back, vomiting, muscle weakness/paralysis, memory loss, seizures, and even coma.[1]

**Traditional Approach:** Treatment of the cause must first be addressed. The fever can be managed with acetaminophen, ice, and cooling blankets. "Vigorous support and avoidance of complications are essential."[2]

**Studies Show:**

- A lethargic, stuporous 8 year-old boy was treated with 2,000 mg of intravenous vitamin C after 4 days of symptoms resulting from viral encephalitis following the mumps — 2 hours after the injection his appetite and energy returned; after 6 hours symptoms began to return; more C was administered both by injection and orally; the child made a full recovery[3]

- A case of viral pneumonia progressed to encephalitis in a 28 year-old woman — after 14 days and treatment with 3 different antibiotics her initial condition was worsening, with an axial temperature of 106.8°F and in a stuporous condition; injections of 4,000 mg of vitamin C were administered every 2 to 3 hours; after 72 hours clinical symptoms were gone[4]

- Many patients recover from comatose encephalitis upon rigorous intravenous vitamin C treatment[5-9]

## Fluoride Poisoning

**Description:** Fluoride in excess damages developing teeth and bones (fluorosis) by pulling out calcium and phosphorus. It can also damage the kidneys, cause genetic defects, and adversely affect the thyroid. Skeletal fluorosis develops from a continual exposure to fluoride (in water, food, and dental products) over many years, since only about 50% of this substance is removed from the blood by the kidneys. The remainder accumulates and, over time, causes much damage. A miscalculation by early researchers substantially overestimated the amount of daily fluoride intake that is safe. A correction has finally been made, and it shows that many people regularly ingest unsafe levels. Since most doctors are not looking for skeletal fluorosis, it is often misdiagnosed as osteoporosis or arthritis.[1]

**Traditional Approach:** *Cecil Medicine, 23rd Edition*, published in 2008, does not provide any treatment recommendations for dental or skeletal fluorosis.

**Studies Show:**

- Dental fluorosis (still considered by many an irreversible condition) can be effectively treated with vitamin C, vitamin D, and calcium[2]

- Vitamin C protocol markedly reduces fluoride levels in the blood, serum, and urine[2]

- Skeletal fluorosis can be reversed as well with vitamin C[3]

- Sodium fluoride induces damage to animal sperm cells, and vitamin C brings about a significant recovery[4]

## Hepatitis, Acute Viral

**Description:** Acute vital hepatitis is a liver infection with a highly variable clinical picture, causing minimal to severe illness. It often resolves over a few months but it is also capable of leading to a state of chronic infection. There are five viruses known to cause acute hepatitis, designated A through E:[1]

1. Hepatitis A is highly contagious, spread largely via the fecal-oral route.

2. Hepatitis B and D are spread mainly through the shared use of contaminated needles or intimate sexual contact.

3. Hepatitis C is predominately spread through needle use and only rarely from intimate sexual contact.

4. Hepatitis E is spread via the fecal-oral route, but is rare in the U.S., and it is not as contagious as type A.

**Traditional Approach:**

1. Hepatitis A: There are no recommended therapies known to shorten or ameliorate the course of illness.[1]

2. Hepatitis B: Some antiviral therapy has been used, but it is controversial — otherwise, there is no recommended therapy.[1]

3. Hepatitis C: Peginterferon alfa and ribavirin have been shown to be of some benefit[1]

4. Hepatitis D: No specific therapies are available.[1]

5. Hepatitis E: "There are no known means of prevention or treatment..."[1]

## Hepatitis, Acute Viral (cont.)

**Studies Show:**

- Intravenous vitamin C was given to an acute hepatitis patient for 24 days at 5,000 mg per day; anemia resolved, white blood cell count and analysis returned to normal, he regained appetite and gained weight, and he lost all of the abdominal fluid accumulated due to his liver failure; most significant was the complete resolution of inflammatory changes in the liver as documented by repeated liver biopsy[2]

- A physician treating many cases of acute hepatitis with intravenous vitamin C reported that he *never* had a case fail to respond to properly-dosed treatment, and he *never* had a case of C-treated acute hepatitis develop chronic hepatitis[3]

- Administration of only 300 to 400 mg of vitamin C daily with other vitamins (B3, B6, & B12) to patients with viral hepatitis resulted in significant improvements in immune protein levels in the blood as well as in immune cell function[4]

- Hospital patients received varying amounts of vitamin C after whole blood transfusions; of the 170 receiving little or no vitamin C, 12 developed hepatitis; of 1,367 receiving 2,000 mg of vitamin C or more per day post-transfusion, only 3 cases of hepatitis developed; representing a huge decrease in the incidence of post-transfusion hepatitis[5]

- Much accelerated resolution of acute hepatitis symptoms were noted with 10,000 mg of vitamin C per day[6]

- Excellent response and clinical resolution were seen in 245 children with acute hepatitis given 10,000 mg of vitamin C daily[7]

## Hepatitis, Acute Viral (cont.)

- Dramatic resolution of acute hepatitis was seen in a 24 year-old patient who received daily 2,000 mg injections of vitamin C for 6 days; the patient reported feeling "completely well" after only the second injection[8]

- A dentist with acute hepatitis B treated himself with 25,000 mg of intravenous vitamin C in conjunction with 20,000 mg by mouth daily for 5 days; extremely elevated liver enzymes (SGOT, SGPT, and LDH) reached near-normal levels; he continued C-treatment for 5 more days, and returned to work at that time[9]

# Herpes

**Description:** Herpesviruses include the herpes simplex virus type 1 (cold sores), type 2 (genital), varicella-zoster virus (chickenpox and shingles), Epstein-Barr virus (mononucleosis), and cytomegalovirus. Herpesviruses often establish latent infection. For reasons not totally understood, they can remain in an inactive state for weeks, months, and even years, and then reactivate during menstruation, times of stress, exposure to UV light, or due to other unexplained causes.[1,2]

**Traditional Approach:** Herpes simplex viruses can be treated with antiviral drugs, the most frequently prescribed being acyclovir. Intravenous administration is often used in severe cases. Otherwise, a protocol of oral antiviral medication is used.[2] As of this writing, there are no recognized treatment protocols for Epstein-Barr or cytomegalovirus.

**Studies Show:**

- Oral vitamin C produces clear remission of symptoms in recurrent herpes labialis (cold sores)[3]

- Vitamin C, in combination with ionic copper, inactivates a host of viruses including cytomegalovirus and herpes simplex virus types 1 and 2[4,5]

- A vitamin C-containing solution used against herpes lesions that erupt on mucous membranes demonstrates statistically significant clinical and antiviral effects in a double-blind, placebo-controlled clinical trial[6]

226 PRIMAL PANACEA

## Hypertension (High Blood Pressure)

**Description:** Blood pressure is a measurement of the force exerted against arterial walls as the heart pumps. The systolic pressure is measured as the heart contracts, and diastolic pressure is the force remaining as the heart rests. Systolic pressure that is regularly over 140 is considered high, as is a diastolic measurement of 90. Obesity, diabetes, arterial narrowings, hormone imbalances, stress, smoking, as well as other factors can cause hypertension. Untreated, this condition increases the chances of atherosclerotic plaques, heart attack, stroke, and kidney disease.[1]

**Traditional Approach:** Lifestyle changes, like dietary changes, increasing exercise, and cessation of smoking, are recommended. If that does not produce the needed results, there are over 100 antihypertensive drugs that may be prescribed[2] — drugs that the patient will often take for the remainder of his/her life.

**Studies Show:**

- Vitamin C deficiency has been shown to play an integral role in the actual causation and sustaining of high blood pressure[3-5]

- Higher blood levels of vitamin C are related to lower blood pressure in humans[6-9]

- Vitamin C, in combination with other antioxidants, reduces blood pressure[10]

- Vitamin C alone is effective in lowering the blood pressure of hypertensive patients, as established in a double-blind, placebo-controlled study[11]

## Lead Poisoning

**Description:** Serious health problems can result from relatively small amounts of lead exposure, and at high levels, lead poisoning can be fatal. Symptoms include: irritability, loss of appetite, weight loss, fatigue, abdominal pain, vomiting, constipation, learning difficulties, muscular weakness, headache, high blood pressure, memory loss, reduced sperm count, abnormal sperm, miscarriage, and premature birth.[1]

**Traditional Approach:** Prevention of further exposure along with chelation therapy is recommended. Chelation agents include calcium disodium ethylenediaminetetraacetic acid ($CaNa_2EDTA$) and 2,3-dimercaptopropanol (dimercaprol). Succimer may be used as well.[2]

**Studies Show:**

- Seventeen workers with chronic lead poisoning were treated with only 100 mg of vitamin C daily — within a week or less, most of the prominent symptoms resolved[3]

- Vitamin C at a daily dose of 250 mg significantly lowers blood lead levels and reverses an enzyme inhibition associated with lead poisoning[4]

- In lead-toxic pregnant women, a combination of vitamin C and calcium phosphate decreased the lead content of their milk by 15% and the lead content of the placenta by 90%, relative to untreated mothers[5]

- Vitamin C is effective in enhancing the chelation of lead already absorbed, preventing lead from being absorbed in the gastrointestinal tract, and enhancing lead elimination from the kidneys in rats[6-11]

## Lead Poisoning (cont.)

- High serum levels of vitamin C are independently linked to a decreased prevalence of elevated lead levels in large population studies[12,13]

- Lower dietary intake of vitamin C may facilitate increased blood lead levels[14]

- Vitamin C reduces the retention of lead in the body in human volunteers[15]

- Pretreatment with vitamin C significantly lowers the concentrations of lead in the femur (bone), kidney, liver, and blood plasma in rats[16]

- The blood lead levels of 75 adult male smokers treated with 1,000 mg of vitamin C daily for only 1 week declined by 81%[17]

## Leprosy

**Description:** Leprosy is caused by the bacterium *Myco-bacterium leprae*. It is actually not very contagious. There are two common forms of this disease, tuberculoid leprosy and lepromatous leprosy. Both forms produce lesions on the skin, but the lepromatous form is most severe, producing large, disfiguring lumps and irregularities. Eventually, all forms of leprosy cause nerve damage in the arms and legs, resulting in a reduction of sensation in the skin and muscle weakness. Often those with long-term leprosy lose some of the use of their hands or feet due to repeated trauma resulting from the lack of sensation.[1]

**Traditional Approach:** A protocol of multiple antimicrobial agents is given for 12 to 24 months, depending on the type of leprosy. The resolution of skin lesions is often delayed as long as 1 to 2 years after cessation of therapy, and some improvement of nerve function may or may not occur.[2]

**Studies Show:**

- Leprosy patients exhibit significant reductions in vitamin C blood levels[3]

- Over half of the 20 leprosy patients treated with intramuscular injections of only 50 to 100 mg of vitamin C had positive results[4]

- Small daily injections of vitamin C in leprosy patients produced an improved sense of well-being, an improved appetite with weight gain, fewer nosebleeds, and an improved tolerance to prescribed anti-leprosy medications[5,6]

- Vitamin C produces a "statistically significant" effect in inhibiting the multiplication of leprosy bacteria in mice[7]

## Malaria

**Description:** Malaria is a relapsing infection caused by protozoa of the genus *Plasmodium*. It is transmitted from person to person by infected mosquitos. The parasites travel to the liver, where they mature and release another form of the parasite (merozoites). As the merozoites enter the bloodstream they infect red blood cells. While inside the blood cell, they multiply for 48 to 72 hours until the cell ruptures. The newly released merozoites then infect more red blood cells. Most symptoms of malaria occur from the rupture of massive numbers of red blood cells. This causes a release of free hemoglobin into the bloodstream, and an anemia results. Symptoms of this disease, including chills, fever, headache, jaundice, muscle pain, nausea, vomiting, and bloody stools, usually manifest in about 10 to 28 days after infection, but can be delayed for up to a year. Once the symptoms appear, they occur in cycles of 48 to 72 hours.[1]

**Traditional Approach:** There are several antimalarial medications, and the one or combination employed can depend on where and when the victim was infected. Hospitalization and aggressive medical support, along with adequate hydration, are sometimes required.[1]

**Studies Show:**

- Small intravenous doses (1,000 mg) of vitamin C prevent chills, lower elevated temperatures, and improve overall sense of well-being in malaria patients — hemoglobin levels and red blood cell counts remain stable during treatment[2]

- Vitamin C injections lower parasite count in blood by 38% and increase survival time by 67% in malaria-infected mice — larger doses increased survival time by 133%[3]

## Malaria (cont.)

- Vitamin C in the presence of copper destroys the parasitic growth of *Plasmodium falciparum*, a microorganism responsible for an especially aggressive form of human malaria[4]

- Malaria-infected red blood cells concentrate 2.5 times more vitamin C than non-infected red blood cells. The vitamin C selectively exerts a destructive pro-oxidant effect inside the infected cells while producing the typical protective antioxidant effects in normal cells[5]

- A small dose of vitamin C, along with iron supplementation, accelerates the normalization of anemia seen with malaria, and it increases the reticulocyte count[6]

- A case of acute blindness after intravenous quinine therapy completely resolved with vitamin C, vitamin B complex, and steroids[7]

- Vitamin C enhances the effect of exifone, an antimalarial drug used against multidrug-resistant strains of *Plasmodium falciparum*[8]

## Measles

**Description:** Measles is a highly contagious disease caused by the rubeola virus. Signs and symptoms include the characteristic rash, cough, runny nose, eye inflammation, and fever. Complications include: ear infection, pneumonia, seizures, and encephalitis. Measles-associated encephalitis is fatal about 10% of the time.[1]

**Traditional Approach:** "There is no specific antiviral therapy with demonstrated efficacy against measles, although ribavirin has been used in some cases."[2]

**Studies Show:**

- Vitamin C produces more rapid recovery of certain lymphocyte subsets affected in measles[3]

- Intramuscular dose (1,000 mg) of vitamin C given every 4 hours to a 10 month-old infant with reddened eyes and throat, high fever (105°F), cough, runny nose, and Koplik's spots (*Koplik's spots are the typical rash spots seen in measles that appear on the mucous membranes inside the mouth prior to skin eruptions*) — after 12 hours cough had subsided, red eyes and throat cleared, and temperature normalized; no external measles rash ever developed, and the baby made a complete and rapid recovery[4]

- Intravenous vitamin C (1,000 mg every 6 hours) provides complete protection from contracting measles during an epidemic — oral vitamin C (1,000 mg in fruit juice every 2 hours) failed to provide complete protection[5]

- Vitamin C successful in treating measles[6]

## Mercury Poisoning

**Description:** For most people, the biggest exposure to mercury comes from amalgam dental fillings. Other sources include vaccinations and seafood. When certain types of seafood are eaten regularly, this can result in a large amount of mercury intake. Intoxication can cause brain, kidney, and lung damage, and it can lead to several diseases. Symptoms of mercury poisoning include: peripheral neuropathy (persistent itching, burning, or pain), shedding of skin, swelling, and hypertension.[1]

**Traditional Approach:** "A patient with mercury poisoning should be immediately removed from the contaminated environment; the source of the mercury must then be identified and removed. Treatment is primarily symptomatic and supportive."[2] [*Translation: There is no effective treatment.*]

**Studies Show:**

- Vitamin C prevents the toxic lowering of oxygen uptake caused by meralluride, an early mercurial diuretic[3]

- Vitamin C infusions ranging from 35,000 to 50,000 mg lessen and often completely block the acute toxic effects of mercury when amalgam fillings were being removed — lower doses (25,000 mg) would occasionally allow some symptoms of acute mercury toxicity to emerge[4]

- Vitamin C added to meralluride given to dogs significantly increased the dose required to cause death[5] — vitamin C in larger doses provides more pronounced protective effects against mercury toxicity[6]

## Mercury Poisoning (cont.)

- Variable doses of both vitamin C and mercury in guinea pigs result in an increased mercury deposition in liver and kidney tissues (*organs of detoxification and excretion*)[7]

- Pretreatment with vitamin C prevents kidney damage otherwise sustained by administration of mercuric chloride in rats[8]

- A moderate pretreatment dose of vitamin C allows 40% of guinea pigs to survive an otherwise 100% lethal dose of mercury cyanide[9]

- Testing with 100% lethal doses of mercury chloride given to guinea pigs shows a:[10]
  - 100% survival with vitamin C pretreatment and continuation of vitamin C for 20 days
  - Almost complete survival with pretreatment only
  - 64% survival with no pretreatment and daily vitamin C treatment for 20 days after lethal injection
  - 68% survival with a single large vitamin C dose after lethal injection

- Vitamin C protects plants from chromosome damage against the genotoxicity of mercuric chloride[11]

- Vitamin C biodegrades organic mercury compounds in rat livers (*biodegradation of mercury greatly lessens mercury toxicity in the body*)[12]

## Mononucleosis

**Description:** Mononucleosis is a viral infection that is usually passed from human to human in saliva. Classically, fever, sore throat, and swollen lymph glands characterize infectious mononucleosis. Other common symptoms include headache, malaise, and loss of appetite. Enlargement of the spleen and/or liver may occur. Typically, the fever lasts about 10 days, and the swollen spleen and lymph nodes return to normal in about four weeks. Fatigue may remain for up to three months.[1]

**Traditional Approach:** "The goal of treatment is to relieve symptoms. Medicines such as steroids (prednisone) and antivirals (such as acyclovir) have little or no benefit."[1] [*Translation: There is no effective treatment.*]

**Studies Show:**

- Large oral doses (20,000 to 30,000 mg daily) of vitamin C resolve mononucleosis in weeks rather than months[2]

- Mononucleosis symptoms completely resolved within 1 week with 3 daily vitamin C injections[3]

- High-dose vitamin C given intravenously has a "striking" influence on the typically prolonged course of infectious mononucleosis[4]

## Mumps

**Description:** Mumps is a contagious viral disease passed through contact with infected saliva. The primary characteristic of the disease is a painful swelling of the salivary glands. However, the infection can spread to the central nervous system, pancreas, and testes. Symptoms include: Swelling of the parotid glands, face pain, sore throat, headache, fever, testicular pain, and scrotal swelling.[1]

**Traditional Approach:** "There is no specific treatment for mumps. Ice or heat packs applied to the neck area and acetaminophen (Tylenol) may help relieve pain."[1]

**Studies Show:**

- A high-dose vitamin C treatment protocol quickly resolved 33 out of 33 cases of mumps — fever was gone after 24 hours, pain was gone after 36 hours, and the parotid swelling was resolved after 48 to 72 hours[2]

- Report on the differing clinical courses of 3 cousins with mumps receiving different therapeutic regimens:[2]
  - Case #1: 7 year-old boy given the "old routine of bed rest, aspirin, and warm camphor oil applications" —had a "rough time" for a week
  - Case #2: 11 year-old boy was allowed to develop his mumps without any therapy to the "point of maximum swelling." At this point he was given 1,000 mg of vitamin C intramuscularly every 2 to 4 hours — entirely well in only 48 hours
  - Case #3: In a 9 year-old girl 1,000 mg intravenous vitamin C given every 4 hours when parotid gland swelling had reached 60% of its anticipated enlargement — completely well in 72 hours

# Mushroom Poisoning

**Description:** Approximately 100 species of mushrooms are known to be poisonous to humans. Fifteen to 20 of these species are usually lethal when consumed.[1] Symptoms of mushroom poisoning vary substantially depending on the toxins present in the offending mushroom. They can include everything from gastric upset to life-threatening organ failure resulting in death. Symptoms of poisoning do not always manifest immediately after ingestion — they can be delayed for days and even weeks.[2]

**Traditional Approach:** "In the absence of a definitive identification of the mushroom, all ingestions should be considered serious and possibly lethal. Once diagnosed, treatment of mushroom poisoning is largely supportive."[3] [*Translation: There is no effective treatment.*]

**Studies Show:**

- A Dr. Bastien developed a protocol for mushroom poisoning that includes daily injections of vitamin C (3,000 mg) combined with 2 antibiotics (nifuroxazide and dihydrostreptomycin)[3]

- Twice Dr. Bastien publicly consumed normally fatal doses of mushrooms (about 70 grams) and used his protocol to successfully treat his own poisoning [3]

- Fifteen mushroom poisoning victims were successfully treated with Dr. Bastien's protocol[3]

- Dr. Bastien's protocol became the treatment of choice at a number of medical centers in France [3]

## Nickel Poisoning

**Description:** The most common nickel toxicity occurs through chronic skin contact with products containing nickel. As many as 30% of people have a skin sensitivity to nickel. Exposure to nickel dust and fumes in the industrial environment has been linked to nose, larynx, and lung cancer. The Environmental Protection Agency identifies nickel dust and nickel subsulfide as class A human carcinogens.[1] Inhalation of nickel carbonyl can result in poisoning symptoms that include headache, irritability, nausea, vertigo, vomiting, and insomnia. Serious intoxications can induce pneumonia-like symptoms, including chest pain, dry cough, sweating, weakness, and rapid heart rate. When toxicity reaches the level that manifests in these symptoms, death may result.[2]

**Traditional Approach:** "There is no specific treatment for nickel-induced dermal sensitivity."[1] Internal toxicity can be treated with chelation therapy (sodium diethyldithiocarbamate) and support therapies such as oxygen, corticosteroids, and bed rest.[2]

**Studies Show:**

- Vitamin C reduces lipid peroxidation (LPO) activity in human platelets exposed to nickel chloride[3]

- Vitamin C protects human platelets from nickel-induced toxicity, increases desired platelet clumping, reduces LPO levels, and increases the levels of vitamin E and glutathione[3]

- Vitamin C reduces the LPO activity in human placental tissue exposed to nickel[4]

- Vitamin C decreases nickel-induced DNA damage in human lymphocyte cultures[5]

## Nickel Poisoning (cont.)

- Pretreatment with vitamin C increases the viability (*percent living*) of human lymphocytes exposed to nickel sulfate[6]

- Vitamin C supplementation (1,000 mg daily) appears to decrease chromosome damage to workers occupationally exposed to nickel[7]

- Vitamin C restores growth rates of rats impaired by toxic doses of nickel[8]

- Activities of multiple enzymes in the liver and kidney of rats poisoned by nickel are restored by vitamin C[8]

- In rats, vitamin C provides protection against nickel-induced LPO (oxidative stress), liver toxicity, and reduced antioxidant levels in the liver[9]

- Vitamin C reduces LPO activity in rats given nickel chloride[10]

- In mice given vitamin C with glutathione, nickel-induced LPO, along with nickel accumulation in the liver, was lessened[11]

- A 20% preparation of topical vitamin C clearly helps the dermatitis seen in nickel-sensitive subjects, while the commonly used 1% hydrocortisone preparation had no significant effect[12]

## Nitrate/Nitrite Toxicity

**Description:** The use of nitrates and nitrites as color stabilizers and preservatives, especially in processed meats, increases the dietary availability of nitrates and nitrites. Peroxynitrite is a highly reactive free radical formed by the combination of superoxide and nitric oxide. Nitrosamines, which can be formed from nitrates and nitrites in the acid of the stomach, can cause cancer.

**Traditional Approach:** Since nitrates and nitrites have been approved for use in food by the FDA, there is no acknowledgment of health risk. Consequently, there is also no perceived requirement for treatment to prevent or lessen toxicity.

**Studies Show:**

- Vitamin C protects against several toxic effects of peroxynitrite[1]

- Vitamin C decreases the peroxynitrite-induced cell death in both human and mouse cells in culture[2]

- Cells are greatly protected from the toxicity of peroxynitrite by vitamin C in combination with other antioxidants (*vitamin E, beta carotene*)[3]

- Vitamin C probably provides "a detoxification pathway" for peroxynitrite[4]

- Vitamin C has a potent antidote effect against several different peroxynitrite-induced oxidation reactions[5]

- Atrial fibrillation, associated with increased formation of peroxynitrite after cardiac bypass surgery, was cut by more than 50% in 43 patients treated with vitamin C for 5 days before and 5 days after surgery[6]

## Nitrate/Nitrite Toxicity (cont.)

- A daily dose of vitamin C has an apparent protective effect against the toxic effects of nitrates and nitrites on the liver in rats[7]

- Vitamin C suppresses nitrate-induced oxidant stress in dogs[8]

- Vitamin C inhibits the conversion of nitrates and nitrites to nitrosamine and other cancer-causing N-nitroso compounds in the stomach[9-12]

- In humans supplementing with vitamin C, the appearance of a monitored nitrosamine in the urine is lessened[13,14]

- Vitamin C helps block the formation of a mutagenic N-nitroso compound when mice are fed high doses of nitrate[15]

## Nitrogen Dioxide Poisoning

**Description:** Nitrogen dioxide ($NO_2$) gas severely irritates the lungs and can cause fluid accumulation there. If inhaled at high concentrations, it can produce pulmonary edema and cause death. Moderate exposure to $NO_2$ may produce shortness of breath, cough (sometimes with blood), and chest pain. Higher concentrations may produce a fatal accumulation of fluid in the lungs. A chronic exposure to $NO_2$ may predispose individuals to chronic obstructive pulmonary diseases, as well as pulmonary infection.[1]

**Traditional Approach:** Treatment should include "removal of the patient from the source of exposure, provision of supplemental oxygen, and, if needed, airway management and ventilatory support. Be aware of the risk of exposure when treating patients and wear a self-contained breathing apparatus (SCBA), when indicated."[2] [*Translation: There is no effective treatment.*]

**Studies Show:**

- Vitamin C and glutathione inhibit nitrogen dioxide's ability to form cancer-causing compounds via its chemical reaction with morpholine[3]

- Vitamin C lessens the mutagenic (mutation-causing) effects of nitrogen dioxide in mice[4]

- Vitamin C, vitamin E, and beta carotene work together to protect against nitrogen dioxide toxicity in guinea pigs[5]

## Ochratoxin Toxicity

**Description:** Ochratoxins are toxic compounds produced by some species of fungi/molds (e.g., *Aspergillus ochraceus* or *Penicillium viridicatum*). Ochratoxin A is the most prevalent of the ochratoxins, and it may be found as a contaminant in cereals, coffee, dried fruit, red wine, meat, and meat products. Dietary exposure to ochratoxin A can damage the kidneys and sometimes cause cancer.[1]

**Traditional Approach:** Toxicity from ochratoxins does not have a specific treatment.

**Studies Show:**

- Vitamin C lessens ochratoxin-induced tumors in the kidneys and livers of rats[2]

- Vitamin C demonstrates an anti-cancer effect in ochratoxin-exposed mouse kidneys[3]

- Vitamin C lessens the toxicity of ochratoxin in laying hens[4]

- A relatively small vitamin C dose significantly lessens sperm abnormalities caused by ochratoxin in mice[5]

## Osteoporosis

**Description:** The healthy body is continually replacing old bone tissue with new. When bone replacement fails to keep up with old bone resorption, osteoporosis results, with the thinning of bone tissue and the loss of bone density. As a person ages, calcium and phosphate may be reabsorbed back into the body from the bones, making the bones more fragile and more prone to fractures, even without injury or trauma. Often, an individual is not aware of a problem until a fracture occurs. By that time osteoporosis is in its advanced stages, and damage is usually severe.[1]

**Traditional Approach:** Once diagnosed, a comprehensive management plan is followed that includes osteoporosis therapy, touted to reduce fracture risk by as much as 50%. Estrogen replacement and bisphosphonate treatment, along with calcitonin and strontium ranelate, may be part of the treatment protocol. In addition, calcium and vitamin D are commonly recommended.[2] (*No mention is made of vitamin C.*)

### Studies Show:

- Vitamin C improves mineralization of calcium into bone tissues, inhibits calcium from being leached from bones into the blood, and reduces oxidative stress in bone tissues[3,4]

- Vitamin C stimulates bone precursor cells to develop into osteoblasts and inhibits osteoclast formation[5,6]

- Oxidative stress is a major cause of osteoporosis[7]

- Vitamin C is essential for the collagen cross-link formation needed to optimize the physical strength of the bones[8]

## Osteoporosis (cont.)

- Vitamin C supplementation appears to reduce the bone loss of osteoporosis[9-14]

- Dietary intake of vitamin C without supplementation provides no significant protection from fracture risk, whereas supplementation does significantly lower fracture risk — the higher the dose, the lower the risk of fractures[15]

- Elderly patients with hip fractures had a "significantly lower" level of vitamin C in the blood than elderly patients who had not sustained such a fracture[16]

- A chronic state of severe vitamin C deficiency (scurvy) appears responsible for loss of bone mass density, and in some instances increased calcium is excreted or deposited into tissues, such as is seen in atherosclerosis[17]

- Postmenopausal women taking vitamin C supplements had greater bone mineral density[18]

- Women between the ages of 55 and 64 years of age who had taken vitamin C supplements for 10 years or more — and had NOT taken estrogens — had a higher bone mineral density than those who had not taken them[19]

## Ozone Toxicity

**Description:** Ozone ($O_3$) is commonly encountered as an air pollutant. As an unstable form of oxygen, $O_3$ leads directly to oxidative stress where it is found. Moderate exposure to this gas will cause irritation to the eyes and can cause inflammation in the airways.

**Traditional Approach:** Because $O_3$ naturally breaks down into oxygen outside of the body, the main intervention is to avoid any additional exposure. As well, injury sustained from exposure to it needs to be addressed.

**Studies Show:**

- Vitamin C prevents ozone-induced bronchial hyperreactivity in guinea pigs[1]
- Vitamin C is efficient in preventing ozone-induced oxidative damage to cultured human skin cells[2]
- Regular supplementation with both vitamin C and vitamin E appears especially important for protecting the developing lungs of children[3]

# Paraquat Poisoning

**Description:** Paraquat is a highly toxic weed killer. Inhalation of this herbicide can damage the lungs. Exposure to the mucous membranes of the mouth, the stomach, the esophagus, or the intestines can cause severe damage on those sites. As well, the kidneys and liver can be damaged by this toxin. Swallowing this substance can result in rapid death. Symptoms after exposure to paraquat can include: difficulty in breathing, nosebleed, stomach pain, vomiting, seizures, and shock. Chronic exposure may lead to pulmonary fibrosis.[1]

**Traditional Approach:** "There is no specific treatment for paraquat poisoning. The goal is to relieve symptoms and treat complications (supportive care)."[1]

**Studies Show:**

- Vitamin C improves survival in paraquat-exposed mice[2]

- Vitamin C appears to be very important in maintaining a high enough total antioxidant status in the blood of paraquat-poisoned patients to substantially support their recoveries[3]

- Vitamin C and N-acetyl cysteine reduce paraquat-induced death of cultured human lung cells[4]

- Vitamin C was able to "drastically reduce" the toxicity of paraquat resulting from toxin-induced oxidative damage on frog embryos[5]

- Vitamin C exerted a dose-dependent inhibition of paraquat accumulation in rabbit kidney preparations[6]

# Pertussis (Whooping Cough)

**Description:** Pertussis is a highly contagious bacterial infection that causes uncontrollable, violent coughing that can last for a month or more. The common name for this disease comes from the "whooping" sound made by those with the disease as they try to take a breath.[1]

**Traditional Approach:** Antibiotic therapy can make the symptoms go away more quickly if started early enough. "Unfortunately, most patients are diagnosed too late, when antibiotics aren't very effective."[1]

**Studies Show:**

- A combination of injected and oral doses of vitamin C reduces coughing, restores appetite, and stops vomiting, and it is especially beneficial in infants[2]

- Vitamin C "definitely shortens" the severest symptoms of pertussis, particularly if relatively "large" doses are used shortly after the first symptoms of the disease appear[3]

- An oral vitamin C protocol was found to "markedly" decrease the intensity, frequency, and length of the characteristic pertussis symptoms[4]

- Very small vitamin C injections (50 to 200 mg, once or twice daily, maximum of 12 injections) to 81 children with pertussis produced the following outcomes:[5]
  - 34 showed a clear improvement of symptoms or "perfect healing"
  - 32 showed a lesser symptom improvement
  - 15 showed an "indeterminate" response

- Daily vitamin C injections (100 to 500 mg) reduced convulsive coughing and accelerated overall rate of recovery in pertussis patients[6]

- Treatment of 26 pertussis-infected infants and children with small daily oral doses of vitamin C were deemed "strikingly effective" in the relief of symptoms in all but 2 patients[7]

## Pesticide/Herbicide Poisoning

**Description:** Many compounds have been and continue to be used for plant and pest eradication. The positive effects of vitamin C on the toxicity of the following chemicals have been studied:

- **Diquat** — moderately toxic, contact herbicide that can be fatal if swallowed, inhaled, or absorbed through the skin in sufficient quantity[1]

- **Endosulfan** — highly neurotoxic insecticide that has now been banned in over 80 countries[2]

- **Phosphamidon** — highly toxic insecticide that acts as an cholinesterase inhibitor[3]

- **Mancozeb** — very low acute toxicity fungicide[4]

- **Dimethoate** — moderately toxic insecticide[5]

- **Malathion** — relatively low toxicity insecticide that has been linked to increased risk of attention deficit hyperactivity disorder[6]

- **Parathion** — highly toxic pesticide banned for use on many food crops[7]

- **Lindane** — highly toxic insecticide that has now been banned for agricultural use in the U.S.[8]

**Studies Show:**

- Treatment results on young boys equally and heavily exposed to pesticide spray from a crop-dusting airplane are as follows:[9]
  - One child given 10,000 mg of vitamin C with a 50 cc syringe every eight hours — discharged to home on the second hospital day.
  - Second child not given vitamin C but only received "supportive care" — developed a chemical burn and dermatitis; died on the fifth day of hospitalization

## Pesticide/Herbacide Poisoning (cont.)

- As long as normal cellular levels of vitamin C are maintained, an otherwise lethal Diquat exposure to liver cells does not klll them[10]

- Low-dose vitamin C lessens toxic effects of endosulfan, phosphamidon, and mancozeb on murine sperm[11]

- Low-dose vitamin C lessens chromosomal abnormalities induced by endosulfan, phosphamidon, and mancozeb in mice[12]

- Vitamin C adequately protects mice from dimethoate-induced chromosomal abnormalities in bone marrow erythrocytes[13]

- Vitamin C significantly lessens both malathion-induced and dimethoate-induced chromosomal abnormalities in mice and lethal mutations in *Drosophila*, a genus of flies[14,15]

- Vitamin C is "very effective in counteracting the growth retardation" and the evidence of toxicity in liver and kidney tissues in rats exposed to parathion and malathion[16]

- Vitamin C blocks the malathion-induced and dimethoate-induced depression of cell division rate in mouse sperm cells[17]

- Vitamin C supplementation to lindane-toxic rats "neutralized the growth retardation and maintained almost normal values" of all liver enzymes studied[18]

- A relatively small dose of vitamin C in rats markedly lessens the ability of lindane and DDT to induce oxidative stress or to suppress the immune system in red blood cells[19]

## Phencyclidine (Angel Dust) Poisoning

**Description:** Phencyclidine (PCP) is a hallucinogenic, neurotoxic drug used almost exclusively for recreation. Depending upon the amount and method of administration, PCP can cause an alcohol-like intoxication to psychotic behavior and convulsions.[1]

**Traditional Approach:** "Management of phencyclidine intoxication mostly consists of supportive care — controlling breathing, circulation, and body temperature — and, in the early stages, treating psychiatric symptoms."[1]

**Studies Show:**

- Vitamin C (2,000 mg) was given intravenously every 6 hours in comatose patients intoxicated with PCP to accelerate their urinary excretion[2]

- Vitamin C is part of a successful treatment protocol for the effects of a low, moderate, or heavy overdose of PCP, with intravenous vitamin C recommended for higher amounts of PCP ingestion[3]

- Vitamin C is effective as an antipsychotic agent when given to men with PCP intoxication — haloperidol and vitamin C together had an even better antipsychotic effect than either one alone[4]

- An 11 day-old PCP-toxic baby was successfully treated with a regimen that included 250 mg of vitamin C every 6 hours[5]

## Phenol Poisoning

**Description:** Also known as hydroxybenzene, phenol is a highly toxic chemical. Ingestion of even a small amount (*a lethal dose is between 3 to 30 grams, but as little as one gram can be fatal*) of phenol-containing chemicals can cause burning of the mucous membranes, weakness, pallor, fluid retention in the lungs, and seizures. Ingestion of larger amounts can result in respiratory, circulatory, cardiac, and renal failure. Skin exposure can result in dermatitis or even third-degree burns. Inhalation can cause respiratory tract irritation and pneumonia.[1,2]

**Traditional Approach:** The treatment of phenol poisoning can involve management of shock with fluids and dopamine, as well as the treatment of arrhythmias with lidocaine and convulsions with diazepam. Oxygen therapy and assisted ventilation may be necessary for respiratory problems. Administration of activated charcoal may be given to ingestion victims.[2] [*Translation: There is no specifically effective treatment.*]

**Studies Show:**

- Vitamin C, along with thiamine and calcium pantothenate, normalized phenol-induced laboratory abnormalities in rats[3]

- Pretreatment with vitamin C reduces the toxicity of 2-amino-5-chlorophenol in rat kidney tissue preparations[4]

- Vitamin C "afforded complete prevention" from several of the measured toxic effects of 4-amino-2,6-dichlorophenol in the rat kidney[5]

- Vitamin C prevents the reduction of activity seen in important liver detoxification enzymes in guinea pigs intoxicated with 2,4-dichlorophenol[6]

## Phenol Poisoning (cont.)

- Vitamin C completely neutralizes eugenol in solution and reduces the toxicity eugenol exerts against some cell lines in culture[7]

- Vitamin C prevents toxicity of p-aminophenol when given to mice[8]

- Vitamin C "completely protected against the cell death" induced by 4-aminophenol in a suspension of rabbit kidney cells[9]

## Pneumonia

**Description:** Pneumonia is a lung infection that may be caused by bacteria, viruses, fungi, or even aspiration of substances into the lungs. The most common type of pneumonia in adults is caused by streptococcal bacteria. Symptoms include a sharp chest pain that gets worse when you breathe deeply or cough, fever, chills, confusion, and excessive sweating.[1]

**Traditional Approach:** Antibiotics are most often prescribed without knowing whether the pathogen is bacterial or viral. Aspirin or acetaminophen is often used to control fever, and the patient is encouraged to drink lots of fluid to facilitate the mobilization of phlegm and secretions. With treatment most uncomplicated cases will improve within two weeks.[1]

**Studies Show:**

- **Streptococcal Pneumonia**

  - In rabbits, intravenous injection of vitamin C about 10 minutes before an intravenous injection of pneumococcal bacteria produced a "substantial" increase in the animals' ability to remove the bacteria from the blood[2]

  - Vitamin C effectively inhibits virulent hemolytic streptococci and pneumococci bacteria[3]

  - Adequate vitamin C intake prevents the pneumonia acquired by C-deficient monkeys[4]

  - Vitamin C was found to be of benefit in the treatment of pneumonia, and it was especially effective in shortening the clinical course of the disease[5-11]

  - Military recruits with influenza, receiving vitamin C supplements, had significantly fewer cases of pneumonia complicating their flu[12]

## Pneumonia (cont.)

- Vitamin C demonstrated "spectacular results" in an elderly patient who developed postoperative pneumonia[13]

- Lambs given intramuscular injections of vitamin C had 83% less pneumonia than control lambs[14]

- The incidence of streptococci in the tonsils of children is inversely related to blood levels of vitamin C — higher levels of C are associated with less tonsillar infection[3]

- Vitamin C (200 mg/kg body weight/day) significantly enhances the ability of mice to clear pneumococcal pneumonia bacteria from their lungs within 24 hours after the infectious challenge[15]

- A randomized double-blind placebo-controlled trial with 674 marine recruits shows that only 2,000 mg of vitamin C daily significantly reduces the incidence of pneumonia[16]

- **Viral Pneumonia**
  - Vitamin C provided "excellent" results in 3 cases of viral pneumonia and 1 case termed a "general viremia"[17]

  - Vitamin C used to treat 42 cases of viral pneumonia produced a "complete clinical and x-ray response" after only 3 to seven vitamin C injections[18]

  - Cyanotic (turning blue) patient with viral pneumonia treated with intramuscular injections of vitamin C every 6 hours appeared to be totally well after 36 hours[19]

# Polio

**Description:** Polio (poliomyelitis) is a viral disease that was epidemic in the U.S. in the 1940s and 1950s. Polio can cause a full or partial permanent paralysis. The virus multiplies in the throat and intestinal tract after entering through the mouth or nose. It then spreads through the body via the blood and lymph systems. Symptoms usually develop within 7 to 14 days after exposure.[1]

**Traditional Approach:** Treatment for polio is limited to symptom relief and supportive care. Once contracted, the infection is allowed to run its course with interventions to provide comfort and, if necessary, provide respiratory-support. The emphasis with this disease is on prevention through the use of vaccination.[1]

**Studies Show:**

- Vitamin C completely inactivates the poliovirus *in vitro,* rendering it non-infectious even when subsequently injected directly into the brains of monkeys[2]

- Small doses of vitamin C produce a significant reduction in the incidence of paralysis in monkeys after poliovirus injection into the brain[3]

- Vitamin C kills poliovirus in infected monkeys[4]

- 60 out of 60 cases of polio cured within 72 hours with high-dose injections of vitamin C (6,000 to 20,000 mg per day) with no residual effects[5]

- Vitamin C (10,000 to 20,000 mg daily) shortens severity and duration of fever and length of illness in polio patients[6]

- Oral vitamin C (10,000 mg per dose) as often as every 3 hours in 5 polio patients produced excellent clinical results[7]

## Polio (cont.)

- Vitamin C, along with hydrogen peroxide, inactivates the poliovirus[8]

- Vitamin C completely cured a 5 year-old girl with a confirmed and very advanced case of polio:[9]
  - Paralyzed in both her lower legs for over 4 days
  - Right leg was completely flaccid (limp)
  - Left leg was determined to be 85% flaccid
  - Pain was noticed especially in the knee and lumbar areas
  - By the 19th day of treatment there was a "complete return of sensory and motor function," and no long-term impairment ever resulted

## PCB Toxicity

**Description:** Polychlorinated biphenyl compounds (PCBs) are organic compounds that were found to be extremely toxic. They were banned from production in the U.S. in 1979. PCBs cause cancer in animals, and they likely cause cancer in humans as well. It appears that PCBs might be responsible for birth defects and adverse developmental effects. They can also negatively impact the endocrine system and the liver. An elevated exposure risk occurs with the consumption of contaminated fish.[1,2]

**Traditional Approach:** Treatment is limited to removal from, or prevention of exposure to, PCBs.

**Studies Show:**

- Increased vitamin C is useful in counteracting PCB toxicity[3,4]

- Vitamin C is needed for the general support and maximum induction of several liver enzyme systems needed to detoxify PCB and other toxins[5-7]

- Supplementing with vitamin C provides "a definite protection" against the toxin-induced changes in the microscopic appearance of rat liver cells[8]

## Pseudomonas Infections

**Description:** *Pseudomonas* is a genus of gram-negative bacteria that is particularly resistant to antibiotics. Found nearly everywhere, it favors moist environments. It is responsible for many nosocomial infections (*infections contracted in a medical treatment facility*), and it is often responsible for sepsis[1] (*a widespread, advanced, life-threatening infection*). "Reports of more resistant strains of *Pseudomonas* organisms to the currently used antimicrobials are causing much concern."[2]

**Traditional Approach:** A variety of antibiotics are employed depending upon the location of the infection.[2]

**Studies Show:**

- Vitamin C, with nitrite, markedly inhibits the growth of *Pseudomonas aeruginosa* in human urine[3]

- A combination of oral and intravenous vitamin C cures *Pseudomonas* in association with severe burns[4]

- The topical application of vitamin C along with antibiotics ensured the absence of *Pseudomonas aeruginosa* from a treated bedsore[5,6]

- *Pseudomonas aeruginosa* becomes "increasingly susceptible" to the effects of 5 different antibiotics when simultaneously exposed to vitamin C[7]

- Vitamin C, in combination with sulfamethoxazole and trimethoprim, kills *Pseudomonas aeruginosa* efficiently *in vitro*[8]

- Vitamin C inhibits the growth of 16 different strains of *Pseudomonas aeruginosa* in the test tube as well as curing mice infected with *Pseudomonas aeruginosa*[9]

- *Pseudomonas aeruginosa* lung infections in cystic fibrosis patients are easily controlled with a combination of vitamin C and antibiotic therapy[9]

# Rabies

**Description:** Rabies is a deadly viral infection that is spread via infected animal saliva that enters the body through a bite or through broken skin. Most cases of human rabies now come from the bite of bats or raccoons. Foxes and skunks have also been known to spread the disease. The incubation time typically runs from 3 to 7 weeks. Once symptoms appear, the disease is almost always fatal.[1]

**Traditional Approach:** A rabies vaccine administered promptly and appropriately almost always prevents the onset of the infection.[1]

**Studies Show:**

- Vitamin C inactivates (kills) the rabies virus[2]
- Vitamin C was found to be effective in the prevention of rabies in guinea pigs[3]

## Radiation Toxicity

**Description:** Radiation is energy transmitted by waves and/or by particles, such as electrons, neutrons, and protons. Sunlight is a natural form of radiation, whereas x-rays, cancer treatment, and nuclear power plants involve man-made radiation. Exposure to small amounts of radiation over a long period of time increases oxidative stress and the risk of cancer. Larger doses of radiation over shorter periods of time can cause burns and/or radiation sickness. If an exposure is large enough, it can cause death immediately.[1,2]

**Traditional Approach:** Treatment of acute radiation toxicity is "generally supportive with blood transfusions and antibiotics."[2] [*Translation: There is no effective treatment.*]

**Studies Show:**

- A small amount of vitamin C substantially increases survival rate from whole body ionizing radiation in rats[3]

- Vitamins C, E, and A reduce the "normal" ionizing radiation damage inflicted on the bone marrow by the radioimmunotherapy used in the treatment of cancer[4]

- After enough vitamin C is administered "the radiation dose given to cancer patients could be increased without increasing acute complications but with an expected increase in tumor-control probability"[5]

- Vitamins C and E successfully treated the symptoms of chronic radiation proctitis in 20 patients receiving courses of pelvic irradiation for cancer in that area of the body:[6]
  - Bleeding, diarrhea, and pain all lessened
  - 7 of 20 reported "return to normal"
  - 10 patients "reported a sustained improvement in their symptoms" 1 year later

## Radiation Toxicity (cont.)

- For patients receiving radiation therapy, "a sufficiently large daily dose of ascorbic acid, given either intravenously or by mouth, can prevent or minimize the fall of white blood cells which follows X-ray exposure" and "also improves considerably the general condition of the patient, and X-ray sickness is very slight or entirely absent"[7]

- Vitamin C lessens free radical load when given prior to irradiation; even when given 20 hours after irradiation it still reduces mutation frequency in human cell studies[8]

- Vitamins C and E reduce chromosome damage induced in mice by gamma or x-ray irradiation[9-11]

- Vitamin C serves to protect against the radiation damage of either accidental or intentional medical exposures[12]

- Irradiation-induced chromosomal damage to mice is reduced by a combination of vitamin C, vitamin E, and beta carotene[13]

- A combination of vitamin C, vitamin E, and beta carotene increases "the efficiency of DNA repair" in the spleen of irradiated mice[14]

- Vitamin C significantly suppresses the X-ray-induced transformation of cultured mouse cells into cancer cells[15]

- Vitamin C and vitamin E taken orally offer significant protection against ultraviolet radiation damage (sunburn) in humans[16,17]

- A topical (versus ingested) application of vitamins C and E provided complete protection against the increase in lipid peroxidation (oxidative stress) induced by UVB (ultraviolet light, type B) exposure in pig skin[18]

## Radiation Toxicity (cont.)

- Injecting a vitamin C derivative prior to UVB exposure significantly reduces a number of the laboratory indices of increased oxidative stress[19]

- Vitamin C supplementation "led to a significant and remarkable reduction of the UVB-induced damage" in a particular biological model[20]

- A stable vitamin C derivative improves human skin cell survival significantly after UVB exposure with fewer large DNA fragments in the debris of cells that were killed[21]

- Vitamin C exhibits a significant protective effect on lipid peroxidation and DNA strand breaks, and it provides a "considerably higher survival rate" in studies with irradiated bacteria[22]

- Vitamin C pretreatment significantly lessens microscopic evidence of chromosomal damage in irradiated mice and irradiated mouse spleen cells[23]

- Vitamin C decreases the incidence and delays the onset of skin cancer lesions caused by UV light exposure in mice[24]

- "Regardless of the detail of the mechanism, the evidence presently available demonstrates that vitamin C is a radioprotective agent"[25]

## Selenium Poisoning

**Description:** Selenium is absorbed via the lungs and the gastrointestinal tract. Chronic (long-term) exposure to high levels of selenium in food and water can produce skin discoloration, deformation and loss of nails, loss of hair, excessive tooth decay and discoloration, lack of mental alertness, and listlessness.

**Traditional Approach:** Removal from the source of exposure, along with "symptomatic and supportive care" are indicated. "Chelating agents are not useful."[1]

**Studies Show:**

- Intramuscular and oral vitamin C along with dimercaprol successfully treated the acute selenium poisoning of a 15 year-old girl — she had intentionally swallowed sodium selenate "many times the minimum lethal dose" for animals. Her blood levels were found to be "at least" 20 times higher than the normal range[2]

- Selenium poisoning in rats lowers vitamin C levels, and the levels of selenides (selenium compounds) in poisoned animals are reduced by vitamin C supplementation[3]

- Vitamin C prevents expected selenium-induced damage to cultured endothelial cells when given in conjunction with selenious acid, a selenium compound[4]

- Increased dietary vitamin C lessens the growth retardation induced by high levels of selenium in chicks[5]

- In mice, vitamin C protects against the selenium-induced loss of hemoglogin, and it significantly decreases the deposition of selenium in the livers and brains of the animals receiving diphenyl diselenide[6]

## Shingles

**Description:** After a case of chickenpox, the virus (*herpes zoster*) can remain dormant in a person's nerves. When the virus becomes active again through a myriad of possible causes, it produces a painful, blistering skin rash. The blisters break, forming small ulcers that dry and form crusts. These fall off in 2 to 3 weeks. Additional symptoms may occur, including swollen glands, joint pain, chills, fever, genital lesions, headache, hearing loss, and abdominal pain.[1]

**Traditional Approach:** Treatment with high doses of an antiviral drug may shorten the course of the disease. All other therapies only provide symptomatic relief.[2]

**Studies Show:**

- Vitamin C injections successfully treated 14 cases of shingles[3]

- A series of eight adults with shingles were successfully treated with 2,000 to 3,000 mg injections of vitamin C every 12 hours, along with 1,000 mg orally every 2 hours — the severe pain associated with the skin lesions (often lasting for weeks) was completely gone in seven of eight patients within 2 hours of the first vitamin C injection[4-6]

- Vitamin C successfully treats 327 of 327 shingle cases — complete resolution of the disease in all patients was seen within 72 hours of the first injection[7]

## Staphylococcal (Staph) Infections

**Description:** The skin and nearly every organ can be infected with *Staphylococcus* (Staph) bacteria. Nosocomial infections (*contracted in a hospital*) are commonly caused by Staph, which are often antibiotic-resistant. The severity of infection can range from mild skin outbreaks (cellulitis, folliculitis, or impetigo) to life- and limb-threatening sepsis. Much of the damage from Staph is produced by the toxins (exotoxins) it releases into the blood and tissues.[1]

**Traditional Approach:** A wide range of anitbiotics are prescribed depending upon where the infection was contracted and where it manifests.[2]

**Studies Show:**

- Vitamin C significantly increases ability of broiler chicken white blood cells to kill *Staphylococcus aureus* in the test tube[3]

- Vitamin C effectively inhibits *Staphylococcus aureus* growth[4]

- Intravenous injections of vitamin C (500 to 700 mg/kg body weight) produced prompt resolution of staphylococcal infections[5]

- Vitamin C renders *Staphylococcus*-related toxin harmless[6]

- After 3 years of failed attempts to heal a skin lesion infected by *Staphylococcus aureus* with conventional therapies, vitamin C therapy provided complete resolution within weeks[7]

- Vitamin C makes antibiotic-resistant *Staphylococcus aureus* treatable with antibiotics[8,9]

- Vitamin C (375 mg/kg body weight/day) allows weight gain and produces lower metabolic rates in burned guinea pigs infected with *Staphylococcus aureus*[10]

## Streptococcal (Strep) Infections

**Description:** There are two types of strep infection. Strep group A causes strep throat, scarlet fever, tonsillitis, ear infections, impetigo, toxic shock syndrome, cellulitis, and necrotizing fasciitis ("flesh-eating disease"). Strep group B causes blood infections, lung infections, skin infections, and bone/joint infections.[1] Strep bacteria are growing increasingly resistant to antibiotics.

**Traditional Approach:** Penicillin and its derivatives, along with cephalosporins and erythromycin, are commonly used antibiotics.[2]

**Studies Show:**

- **General Infections**
  - Vitamin C had a killing effect ("bactericidal") on *Streptococcus faecalis* in urine[3]
  - Intravenous vitamin C (500 to 700 mg/kg body weight) cures "hemolytic streptococcus" infections[4]
  - Vitamin C-deficient guinea pigs are significantly more likely to contract severe streptococcal infections that often result in death[5]
- **Kidney Infections**
  - Children with streptococcal kidney infections have significantly lower levels of vitamin C in the plasma and red blood cells and significant laboratory evidence of increased oxidative stress[6]
- **Middle Ear Infections**
  - Intramuscular injections of vitamin C provided a striking success in treating 10 patients with otitis media, a middle ear infection, over a one-year period — "all showed signs of improvement within 12 hours and had resolved within 4 to 5 days" — furthermore "the results were too striking" to even question "the therapeutic effect of the parenteral administration" of vitamin C[7]

## Streptococcal (Strep) Infections (cont.)

- **Rheumatic Fever**
  - Vitamin C produced dramatic and rapid resolution of advanced rheumatic fever in seven patients[8]
  - Low-dose daily vitamin C supplementation in 335 students over several months compared to a larger, but similar group of non-supplementers produced the following results:[9]

    | Group | Rheumatic Fever | Pneumonia |
    |-------|-----------------|-----------|
    | Control | 16 cases | 17 cases |
    | Vitamin C | 0 cases | 0 cases |

- **Scarlet Fever**
  - Intravenous and oral vitamin C together produced dramatic, successful responses in several cases of scarlet fever[10]
  - Vitamin C administration produced a very rapid clinical response in 3 cases of scarlet fever[11]

- **Tonsillitis / Throat Infections**
  - Vitamin C supplementation lessened the incidence of positive beta-hemolytic streptococci throat cultures in a double-blind, placebo-controlled trial with 868 children[12]

## Strychnine Poisoning

**Description:** Strychnine poisoning can occur by inhalation, swallowing, or absorption through the eyes or mouth. Within minutes of exposure the muscles begin to spasm, starting with the head and neck and then moving to the other muscles throughout the body, resulting in nearly continuous convulsions. Death can ensue within 2 to 3 hours, caused by an inability to breathe secondary to a poisoning of the nerves that control breathing, or ultimately by exhaustion from the convulsions.[1]

**Traditional Approach:** "There is no specific antidote for strychnine." If caught in time, activated charcoal is given by mouth to absorb any strychnine still remaining in the gut. Anticonvulsants and muscle relaxants are given to counteract convulsions and muscle rigidity. If the patient survives past 24 hours, recovery is probable.[1]

**Studies Show:**

- Vitamin C "in very high doses shows protection against strychnine" (*in vitro*)[2]

- Strychnine toxicity is greatly increased in scurvy-stricken (vitamin C-deficient) guinea pigs[3]

- Vitamin C "completely counteracted the convulsive and lethal actions of strychnine," and the protective action of vitamin C was "directly dependent on the plasma ascorbic acid level" (*in vivo* - mice)[3]

- Vitamin C significantly lessens the ability of strychnine to produce a tetanus-like condition in young chicks[4]

## Tetanus

**Description:** Tetanus, commonly called "lockjaw," is caused by the bacteria, *Clostridium tetani*. The spores of this bacteria can be found in soil all over the globe. The infection typically starts when these spores enter a wound in the skin. Once inside an oxygen-deprived environment, the spores release the bacteria, which then express a very potent exotoxin called teta-nospasmin. This toxin affects the nervous system, causing severe muscle spasms. The symptoms of infection often appear from 1 to 3 weeks after the introduction of the spores into the body. Without treatment, about 1 in 4 victims will die from tetanus.[1]

**Traditional Approach:** Tetanus antitoxin is adminis-tered, along with the provision of respiratory support, autonomic nervous system support, passive and active immunization, surgical cleaning of the portal wound, and antibiotics. Despite antitoxin treatment, "there may be clinical progression for about two weeks," and there might be as high as a 60% mor-tality rate, even with expert care.[2]

**Studies Show:**

- Vitamin C neutralizes tetanus toxin in the test tube[3]

- Vitamin C added to growing cultures of tetanus bacteria reduces the toxicity of those cultures in proportion to the amount of vitamin C added[4]

- Vitamin C cured tetanus in a 6 year-old boy already demonstrating very advanced muscle spasms and other symptoms from the production of tetanus toxin and the progression of the infection[5]

- Vitamin C, without tetanus antitoxin (*which carries its own toxicity*), completely neutralizes tetanus toxin in rats injected with twice the minimal lethal amount[6]

## Tetanus (cont.)

- In an animal model, adequate doses of vitamin C given prior to tetanus toxin administration prove completely protective in preventing any manifestation of toxicity[7]

- Intravenous vitamin C (22,000 to 24,000 mg per day) cured a 6 year-old boy with tetanus — the toxicity of the antitoxin *delayed* recovery[8]

- Effectiveness and dose-dependent relationship of vitamin C in the treatment of tetanus — control group received antitoxin alone, all C-group subjects received antitoxin and only 1,000 mg vitamin C intravenously daily[9]

| Group | Outcome |
| --- | --- |
| Ages 1-12 w/no vitamin C | 75% died |
| Ages 1-12 w/1,000 mg vitamin C | 0% died |
| Ages 13-30 w/no vitamin C | 68% died |
| Ages 13-30 w/1,000 mg vitamin C | 37% died |

## Toxic Drugs

**Description:** Nearly all of the drugs prescribed today
have an associated toxicity. Here is a list of common
drugs with known toxicities that have been successfully neutralized with vitamin C alone, or with
vitamin C in conjunction with other substances. A
short description of each drug will appear with each
entry on the list.

**Studies Show:**

- **Acetaminophen** (*This pain reliever/fever reducer
  goes by numerous names but the most common is
  probably Tylenol®*)[1] Overdose with this drug is a
  common cause of liver failure and can be fatal. Even
  at the maximum recommended daily adult dose size
  of 4,000 mg, rare cases of acute liver injury have
  been seen.[2]
  - Vitamin C (1,000 mg/kg body size) given
    either 1 hour before or 1 hour after a dose of
    acetaminophen that kills a large number of liver
    cells had a pronounced protective effect in mice[3]
  - Vitamin C, N-acetyl cysteine, and DL-methionine
    allowed the clinical recovery of a "moribund
    and cyanotic" cat that ingested a fatal dose of
    acetaminophen 14 hours earlier[4]
- **Acetanilide, aniline, and antipyrine**
  - Vitamin C supplementation substantially reduces
    the half-life of acetanilide, aniline, and antipyrine
    seen in vitamin C-depleted guinea pigs because
    vitamin C repletion increases the hydroxylation
    rate for each chemical[5]

## Toxic Drugs (cont.)

- **Arsphenamine** This drug contains organic arsenic and was the first modern chemotherapeutic agent (1910s). It was used to treat syphilis and trypanosomal infections. Because of the serious side effects and toxicity, the arsenical compounds were replaced by penicillin in the 1940s[6]
  - A diet rich in vitamin C inhibits the toxic reaction to an arsphenamine compound (neoarsphenamine) in guinea pigs[7]
  - Intravenous vitamin C shortened the recovery time of 3 patients with arsphenamine-related dermatitis[8]

- **Chloroform** was used for general anesthesia in the 1800s because of its ability to depress the central nervous system. It was soon replaced with ether because of its cardiac toxicity and the associated fatal cardiac arrhythmias. Today, chloroform is used to produce the non-stick substance known as Teflon®[9]
  - Vitamin C neutralizes chloroform toxicity in mice given a dose that would otherwise kill 50% of them:[10]
    - 400 mg/kg body weight reduced death rate to 40%
    - 600 mg/kg body weight reduced death rate to only 10%
    - 1,000 mg/kg body weight produced 100% survival rate

- **Cisplatin** is a chemotherapy drug used to treat a wide variety of cancers. This drug can cause chromosomal damage in immune cells, as well as severe kidney damage[11]

## Toxic Drugs (cont.)

- Vitamin C reduced the ability of cisplatin to induce chromosomal damage in human lymphocyte cultures[12]
- Vitamin C protects against cisplatin-induced chromosomal damage in mouse bone marrow cells[13]
- Vitamin C protects rat kidneys from the toxic effects of cisplatin in a dose-dependent manner[14]
- Vitamin C, when administered with vitamin E, provides even more protection from cisplatin-induced kidney toxicity in the rat[15]
- Antioxidant treatment, including vitamin C, lessens cisplatin-induced hearing damage caused by increased oxidative stress in rats[16,17]
- Vitamin C protects against cisplatin-induced LPO and other indicators of oxidative stress in blood platelets[18]

• **Cyclophosphamide** (*also known as Cytoxan®*) is a chemotherapy drug used to treat a host of cancers. It can be administered in pill form or by intravenous infusion.[19] As with all chemo drugs, there are serious side effects and toxicity associated with it

- Vitamin C and theophylline therapy allows a patient to survive acute cyclophosphamide toxicity[20]
- Vitamin C supplementation normalizes elevated levels of 2 common liver enzymes (SGOT and SGPT) induced by cyclophosphamide[21]
- Co-administration of vitamin C with cyclophosphamide treatment corrects significant lipid abnormalities, including substantial increases in total cholesterol/triglycerides and reduction of HDL-cholesterol caused by this drug in rats[22]

## Toxic Drugs (cont.)

- – Vitamin C is effective in reducing the microscopic evidence of cyclophosphamide-induced chromosomal damage in mice[23]
- – Vitamin C exhibits "a significant antimutagenic effect" against the toxicity of cyclophosphamide in mice and larger vitamin C doses have the most striking antitoxic effects[24]
- – Vitamin C (800 mg/kg body weight) significantly lowered the cyclophosphamide-induced chromosomal abnormalities in pregnant mice[25]
- – Vitamin C (up to 1,600 mg/kg body weight) reduces chromosomal damage from cyclophosphamide in pregnant mice[26]
- – Vitamin C (3,340 mg/kg body weight) had no toxic effects and produced "a protective effect against the toxic manifestations of cyclophosphamide" in pregnant mice, with all offspring being morphologically normal[27]

- • **Cyclosporine** is generally given to suppress immune response. It is prescribed for organ transplant patients, rheumatoid arthritis sufferers, and to treat psoriasis. It can cause a wide array of side effects[28]
  - – Vitamins C and E lessen cyclosporine-induced kidney damage and increase oxidative stress in rabbits treated with cyclosporine[29]
  - – Vitamin C and N-acetyl cysteine lessen cyclosporine-induced cell death in human lymphocyte cultures[30]
  - – Vitamins C (equivalent to 100,000 mg per day for a 200-pound man) and E prolong the survival of transplanted hearts in rats given cyclosporine[31,32]

## Toxic Drugs (cont.)

- **Digoxin** (*also known as Lanoxin®*) is prescribed
  to control heart rate and improve heart function.
  Digoxin toxicity can be fatal[33]
  - Vitamin C significantly suppresses
    manifestations of digoxin-induced toxicity in goat
    liver tissue[34]
- **Doxorubicin** (*also known as Adriamycin®*) This
  chemotherapeutic drug is used to fight various
  cancers, and it is administered intravenously. It can
  cause severe heart damage even years after the
  discontinuation of the drug. An exceptionally potent
  chemotherapy agent, it is also exceptionally toxic[35]
  - Vitamins C and E lessen the amount of lipid
    peroxidation initiated by doxorubicin in rats[36]
  - Vitamin C significantly prolongs the lifespans of
    mice and guinea pigs treated with doxorubicin,
    while preserving the antitumor effect of the
    drug[37]
  - Vitamin C improves the cancer cell-killing ability
    of doxorubicin in cultured human breast cancer
    cells[38]
  - Benzylideneascorbate, a derivative of vitamin C,
    very effectively decreases the heart enzyme
    elevations associated with doxorubicin-induced
    toxicity in mice[39]
  - In animals tested, vitamin C significantly
    prolongs the lifespan and reduces the
    doxorubicin-induced cardiac toxicity without
    diminishing doxorubicin's antitumor activity[40]
  - When injected under the skin of pigs, vitamin C
    combined with the doxorubicin decreases ulcer
    incidence from 87% to 27%[41]
  - Vitamin C "significantly decreased the frequency"
    of doxorubicin-induced chromosome damage in
    rat bone marrow cells[42]

## Toxic Drugs (cont.)

- – Vitamin C protection against doxorubicin-induced chromosome damage is "dependent on the dose used" in rat bone marrow cells[43]

- **Iproniazid** was used as an antidepressant starting in the late 1950s. It is no longer used, as it was found to cause liver damage[44]
  - – Vitamin C significantly inhibits the iproniazid-induced increase in free radicals seen in rats[45]
  - – Administration of vitamin C "remarkably" lowers iproniazid-induced cell death in the liver of rats "both quantitatively and qualitatively"[46]

- **Isoproterenol** (*also known as Isuprel®*) is similar in structure to adrenaline. A beta receptor activator, it is used to treat heart block and bradycardia. A potent cardiac stimulant, this drug has resulted in cardiac arrest[47]
  - – In cultured rat heart cells, vitamin C lessens isoproterenol-induced damage[48-51]
  - – Isoproterenol toxicity results in the gradual accumulation of calcium inside rat heart cells; vitamin C blocks much of this intracellular increase[52]
  - – Magnesium ascorbate, a mineral salt of vitamin C, demonstrates protective effects against isoproterenol-induced cardiac toxicity in rats[53]

- **Neoarsphenamine** is an arsenic-containing drug that was used from 1912 into the 1940s for the treatment of syphilis. At that time this drug was replaced with penicillin because of neoarsphenamine's serious side effects.[54]
  - – Guinea pigs on a low vitamin C diet have a dramatic toxic response to neoarsphenamine; when given much larger amounts of vitamin C these animals are protected from such toxicity[55]

## Toxic Drugs (cont.)

- Vitamin C significantly reduces the toxicity of neoarsphenamine in rats[56]
- A high blood concentration of vitamin C is necessary to produce a detoxifying effect on circulating neoarsphenamine[57]
- Addition of vitamin C to a skin patch used to test for allergic sensitivity to neoarsphenamine can completely eliminate the skin reaction, even in patients who were already known to be highly sensitive to the drug — the authors suggest that if enough vitamin C was given along with the neoarsphenamine when treating their syphilis patients, most of the toxic reactions that might otherwise occur could be greatly lessened or prevented[58]
- After vitamin C was added to their neoarsphenamine treatment for syphilis, the infection appeared eradicated in 10 of 14 patients who had been ill between 8 months and 20 years[59]

• **Sulfa drugs** are a class of medicines that contain the sulfonamide group. Sulfa drugs have been used for antimicrobial, diuretic, anticonvulsant, and dermatological applications. These drugs have a variety of adverse effects, some life-threatening[60]

- A tiny dose of vitamin C produced "astounding" results from  sulfapyridine-induced side effects in a 5 year-old boy[61]
- Vitamin C produced "a rapid and uneventful recovery" from sulfanilamide toxicity in a middle-aged female who developed a rash over her entire body and "mucous membranes" from the use of a "sulfa ointment" for a sore on her hand[62]

## Toxic Drugs (cont.)

- – Vitamin C protects against sulfanilamide-induced birth defects in chicken embryos[63]

- **Tetracycline** is a popular antibiotic prescribed for respiratory infections, acne, urinary infections, and the infection associated with stomach ulcers (*Helicobacter pylori*)[64]

  - – A vitamin C injection prevented kidney damage induced by intravenous administration of tetracycline in both rats and dogs[65]

- **Valproic acid** is prescribed for migraine headaches, bipolar disorder, and certain types of seizures. This drug can cause serious life-threatening damage to the liver and the pancreas[66]

  - – Vitamins C and E demonstrated a protective effect against the cellular damage induced by valproic acid in rat liver cells[67]

## Trichinosis

**Description:** Trichinosis is an infection caused by the ingestion of a roundworm (*Trichinella spiralis*). These worms can be found in multiple animal meats, including pork, horse, and several wild animals. Adequate cooking will kill these parasites.[1]

**Traditional Approach:** "Mebendazole or albendazole can be used to treat infections in the intestines. There is no specific treatment for trichinosis once the larvae have invaded the muscles. The cysts remain viable for years. Pain killers can help relieve muscle soreness."[1]

**Studies Show:**

- Vitamin C, in combination with vitamins A, E, and an antiparasite drug (mebendazole), resulted in the number of larvae in the muscles of rats being "highly decreased" relative to no treatment[2]

- A daily dose of vitamin C (equivalent to about 35,000 mg for a 150-pound man) to trichinosis-infected rats produced a 40% reduction in worm (larvae) count in the muscles after 30 days of treatment — this significant decrease took place with vitamin C treatment alone, since no traditional antiparasite medications were given[3]

## Trypanosomal Infections

**Description:** Trypanosomal infections are caused by protozoa and are commonly transmitted by insects. The most common infection is known as sleeping sickness, which is carried by the tsetse fly. Within days of the bite from an infected insect, a nodule forms on the skin which persists for up to two weeks. After this incubation period, the trypanosomes begin to invade the circulatory and lympatic systems, and fever, headache, dizziness, and weakness frequently occur. Six months to several years later, the disease passes from the hemolymphatic state to a meningoencephalitic stage as the parasites reach the central nervous system.[1]

**Traditional Approach:** Suramin is the drug of choice before any central nervous system involvement. After that time the drug is ineffective because it does not sufficiently cross the blood-brain barrier. Melarsoprol, an arsenic-containing drug, is then used. Both drugs are highly toxic.[1]

**Studies Show:**

- A small dose of vitamin C (approximately 20 mg/kg body weight), raises the natural resistance of guinea pigs to *Trypanosoma brucei* infection[2]

- Addition of vitamin C to the gentian violet treatment of blood deliberately infected with *Trypanosoma cruzi* before transfusion allows sterilization with less gentian violet than is typically needed[3]

- Vitamin C, along with glutathione, readily kills trypanosomes in culture[4]

- Vitamin C (100 mg/kg body weight) prevents the elevation in liver enzymes that otherwise results from the infections of rabbits with *Trypanosoma brucei brucei*[5]

## Tuberculosis

**Description:** The bacteria *Mycobacterium tuberculosis* causes pulmonary tuberculosis (TB). The disease is transmitted in the droplets discharged in a cough or sneeze of an infected person. This first infection is called primary TB, and most people recover from it without further evidence of the disease. In some individuals, however, the infection can become dormant for several years and then reactivate.[1]

**Traditional Approach:** The active disease is usually treated with a combination of drugs. The four most common drugs are isoniazid, rifampin, pyrazinamide, and ethambutol. Additional drugs used include amikacin, ethionamide, moxifloxacin, para-aminosalicylic acid, and streptomycin. Medications may have to be taken for six months or longer.[1]

**Studies Show:**

- Vitamin C protects guinea pigs injected with toxic doses of tuberculin:[2]
  - 81% of injected animals not receiving vitamin C died
  - Only 17% of infected animals that received vitamin C died
- Small vitamin C injections produce positive responses in temperature, weight, general well-being, appetite, and some blood tests in tuberculosis patients[3]
- Vitamin C-treated individuals (74 tuberculosis patients) showed a "marked increase" in hemoglobin content and red blood cell counts[4]
- A "significant and progressive" deficiency of vitamin C is seen in guinea pigs infected with tuberculosis, and daily vitamin C administration causes significant weight gain, along with a reduction in the clinical invasiveness of tuberculous lesions[5,6]

## Tuberculosis (cont.)

- Daily oral dosing of vitamin C significantly inhibits the skin reaction to subcutaneous injections of tuberculin in tuberculous guinea pigs[6]

- 150 mg of vitamin C supplementation daily, along with whatever was already present in the diet, appeared to reduce tuberculous lesions in the respiratory passages, intestines, and rectum[7]

- Vitamin C prevents tuberculosis bacteria growth in artificial medium that otherwise supports growth[8]

- 100 mg vitamin C injections controlled the coughing up of blood in 140 tuberculous patients[9]

- More highly-dosed vitamin C (15,000 mg daily) administered to very advanced tuberculosis patients resulted in the following:[10]
  - Still alive a half year later (5 of 6)
  - Gained from 20 to 70 pounds in the process
  - No longer bedridden
  - Considered to have undergone an enormous degree of improvement in their general condition
  - Total vitamin C dosing was roughly 3,000,000 mg per patient with no evidence of any toxicity or side effect

- Daily supplementation of vitamins and minerals that included vitamin C resulted in an "appreciably lower" incidence of new cases of tuberculosis when compared to a non-supplemented control group[11]

- Three times more vitamin C than normal was required to maintain normal plasma levels in 2 patients with active tuberculosis[12]

- All 28 men — from a group of 1,100 free from the disease upon first examination — who developed X-ray evidence of pulmonary tuberculosis were also found to have low plasma levels of vitamin C[13]

## Tuberculosis (cont.)

- Increased amounts of vitamin C seem to decrease the severity and extent of tuberculous lesions in the lungs of infected guinea pigs[14]

- Daily urinary excretion of vitamin C correlated with the activity level of the infection in tuberculous patients: the lowest levels of urinary vitamin C (indicating low body levels) were associated with the greatest disease activity[15]

- Daily vitamin C injections control the clinical course of tuberculosis in guinea pigs very well — they grew at a "normal rate" and "behaved in every way just as the controls" over a five-month period[16]

- Individuals who had a dietary vitamin C intake greater than 90 mg daily and who consumed "more than the average" amount of fruits, vegetables, and berries had a significantly lower risk of contracting tuberculosis[17]

- "Massive daily doses" of vitamin C "will also cure tuberculosis by removal of the organisms' polysaccharide coat," according to Dr. Klenner[18]

- Tuberculous guinea pigs fed with large amounts of orange juice survived twice as long as animals fed only the normal diet (this preceding the discovery of vitamin C)[19]

- The vitamin C level in the body appears to determine the likelihood of contracting intestinal tuberculosis[20]

- A combination of injected and oral vitamin C with high amounts of citrus juice eliminated fever, stopped the characteristic tuberculosis cough, and resulted in a ten-pound weight gain in an active tuberculosis patient[21]

## Tuberculosis (cont.)

- Vitamin C added to a tuberculosis bacteria culture medium inhibits growth[22]

- A small oral dose of only 150 mg vitamin C daily produced a clear improvement in 88% of children and 61% of adults with tuberculosis, showing the fixed dose had a greater effect in a smaller body[23]

- A minimum of twice as much vitamin C is needed on a daily basis by tuberculosis patients to maintain the same plasma levels as normal subjects in a study on Navajo Indians with tuberculosis[24]

- Only 250 mg of vitamin C daily improves the overall "blood picture" of the treated tuberculosis patients[25]

- Daily injections of vitamin C are adequate to protect tuberculous guinea pigs against otherwise lethal doses of tuberculin that would have readily killed the unsupplemented control animals[26]

## Typhoid Fever

**Description:** Typhoid fever is a bacterial infection caused by *Salmonella typhi*. The disease spreads through contaminated food, drink, or water. Symptoms include: high fever, abdominal pain, diarrhea, bloody stools, chills, delirium, nosebleeds, severe fatigue, and weakness.[1]

**Traditional Approach:** Intravenous fluids are given to combat dehydration, and antibotic therapy is given as well. With treatment, symptoms usually improve in 2 to 4 weeks.[1]

**Studies Show:**

- Vitamin C rapidly kills typhoid bacteria *in vitro*[2]
- Injected and oral vitamin C treated 106 cases of typhoid fever with great success[2]
- Intravenous vitamin C and adrenal gland extract demonstrated significant success in reducing the length of illness as well as the mortality rate in 18 cases of typhoid — treatment was "dramatic from the first injection"[3]
- Using vitamin C as the sole therapy for typhoid fever would eliminate the anemia that often accompanies the use of chloramphenicol (one of the first-line antibiotics used in the treatment of typhoid fever)[4]
- High levels of vitamin C improves the resistance of chicks to typhoid[5]

# Vanadium Poisoning

**Description:** All vanadium compounds appear to be toxic. The biggest danger to humans is in breathing fumes or dust that contain this element.[1] Vanadium poisoning can adversely affect the heart, blood vessels, G.I. tract, kidneys, reproductive system, and lungs.[2] The toxicity caused by this metal appears to be secondary to oxidative damage.[3]

**Traditional Approach:** No generally accepted protocols specific for vanadium poisoning were found, although dimercaprol and vitamin C "may have value."[4]

**Studies Show:**

- Vitamin C has a significant protective, antidote effect against an otherwise lethal dose of a vanadium-containing compound in mice[5]

- In the investigation of 18 different antidotes, vitamin C "appeared to be the most promising" as an antidote against 2 vanadium compounds in a mouse model[6]

- Vitamin C is very effective in preventing vanadium intoxication when administered immediately after the vanadium in mice[7]

- Pretreatment with vitamin C significantly reduces the clinical toxicity of vanadium in mice as evidenced by less respiratory depression and limb paralysis[8]

- Vitamin C reduces growth retardation related to the administration of vanadium in chicks[9]

- Vitamin C protects hens from the toxic effects of vanadium in decreasing egg production and body weight[10]

## Vanadium Poisoning (cont.)

- Vitamin C protects the eggs of laying hens from the decreased albumin (egg white) quality associated with excess dietary vanadium.[11]

- Vitamin C increases the urinary elimination of administered vanadium in mice[12]

- Vitamin C appears to be one of the natural reducing agents of vanadium[13]

- Vitamin C chemically reduces vanadium compounds more effectively than glutathione, another important antioxidant, for the same vanadium compounds[14]

- Vitamin C at least partially reverses the vanadium inhibition of an important enzyme that helps neurons communicate in the brain[15]

## Venoms

**Description:** More than 200 out of approximately 2,900 snake species have caused fatal bites in humans. At least eight of about 50 spiders in the U.S. can cause serious disease and/or death. These are the widow, brown recluse, hobo, wolf, fishing, green lynx, jumping, and yellow sac spiders.[1] Many marine organisms (for example: jelly fish and anemones) have venomous stings or bites.[2]

**Traditional Approach:** Unless the identity of a biting snake is known, antivenin therapy is of little use, and even then, the effectivness of antivenins is not clear-cut.[1] Many of the treatment protocols are venom-specific. Mostly supportive care that addresses particular symptoms is employed.

**Studies Show:**

- **Dosing Notes**
  - Vitamin C "is a non-toxic, non-specific antitoxin that may be used for any type of venomous bite without having to await identification of the culprit"[3]
  - Dr. Fred Klenner noted that the amount of vitamin C administered to a patient "is the all important factor" in assuring a positive clinical response for the toxin or infection being treated[4]
    1. "Never give less than 350 mg/kg body weight," repeated every hour for 6 to 12 doses depending upon clinical improvement
    2. Doses can be spaced from 2 to 4 hours when improvement is apparent until the patient recovers
    3. Doses can be as high as 1,200 mg/kg body weight for the critically ill person, such as a patient comatose with viral encephalitis

## Venoms (cont)

- **Black Widow Spider**
  - A 3$^1$/$_2$ year-old girl bitten by a black widow spider fully recovers after multiple administrations of high-dose vitamin C — some by injection and more by mouth over a period of 4 days[5]
  - "Eight proven cases of black widow bite" were cured with high-dose vitamin C[5]
- **Puss Caterpillar**
  - High-dose intravenous vitamin C given by syringe as rapidly as possible saved a cyanotic puss caterpillar bite victim[6]

- **Snake Bite**
  - High-dose intravenous vitamin C cures a 4 year-old child who received a "full strike" from a highland moccasin[7]
  - Snake bite victim who had already been ineffectively treated at another emergency room was treated with 15,000 mg of vitamin C intravenously twice daily, along with 5,000 mg of oral vitamin C every 4 hours; penicillin was given as well, and the patient was back to work in seven days[8]

# Cited References

## CHAPTER ONE

1. "Living Proof?" *60 Minutes*, New Zealand.
2. "Why Can't We Try?" *60 Minutes*, New Zealand.
3. Todar K, *Todar's Online Textbook of Bacteriology* 2008. Published online at www.textbookofbacteriology.net
4. Salaman MK, "Resistant Bacterial Infections Treated with Vitamin C" Published online at www.thenhf.com/article.php?id-1980, Jan 14, 2004.
5. Galloway T, Seifert M, "Bulbar poliomyelitis: favorable results in its treatment as a problem in respiratory obstruction" *Journal of the American Medical Association* 1949 141(1):1-8.
6. Landwehr R, "The origin of the 42-year stonewall of vitamin C" *Journal of Orthomolecular Medicine* 1991 6(2):99-103.
7. Holden M, Resnick R, "The *in vitro* action of synthetic crystalline vitamin C (ascorbic acid) on herpes virus" *Journal of Immunology* 1936 31:455-462.
8. Holden M, Molloy E, "Further experiments on the inactivation of herpes virus by vitamin C (L-ascorbic acid)" *Journal of Immunology* 1937 33:251-257.
9. Sagripanti J, et al, "Mechanism of copper-mediated inactivation of herpes simplex virus" *Antimicrobial Agents and Chemotherapy* 1997 41(4):812-817.
10. White L, et al, "*In vitro* effect of ascorbic acid on infectivity of herpesviruses and paramyxoviruses" *Journal of Clinical Microbiology* 1986 24(4):527-531.
11. Zureick M, "Treatment of shingles and herpes with vitamin C intravenously" *Journal des Praticiens* 1950 64:586.
12. Cathcart R, "Vitamin C in the treatment of acquired immune deficiency syndrome (AIDS)" *Medical Hypotheses* 1984 14(4):423-433.
13. Landwehr R, "The origin of the 42-year stonewall of vitamin C" *Journal of Orthomolecular Medicine* 1991 6(2):99-103.
14. Klenner F, "Significance of high daily intake of ascorbic acid in preventive medicine" *Journal of the International Academy of Preventive Medicine* 1974 1(1):45-69.

## CHAPTER TWO

1. Klenner F, "Observations of the dose and administration of ascorbic acid when employed beyond the range of a vitamin in human pathology" *Journal of Applied Nutrition* 1971 23(3&4):61-88.
2. Klenner F, "The black widow spider: case history" *Tri-State Medical Journal* Dec 1957 pp.15-18.
3. Klenner F, "Observations of the dose and administration of ascorbic acid when employed beyond the range of a vitamin in human pathology" *Journal of Applied Nutrition* 1971 23(3&4):61-88.
4. Klenner F, "Significance of high daily intake of ascorbic acid in preventive medicine" *Journal of the International Academy of Preventive Medicine* 1974 1(1):45-69.

5. Klenner F, "Case history: cure of a 4-year-old child bitten by a mature highland moccasin with vitamin C" *Tri-State Medical Journal* July 1954.

6. Smith L, *The Clinical Experiences of Frederick R. Klenner, M.D.: Clinical Guide to the Use of Vitamin C* 1988 Portland, OR: Life Sciences Press.

7. Laing M, "A cure for mushroom poisoning" *South African Medical Journal* 1984 65(15):590.

8. Khaw K, et al, "Relation between ascorbic acid and mortality in men and women in EPIC-Norfolk prospective study: a prospective population study, European Prospective Investigation into Cancer and Nutrition" *Lancet* 2001 357(9257):657-663.

## CHAPTER THREE

1. Osborn T, Gear J, "Possible relation between ability to synthesize vitamin C and reaction to tubercle bacillus" *Nature* 1940 145:974.

2. Khaw K, et al, "Relation between ascorbic acid and mortality in men and women in EPIC-Norfolk prospective study: a prospective population study. European Prospective Investigation into Cancer and Nutrition" *Lancet* 2001 357(9257):657-663.

3. Nishikimi M, et al, "Occurrence in humans and guinea pigs of the gene related to their missing enzyme L-gulonolactone oxidase" *Archives of Biochemistry and Biophysics* 1988 267(2):842-846.

4. *Wikipedia* http://en.wikipedia.org/wiki/Hunza_people

5. Cummings M, "Can some people synthesize ascorbic acid?" *The American Journal of Clinical Nutrition* 1981 34(2):297-298.

6. Kline A, Eheart M, "Variation in the ascorbic acid requirements for saturation of nine normal young women" *Journal of Nutrition* 1944 28:413-419.

7. Pijoan M, Lozner E, "Vitamin C economy in the human subject" *Bulletin of the Johns Hopkins Hospital* 1944 75:303-314.

8. Chatterjee G, Pal D, "Metabolism of L-ascorbic acid in rats under *in vivo* administration of mercury: effect of L-ascorbic acid supplementation" *International Journal for Vitamin and Nutrition Research* 1975 45(3):284-292.

9. Stone I, "*Homo sapiens ascorbicus*, a biochemically corrected robust human mutant" *Medical Hypotheses* 1979 5(6):711-721.

10. Conney A, et al, *Annals of the New York Academy of Sciences* 1961 92:115.

## CHAPTER FOUR

1. *American Heart Association Heart Disease and Stroke Statistics – 2010 Update* Dallas, Texas: American Heart Association 2010.

2. Levy T, *Curing the Incurable. Vitamin C, Infectious Diseases, and Toxins* 2004, MedFox Publishing, Henderson, NV.

3. Clark E, Clark E, "On the reaction of certain cells in the tadpole's tail toward vital dyes" *The Anatomical Record* (1918) 15:151.

4. Clark E, Clark E, "Further observations on living lymphatic vessels in the transparent chamber in the rabbit's ear—their relation to the tissue spaces" *American Journal of Anatomy* 1933 52:273-305.

5. Laguesse E, "La structure lamelleuse et le developpement du tissu conjonctif lache chez les mammiferes en general et chez l'homme en particulier" *Arch de Biol* 1921 31:173-298.

6. Bensley S, "On the presence, properties and distribution of the intercellular ground substance of loose connective tissue" *The Anatomical Record* 1934 60:93-109.

7. McMasters P, Parsons R, 'Physiological conditions existing in connective tissue. II. The state of the fluid in the intradermal tissue" *Journal of Experimental Medicine* 1939 69:265-282.

8. Wolbach S, Howe P, "Intercellular substances in experimental scorbutus" *Archives of Pathology and Laboratory Medicine* 1926 1(1):1-24.

9. Kefalides N, "Isolation and characterization of the collagen from glomerular basement membrane" *Biochemistry* 1968 7(9):3103-3112.

10. Gore I, et al, "Endothelial changes produced by ascorbic acid deficiency in guinea pigs" *Archives of Pathology* 1965 80(4):371-376.

11. Pauling L, "Vitamin C and longevity" *Agressologie* 1983 24(7):317-319.

12. Pirani C, Catchpole H, "Serum glycoproteins in experimental scurvy" *A.M.A. Archives of Pathology* 1951 51:597-601.

13. Fisher E, et al, "Interaction of ascorbic acid and glucose on production of collagen and proteoglycan by fibroblasts" *Diabetes* 1991 40(3):371-376.

14. Wolbach, S. and P. Howe (1926) Intercellular substances in experimental scorbutus. Archives of Pathology and Laboratory Medicine 1(1):1-24.

15. Gersh I, Catchpole H, "The organization of ground substance and basement membrane and its significance in tissue injury, disease and growth" *American Journal of Anatomy* 1949 85:457-521.

16. Pirani C, Catchpole H, "Serum glycoproteins in experimental scurvy" *A.M.A. Archives of Pathology* 1951 51:597-601.

17. Fisher E, et al, "Interaction of ascorbic acid and glucose on production of collagen and proteoglycan by fibroblasts" *Diabetes* 1991 40(3):371-376.

18. Katz E, "Reduction of cholesterol and Lp(a) and regression of coronary artery disease: a case study" *Journal of Orthomolecular Medicine* 1996 11(3):173-179.

19. Ibid.

20. Horlick L, Katz L, "Retrogression of atherosclerotic lesions on cessation of cholesterol feeding in the chick" *Journal of Laboratory and Clinical Medicine* 1949 34:1427-1442.

21. Levy T, *Curing the Incurable. Vitamin C, Infectious Diseases, and Toxins* 2004, MedFox Publishing, Henderson, NV.

22. Beck J, et al, "Dental infections and atherosclerosis" *American Heart Journal* 1999 138(5 Pt 2):S528-533.

23. Muhlestein J, "Infectious agents, antibiotics, and coronary artery disease" *Current Interventional Cardiology Reports* 2000 2(4):342-348.

24. Emingil G, et al, "Association between periodontal disease and acute myocardial infarction" *Journal of Periodontology* 2000 71(12):1882-1886.

25. Huggins H, Levy T, *Uninformed Consent: The Hidden Dangers in Dental Care* 1999 Charlottesville, VA: Hampton Roads Publishing Company, Inc.

26. Kulacz R, Levy T, *The Roots of Disease. Connecting Dentistry and Medicine* 2002 Philadelphia, PA: Xlibris Corporation.

27. Ibid.

28. Leren P, "The Oslo Diet Heart Study: eleven-year report" *Circulation* 1970 42(5):935-942.

29. Coronary Drug Project Research Group, "Clofibrate and niacin in coronary heart disease" *Journal of the American Medical Association* 1975 231(4):360-381.

30. Carlson L, et al, "Reduction of myocardial reinfarction by the combined treatment with clofibrate and nicotinic acid" *Atherosclerosis* 1977 28(1):81-86.

31. Lipid Research Clinics Program, "The Lipid Research Clinics Coronary Primary Prevention Trial results. I. Reduction in incidence of coronary heart disease" *Journal of the American Medical Association* 1984 251(3):351-374.

32. Frick M, et al, "Helsinki Heart Study: primary-prevention with gemfibrozil in middle-aged men with dyslipemia" *The New England Journal of Medicine* 1987 317(20):1237-1245.

33. Dorr A, et al, "Colestipol hydrochloride in hypercholesterolemic patients-effect on serum cholesterol and mortality" *Journal of Chronic Disease* 1978 31(1):5-14.

34. Buchwald H, et al, "Effect of partial ileal bypass on mortality and morbidity from coronary heart disease in patients with hypercholesterolemia. Report of the Program on the Surgical Control of Hyperlipidemias (POSCH)" *The New England Journal of Medicine* 1990 323(14):946-955.

35. Brophy J, Brassard P, Bourgault C, "The benefit of cholesterol-lowering medications after coronary revascularization: a population study". *American Heart Journal* 2005 150(2):282-286.

36. Willis G, "An experimental study of the intimal ground substance in atherosclerosis" *Canadian Medical Association Journal* 1953 69:17-22.

37. Ibid.

38. Duff G, "Experimental cholesterol arteriosclerosis and its relationship to human arteriosclerosis" *Archives of Pathology* 1935 20:81-123, 259-304.

39. Turley S, West C, Horton B, "The role of ascorbic acid in the regulation of cholesterol metabolism and in the pathogenesis of atherosclerosis" *Atherosclerosis* 1976 24(1-2):1-18.

40. Ginter E, "Ascorbic acid in cholesterol and bile acid metabolism" *Annals of the New York Academy of Sciences* 1975 258:410-421.

41. Ginter E, et al, "Lowered cholesterol catabolism in guinea pigs with chronic ascorbic acid deficiency" *American Journal of Clinical Nutrition* 1971 24(10):1238-1245.

42. Banerjee S, Singh H, "Cholesterol metabolism in scorbutic guinea pigs" *Journal of Biological Chemistry* 1958 233(1):336-339.

43. Maeda N, et al, "Aortic wall damage in mice unable to synthesize ascorbic acid" *Proceedings of the National Academy of Sciences of the United States of America* 2000 97(2):841-846.

44. Dent F, Hayes R, Booker W, "Further evidence of cholesterol-ascorbic acid antagonism in blood; role of adrenocortical hormones" *Federation Proceedings* 1951 18:291.

45. Booker W, et al, "Cholesterol-ascorbic acid relationship; changes in plasma and cell ascorbic acid and plasma cholesterol following administration of ascorbic acid and cholesterol" *American Journal of Physiology* 1957 189:75-77.

46. Sitaramayya C, Ali T, "Studies on experimental hypercholesterolemia and atherosclerosis" *Journal of Physiology and Pharmacology* 1962 6:192-204.

47. Sadava D, et al, "The effect of vitamin C on the rapid induction of aortic changes in rabbits" *Journal of Nutritional Science and Vitaminology* 1982 28(2):85-92.

48. Ginter E, Kajaba T, Nizner O, "The effect of ascorbic acid on cholesterolemia in healthy subjects with seasonal deficit of vitamin C" *Nutrition and Metabolism* 1970 2(2):76-86.

49. Ginter E, et al, "Effect of ascorbic acid on plasma cholesterol in humans in a long-term experiment" *International Journal for Vitamin and Nutrition Research* 1977 47(2):123-134.

50. Ginter E, "Marginal vitamin C deficiency, lipid metabolism, and atherogenesis" *Advances in Lipid Research* 1978 16:167-220.

51. Sokoloff B, et al, "Aging, atherosclerosis and ascorbic acid metabolism" *Journal of the American Geriatrics Society* 1966 14(12):1239-1260.

52. Willis G, "An experimental study of the intimal ground substance in atherosclerosis" *Canadian Medical Association Journal* 1953 69:17-22.

53. Datey K, et al, "Ascorbic acid and experimental atherosclerosis" *Journal of the Association of Physicians of India* 1968 16(9):567-570.

54. Stamler J, Stamler R, Liu K, "High blood pressure" In: Connor W, Bristow J (eds.), *Coronary Heart Disease: Prevention, Complications, and Treatment* 1985 Philadelphia, PA: J.P. Lippincott Company.

55. Hjerkinn E, et al, "Markers of endothelial cell activation in elderly men at high risk for coronary heart disease" *Scandinavian Journal of Clinical and Laboratory Investigation* 2005 65(3):201-209.

56. Kempler P, "Learning from large cardiovascular clinical trials: classical cardiovascular risk factors" *Diabetes Research and Clinical Practice* 2005 68(Suppl 1):S43-47.

57. Bates C, et al, "Does vitamin C reduce blood pressure? Results of a large study of people aged 65 or older" *Journal of Hypertension* 1998 16(7):925-932.

58. Fotherby M,et al, "Effect of vitamin C on ambulatory blood pressure and plasma lipids in older persons" *Journal of Hypertension* 2000 18(4):411-415.

59. May J, "How does ascorbic acid prevent endothelial dysfunction?" *Free Radical Biology & Medicine* 2000 28(9):1421-1429.

60. Moran J, et al, "Plasma ascorbic acid concentrations relate inversely to blood pressure in human subjects" *The American Journal of Clinical Nutrition* 1993 57(2):213-217.

61. Ness A, et al, "Vitamin C status and blood pressure" *Journal of Hypertension* 1996 14(4):503-508.

62. Ness A, Chee D, Elliott P, "Vitamin C and blood pressure—an overview" *Journal of Human Hypertension* 1997 11(6):343-350.

63. Sakai N, et al, "An inverse relationship between serum vitamin C and blood pressure in a Japanese community" *Journal of Nutritional Science and Vitaminology* 1998 44(6):853-867.

64. Duffy S, et al, "Treatment of hypertension with ascorbic acid" *Lancet* 1999 354(9195):2048-2049.

65. Galley H, et al, "Combination oral antioxidant supplementation reduces blood pressure" *Clinical Science* 1997 92(4):361-365.

66. Blanck T, Peterkofsky B, "The stimulation of collagen secretion by ascorbate as a result of increased proline hydroxylation in chick embryo fibroblasts" *Archives of Biochemistry and Biophysics* 1975 171(1):259-267.

67. Wendt M, et al, "Ascorbate stimulates type I and type III collagen in human Tenon's fibroblasts" *Journal of Glaucoma* 1997 6(6):402-407.

68. May J, Qu Z, "Transport and intracellular accumulation of vitamin C in endothelial cells: relevance to collagen synthesis" *Archives of Biochemistry and Biophysics* 2005 434(1):178-186.

69. Dahl-Jorgensen K, Larsen J, Hanssen K, "Atherosclerosis in childhood and adolescent type I diabetes: early disease, early treatment?" *Diabetologia* 2005 48(8):1445-1453.

70. Haffner S, "Rationale for new American Diabetes Association Guidelines: are national cholesterol education program goals adequate for the patient with diabetes mellitus?" *The American Journal of Cardiology* 2005 96(4A):33E-36E.

71. Online article: http://www.diabetes.org/living-with-diabetes/complications/heart-disease/

72. Kodama M, et al, "Diabetes mellitus is controlled by vitamin C treatment" *In Vivo* 1993 7(6A):535-542.

73. Dou C, Xu D, Wells W, "Studies on the essential role of ascorbic acid in the energy dependent release of insulin from pancreatic islets" *Biochemical and Biophysical Research Communications* 1997 231(3):820-822.

74. Ginter E, et al "Hypocholesterolemic effect of ascorbic acid in maturity-onset diabetes mellitus" *International Journal for Vitamin and Nutrition Research* 1978 48(4):368-373.

75. Som S, et al, "Ascorbic acid metabolism in diabetes mellitus" *Metabolism: Clinical and Experimental* 1981 30(6):572-577.

76. Stankova L, et al, "Plasma ascorbate concentrations and blood cell dehydroascorbate transport in patients with diabetes mellitus" *Metabolism: Clinical and Experimental* 1984 33(4):347-353.

77. Mooradian A, Morley J, "Micronutrient status in diabetes mellitus" *The American Journal of Clinical Nutrition* 1987 45(5):877-895.

78. Simon J, "Vitamin C and cardiovascular disease: a review" *Journal of the American College of Nutrition* 1992 11(2):107-125.

79. Bigley R, et al, "Interaction between glucose and dehydroascorbate transport in human neutrophils and fibroblasts" *Diabetes* 1983 32(6):545-548.

80. Kapeghian J, Verlangieri A, "The effects of glucose on ascorbic acid uptake in heart endothelial cells: possible pathogenesis of diabetic angiopathies" *Life Sciences* 1984 34(6):577-584.

81. Khatami M, Li W, Rockey J, "Kinetics of ascorbate transport by cultured retinal capillary pericytes. Inhibition by glucose" *Investigative Ophthalmology & Visual Science* 1986 27(11):1665-1671.

82. Sagun K, Carcamo J, Golde D, "Vitamin C enters mitochondria via facilitative glucose transporter 1 (Glut1) and confers mitochondrial protection against oxidative injury" *The FASEB Journal: Official Publication of the Federation of American Societies for Experimental Biology* 2005 19(12):1657-1667.

83. Wilson J, "Regulation of vitamin C transport" *Annual Review of Nutrition* 2005 25:105-125.

84. Cunningham J "The glucose/insulin system and vitamin C: implications in insulin-dependent diabetes mellitus" *Journal of the American College of Nutrition* 1998 17(2):105-108.

85. Belting C, Hinkler J, Dummett C, "Influence of diabetes mellitus on the severity of periodontal disease" *Journal of Periodontology* 1964 35:476.

86. Kodama M, et al, "Diabetes mellitus is controlled by vitamin C treatment" *In Vivo* 1993 7(6A):535-542.

## CHAPTER FIVE

1. Rowland JH, et al, "Cancer Survivors — United States, 2007" *Morbidity & Mortality Weekly Report* 2011 60(9):269-272.

2. Online article: http://www.cancer.org/Cancer/CancerCauses/index

3. Ibid.

4. Khaw K, et al, "Mortality in men and women in EPIC-Norfolk prospective study: a prospective population study. European Prospective Investigation into Cancer and Nutrition" *Lancet* 2001 357(9257):657-663.

5. Kromhout D, et al, "Saturated fat, vitamin C and smoking predict long-term population all-cause mortality rates in the Seven Countries Study" *Int J Epidemiol.* 2000 Apr;29(2):260-5.

6. Riordan HD, et al, "Intravenous Vitamin C as a Chemotherapy Agent: A Report on Clinical Cases" *Puerto Rico Health Sci J* 2004 23-2:115.

7. Riordan HD, et al, "Intravenous Vitamin C as a Chemotherapy Agent: A Report on Clinical Cases" *Puerto Rico Health Sci J* 2004 23-2:117.

8. Riordan HD, et al, "Intravenous Vitamin C as a Chemotherapy Agent: A Report on Clinical Cases" *Puerto Rico Health Sci J* 2004 23-2:115.

9. Jackson JA, et al, "Sixteen-Year History with High Dose Intravenous Vitamin C Treatment for Various Types of Cancer and Other Diseases" *J Orthomol Med* 2002 17-2:117-119.

10. Padayatty SJ, et al, "Intravenously administered vitamin C as cancer therapy: three cases" *Canadian Med Assoc Journal* March 28, 2006 174(7).

11. Jackson JA, Riordan, HD, Schultz M, "High-dose intravenous vitamin C in the treatment of a patient with adenocarcinoma of the kidneys – a case study" *J Orthomol Med* 1990 5-1: 5-7.

12. Jackson JA, et al, "High-dose intravenous vitamin C and long time survival of a patient with cancer of the head of the pancreas" *J Orthomol Med* 1995 10-2:87-88.

13. Riordan NH, Jackson JA, Riordan HD "Intravenous vitamin C in a terminal cancer patient" *J Orthomol Med* 1996 11-2:80-82.

14. Riordan HD, et al, "High-dose intravenous vitamin C in the treatment of a patient with renal cell carcinoma of the kidney" *J Orthomol Med* 1998 13-2:72-73.

15. Online article: http://www.oasisofhope.com/irt_ch17_survival_statistics.php

16. Online article: http://www.oasisofhope.com/irt_ch14_diet_exercise.php

17. Online article: http://www.oasisofhope.com/irt_ch16_caring_spirit.php

18. Online article: http://www.oasisofhope.com/alternative-cancer-treatments.php

19. Pauling L, "Vitamin C and longevity" *Agressologie* (1983) 24(7):317-319.

20. Pirani C, Catchpole H, "Serum glycoproteins in experimental scurvy" *A.M.A. Archives of Pathology* (1951) 51:597-601.

21. Fisher E, et al, "Interaction of ascorbic acid and glucose on production of collagen and proteoglycan by fibroblasts" *Diabetes* 1991 40(3):371-376.

22. Wolbach, S. and P. Howe (1926) Intercellular substances in experimental scorbutus. Archives of Pathology and Laboratory Medicine 1(1):1-24.

23. Gersh I, Catchpole H, "The organization of ground substance and basement membrane and its significance in tissue injury, disease and growth" *American Journal of Anatomy* 1949 85:457-521.

24. Pirani C, Catchpole H, "Serum glycoproteins in experimental scurvy" *A.M.A. Archives of Pathology* (1951) 51:597-601.

25. Fisher E, et al, "Interaction of ascorbic acid and glucose on production of collagen and proteoglycan by fibroblasts" *Diabetes* 1991 40(3):371-376.

26. Tian J, et al, "Metalloporphyrin synergizes with ascorbic acid to inhibit cancer cell growth through fenton chemistry" *Cancer Biother Radiopharm* 2010 Aug 25(4):439-48.

27. Riordan NH, Riordan HD, Jackson JA, "Intravenous ascorbate as a tumor cytotoxic chemo-therapeutic agent" *Med Hypoth* 1994 44-3: 7-213.

28. Casciari JP, et al, "Cytotoxicity of ascorbate, lipoic acid and other antioxidants in hollow fibre *in vitro* tumors" *Brit J Canc* 01 84-11:1544-1550.

29. Kurbacher, et al, "Ascorbic acid (vitamin C) improves the antineoplastic activity of doxorubicin, cisplatin, and paclitaxel in human breast carcinoma cells *in vitro*" *Cancer Letters* 1996 103(2):183-189.

30. Shimpo K, et al, "Ascorbic acid and adriamycin toxicity" *The American Journal of Clinical Nutrition* 1991 54(6 Suppl):1298S-1301S.

31. Padayatty SJ, et al, "Intravenously administered vitamin C as cancer therapy: three cases" *Canadian Med Assoc Journal* March 28, 2006; 174 (7).

## CHAPTER SIX

1. Jomova K, Valko M, "Advances in metal-induced oxidative stress and human disease" *Toxicology* 2011 Mar 14.

2. Gabbay KH, et al, "Ascorbate synthesis pathway: dual role of ascorbate in bone homeostasis" *J Biol Chem* 2010 Jun 18 285(25):19510-20.

3. Yalin S, et al "Is there a role of free oxygen radicals in primary male osteoporosis?" *Clin Exp Rheumatol* 2005 Sep-Oct 23(5):689-92.

4. Park JB, "The Effects of Dexamethasone, Ascorbic Acid, and β-Glycerophosphate on Osteoblastic Differentiation by Regulating Estrogen Receptor and Osteopontin Expression" *J Surg Res* 2010 Oct 8.

5. Hie M, Tsukamoto I, "Vitamin C-deficiency stimulates osteoclastogenesis with an increase in RANK expression" *J Nutr Biochem* 2011 Feb 22(2):164-71.

6. Sheweita SA, Khoshhal KI, "Calcium metabolism and oxidative stress in bone fractures: role of antioxidants" Curr Drug Metab 2007 Jun 8(5):519-25.

7. Saito M, "Nutrition and bone health. Roles of vitamin C and vitamin B as regulators of bone mass and quality" Clin Calcium 2009 Aug 19(8):1192-9.

8. Maehata Y, et al, "Type III collagen is essential for growth acceleration of human osteoblastic cells by ascorbic acid 2-phosphate, a long-acting vitamin C derivative" Matrix Biol 2007 Jun 26(5):371-81.

9. Hie M, Tsukamoto I, "Vitamin C-deficiency stimulates osteoclastogenesis with an increase in RANK expression" J Nutr Biochem 2011 Feb 22(2):164-71.

10. Chuin A, et al, "Effect of antioxidants combined to resistance training on BMD in elderly women: a pilot study" Osteoporos Int 2009 Jul 20(7):1253-8.

11. Sahni S, et al, "High vitamin C intake is associated with lower 4-year bone loss in elderly men" J Nutr 2008 Oct 138(10):1931-8.

12. Pasco JA, et al, "Antioxidant vitamin supplements and markers of bone turnover in a community sample of nonsmoking women" J Womens Health (Larchmt) 2006 Apr 15(3):295-300.

13. Sugiura M, et al, "Dietary patterns of antioxidant vitamin and carotenoid intake associated with bone mineral density: findings from post-menopausal Japanese female subjects" Osteoporos Int 2011 Jan 22(1):143-52.

14. Ruiz-Ramos M, et al, "Supplementation of ascorbic acid and alpha-tocopherol is useful to preventing bone loss linked to oxidative stress in elderly" J Nutr Health Aging 2010 Jun 14(6):467-72.

15. Zinnuroglu M, et al, "Prospective evaluation of free radicals and antioxidant activity following 6-month risedronate treatment in patients with postmenopausal osteoporosis" Rheumatol Int 2011 Jan 8.

16. Sahni S, et al, "Protective effect of total and supplemental vitamin C intake on the risk of hip fracture — a 17-year follow-up from the Framingham Osteoporosis Study" Osteoporos Int 2009 Nov 20(11):1853-61.

17. Falch JA, Mowé M, Bøhmer T, "Low levels of serum ascorbic acid in elderly patients with hip fracture" Scand J Clin Lab Invest 1998 May 58(3):225-8.

18. Bourne G, "Vitamin C and repair of injured tissues" Lancet 1942 2:661-664.

19. Morton D, Barrett-Connor E, Schneide D, "Vitamin C supplement use and bone mineral density in postmenopausal women" Journal of Bone and Mineral Research 2001 16(1):135-140.

20. Leveille S, et al, "Dietary vitamin C and bone mineral density in postmenopausal women in Washington State, USA" Journal of Epidemiology and Community Health 1997 51(5):479-485.

21. Khodyrev VN, et al, "The influence of the vitamin-mineral complex upon the blood vitamin, calcium and phosphorus of patients with ostreoarthrosis" Vopr Pitan 2006 75(2):44-7.

22. Yudoh K, et al, "Potential involvement of oxidative stress in cartilage senescence and development of osteoarthritis: oxidative stress induces chondrocyte telomere instability and downregulation of chondrocyte function" Arthritis Res Ther 2005 7(2):R380-91.

23. Lau H, Massasso D, Joshua F, "Skin, muscle and joint disease from the 17th century: scurvy" Int J Rheum Dis. 2009 Dec 12(4):361-5.

24. Kumar V, Choudhury P, "Scurvy — a forgotten disease with an unusual presentation" Trop Doct 2009 Jul 39(3):190-2.

25. Vitale A, et al, "Arthritis and gum bleeding in two children" J Paediatr Child Health 2009 Mar 45(3):158-60.

26. Regan EA, Bowler RP, Crapo JD, "Joint fluid antioxidants are decreased in osteoarthritic joints compared to joints with macroscopically intact cartilage and subacute injury" Osteoarthritis Cartilage 2008 Apr 16(4):515-21.

27. Choi HK, et al, "Dietary risk factors for rheumatic diseases" Curr Opin Rheumatol 2005 Mar 17(2):141-6.

28. Pattison DJ, et al, "Vitamin C and the risk of developing inflammatory polyarthritis: prospective nested case-control study" *Ann Rheum Dis* 2004 Jul 63(7):843-7.

29. Jaswal S, et al, "Antioxidant status in rheumatoid arthritis and role of antioxidant therapy" *Clin Chim Acta* 2003 Dec 338(1-2):123-9.

30. Wang Y, et al, "Effect of antioxidants on knee cartilage and bone in healthy, middle-aged subjects: a cross-sectional study" *Arthritis Res Ther* 2007 9(4):R66.

31. Sakai A, et al, "Large-dose ascorbic acid administration suppresses the development of arthritis in adjuvant-infected rats" *Arch Orthop Trauma Surg* 1999 119(3-4):121-6.

32. Gray SL, et al, "Antioxidant vitamin supplement use and risk of dementia or Alzheimer's disease in older adults" *J Am Geriatr Soc* 2008 Feb 56(2):291-5.

33. Fotuhi M, et al, "Better cognitive performance in elderly taking antioxidant vitamins E and C supplements in combination with nonsteroidal anti-inflammatory drugs: the Cache County Study" *Alzheimers Dement* 2008 May 4(3):223-7.

34. Cornelli U, "Treatment of Alzheimer's disease with a cholinesterase inhibitor combined with antioxidants" *Neurodegener Dis* 2010 7(1-3):193-202.

35. Harrison FE, et al, "Vitamin C deficiency increases basal exploratory activity but decreases scopolamine-induced activity in APP/PSEN1 transgenic mice" *Pharmacol Biochem Behav* 2010 Feb 94(4):543-52.

36. Harrison FE, et al, "Antioxidants and cognitive training interact to affect oxidative stress and memory in APP/PSEN1 mice" *Nutr Neurosci* 2009 Oct 12(5):203-18.

37. Harrison FE, et al, "Ascorbic acid attenuates scopolamine-induced spatial learning deficits in the water maze" *Behav Brain Res* 2009 Dec 28 205(2):550-8.

38. Harrison FE, May JM, "Vitamin C function in the brain: vital role of the ascorbate transporter SVCT2" *Free Radic Biol Med* 2009 Mar 15 46(6):719-30.

## CHAPTER SEVEN

1. Hayashi T, et al, "Fatal water intoxication in a schizophrenic patient--an autopsy case" *J Clin Forensic Med.* 2005 Jun;12(3):157-9. Epub 2005 Mar 16.

2. Levy T, *Curing the Incurable. Vitamin C, Infectious Diseases, and Toxins* 2004, MedFox Publishing, Henderson, NV.

3. Lazarou J, Pomeranz BH, Corey PN, "Incidence of adverse drug reactions in hospitalized patients: a meta-analysis of prospective studies" *JAMA* 1998 279:10-15.

4. Casciari J, et al, "Cytotoxicity of ascorbate, lipoic acid, and other antioxidants in hollow fibre *in vitro* tumours" *British Journal of Cancer* 2001 84(11):1544-1550.

5. Kalokerinos A, Dettman I, Dettman G, "Ascorbate—the proof of the pudding! A selection of case histories responding to ascorbate" *Australas Nurses J.* 1982 Mar;11(2):18-21.

6. Cathcart R, "Vitamin C, titrating to bowel tolerance, anascorbemia, and acute induced scurvy" *Medical Hypotheses* 1981 7(11):1359-1376.

7. Cathcart R, "Vitamin C in the treatment of acquired immune deficiency syndrome (AIDS)" *Medical Hypotheses* 1984 14(4):423-433.

8. Cathcart R, "Vitamin C: the nontoxic, nonrate-limited, antioxidant free radical scavenger" *Medical Hypotheses* 1985 18(1):61-77.

9. Cathcart R, "The third face of vitamin C" *Journal of Orthomolecular Medicine* 1993 7(4):197-200.

10. Creagan E, et al, "Failure of high-dose vitamin C (ascorbic acid) therapy to benefit patients with advanced cancer. A controlled trial" *The New England Journal of Medicine* 1979 301(13):687-690.

11. Moertel C, et al, "High-dose vitamin C versus placebo in the treatment of patients with advanced cancer who have had no prior chemotherapy. A randomized double-blind comparison" *The New England Journal of Medicine* 1985 312(3):137-141.

12. Ludvigsson J, Hansson L, Stendahl O, "The effect of large doses of vitamin C on leukocyte function and some laboratory parameters" *International Journal of Vitamin and Nutrition Research* 1979 49(2):160-165.

13. Bussey H, et al, "A randomized trial of ascorbic acid in polyposis coli" *Cancer* 1982 50(7):1434-1439.

14. McKeown-Eyssen G, et al, "A randomized trial of vitamins C and E in the prevention of recurrence of colorectal polyps" *Cancer Research* 1988 48(16):4701-4705.

15. Taylor A, et al, "Relationship in humans between ascorbic acid consumption and levels of total and reduced ascorbic acid in lens, aqueous humor, and plasma" *Current Eye Research* 1991 10(8):751-759.

16. Osilesi O, et al, "Blood pressure and plasma lipids during ascorbic acid supplementation in borderline hypertensive and normotensive adults" *Nutrition Research* 1991 11:405-412.

17. Lux B, May P, "Long-term observation of young cystinuric patients under ascorbic acid therapy" *Urologia Internationalis* 1983 38(2):91-94.

18. Melethil S, Mason D, Chang C, "Dose-dependent absorption and excretion of vitamin C in humans" *International Journal of Pharmacology* 1986 31:83-89.

19. Brox A, Howson-Jan K, Fauser A, "Treatment of idiopathic thrombocytopenic purpura with ascorbate" *British Journal of Haematology* 1988 70(3):341-344.

20. Godeau B, Bierling P, "Treatment of chronic autoimmune thrombocytopenic purpura with ascorbate" *British Journal of Haemotology* 1990 75(2):289-290.

21. Reaven P, et al, "Effect of dietary antioxidant combinations in humans. Protection of LDL by vitamin E but not by beta-carotene" *Arteriosclerosis and Thrombosis* 1993 13(4):590-600.

22. Sharma D, Mathur R, "Correction of anemia and iron deficiency in vegetarians by administration of ascorbic acid" *Indian Journal of Physiology and Pharmacology* 1995 39(4):403-406.

23. Bass W, et al, "Evidence for the safety of ascorbic acid administration to the premature infant" *American Journal of Perinatology* 1998 15(2):133-140.

24. Maikranz P, et al, "Gestational hypercalciuria causes pathological urine calcium oxalate supersaturations" *Kidney International* 1989 36(1):108-113.

25. Curhan G, et al, "Intake of vitamins B6 and C and the risk of kidney stones in women" *Journal of the American Society of Nephrology* 1999 10(4):840-845.

26. Gerster H, "No contribution of ascorbic acid to renal calcium oxalate stones" *Annals of Nutrition & Metabolism* 1997 41(5):269-282.

27. Padayatty SJ, et al, "Vitamin C: intravenous use by complementary and alternative medicine practitioners and adverse effects" PLoS One. 2010 Jul 7;5(7):e11414.

28. Heaney ML, et al, "Vitamin C antagonizes the cytotoxic effects of antineoplastic drugs" *Cancer Res* 2008 Oct 1 68(19):8031-8.

29. Challem J, "Medical Journal Watch" *Alternative and Complementary Therapies* 2009 February 15(1): 42-46.

## *CHAPTER EIGHT*

1. Lazarou J, Pomeranz BH, Corey PN, "Incidence of adverse drug reactions in hospitalized patients: a meta-analysis of prospective studies" *JAMA* 1998 Apr 15 279(15):1200-5.

2. Online article: http://www.wrongdiagnosis.com/a/adverse_reaction/prevalence.htm

3. *Kaiser Family Foundation Newsletter* May 2007 Menlo Park, CA 94025.

4. Lai M, et al, "2005 Annual Report of the American Association of Poison Control Centers' National Poisoning and Exposure Database" *Clinical Toxicology* 2006 (44):803-932.

5. Bronstein A, et al, "2006 Annual Report of the American Association of Poison Control Centers' National Poison Data System (NPDS)" *Clinical Toxicology* 2007 (45):815-917.

6. Bronstein A, et al, "2007 Annual Report of the American Association of Poison Control Centers' National Poison Data System (NPDS): 25th Annual Report" *Clinical Toxicology* 2008 (46):927-1057.

7. Bronstein A, et al, "2008 Annual Report of the American Association of Poison Control Centers' National Poison Data System (NPDS): 26th Annual Report" *Clinical Toxicology* 2009 (47):911-1084.

8. Bronstein A, "2009 Annual Report of the American Association of Poison Control Centers' National Poison Data System (NPDS): 27th Annual Report" *Clinical Toxicology* 2010 (48):979-1178.

9. HHS1 FDA, Department of Health & Human Services, *Prescription Drug Fee Rates for Fiscal Year 2010* Docket No. FDA-2009-N-0339 page 38451.

10. Cauchon D, "FDA Advisers Tied to Industry" *USA Today* September 25, 2000.

## CHAPTER NINE

1. Groff JL, Gropper SS, Hunt SM, "Advanced Nutrition and Human Metabolism" *West Publishing Co* 1995, pages 222-237.

2. "Bio-Technology Breakthrough Promises Nearly 100% Bioavailability" *USA Today* December 19, 2006.

3. Bangham, A., Standish M, Watkins J, "Diffusion of univalent ions across the lamellae of swollen phospholipids" *Journal of Molecular Biology* 1965 13(1):238-252.

4. Gregoriadis G. [ed.] *Liposome Technology. Third edition. Volume II: Entrapment of Drugs and Other Materials into Liposomes*, New York, NY: Informa Healthcare USA, Inc. 2007.

5. Hickey S., Roberts H, Miller N, "Pharmacokinetics of oral vitamin C" *Journal of Nutritional & Environmental Medicine* July 31, 2009.

6. Cathcart R, "Vitamin C, titrating to bowel tolerance, anascorbemia, and acute induced scurvy" *Medical Hypotheses* 1981 7(11):1359-1376.

## Resource B

1. Siegel B, "Enhanced interferon response to murine leukemia virus by ascorbic acid" *Infection and Immunity* 1974 10(2):409-410.

2. Siegel B, "Enhancement of interferon production by poly(rI)-poly(rC) in mouse cell cultures by ascorbic acid" *Nature* 1975 254(5500):531-532.

3. Geber W, Lefkowitz S, Hung C, "Effect of ascorbic acid, sodium salicylate, and caffeine on the serum interferon level in response to viral infection" *Pharmacology* 1975 13(3):228-233.

4. Dahl H ,Degre M, "The effect of ascorbic acid on production of human interferon and the antiviral activity *in vitro*. Acta Pathologica et Microbiologica Scandinavica. Section B" *Microbiology* 1976 84(5):280-284.

5. Stone I, "The possible role of mega-ascorbate in the endogenous synthesis of interferon" *Medical Hypotheses* 1980 6(3):309-314.

6. Karpinska T, Kawecki Z, Kandefer-Szerszen M, "The influence of ultraviolet irradiation, L-ascorbic acid and calcium chloride on the induction of interferon in human embryo fibroblasts" *Archivum Immunologiae et Therapiae Experimentalis* 1982 30(1-2)33-37.

7. Nungester W, Ames A, "The relationship between ascorbic acid and phagocytic activity" *Journal of Infectious Diseases* 1948 83:50-54.

8. Goetzl E, et al, "Enhancement of random migration and chemotactic response of human leukocytes by ascorbic acid" *The Journal of Clinical Investigation* 1974 53(3):813-818.

9. Sandler J, Gallin J, Vaughan M, "Effects of serotonin, carbamylcholine, and ascorbic acid on leukocyte cyclic GMP and chemotaxis" *The Journal of Cell Biology* 1975 67(2 Pt 1):480-484.

10. Boxer L, et al, "Correction of leukocyte function in Chediak-Higashi syndrome by ascorbate" *The New England Journal of Medicine* 1976 295(19):1041-1045.

11. Ganguly R, Durieux M, Waldman R, "Macrophage function in vitamin C-deficient guinea pigs" *The American Journal of Clinical Nutrition* 1976 29(7):762-765.

12. Anderson R, Dittrich O, "Effects of ascorbate on leucocytes. Part IV. Increased neutrophil function and clinical improvement after oral ascorbate in 2 patients with chronic granulomatous disease" *South African Medical Journal* 1979 56(12):476-480.

13. Anderson R, Theron A, "Effects of ascorbate on leucocytes. Part III. *In vitro* and *in vivo* stimulation of abnormal neutrophil motility by ascorbate" *South African Medical Journal* 1979 56(11):429-433.

14. Anderson R, et al, "The effects of increasing weekly doses of ascorbate on certain cellular and humoral immune functions in normal volunteers" *The American Journal of Clinical Nutrition* 1980 33(1):71-76.

15. Anderson R, et al, "The effect of ascorbate on cellular humoral immunity in asthmatic children" *South African Medical Journal* 1980 58(24):974-977.

16. Dallegri F, Lanzi G, Patrone F, "Effects of ascorbic acid on neutrophil locomotion" *International Archives of Allergy and Applied Immunology* 1980 61(1):40-45.

17. Corberand J, et al, "Malignant external otitis and polymorphonuclear leukocyte migration impairment. Improvement with ascorbic acid" *Archives of Otolaryngology* 1982 108(2):122-124.

18. Patrone F, et al, "Effects of ascorbic acid on neutrophil function. Studies on normal and chronic granulomatous disease neutrophils" *Acta Vitaminologica et Enzymologica* 1982 4(1-2):163-168.

19. Cunningham-Rundles S, "Effects of nutritional status on immunological function" *The American Journal of Clinical Nutrition* 1982 35(5 Suppl):1202-1210.

20. Oberritter H, et al, "Effect of functional stimulation on ascorbate content in phagocytes under physiological and pathological conditions" *International Archives of Allergy and Applied Immunology* 1986 81(1):46-50.

21. Levy R, Schlaeffer F, "Successful treatment of a patient with recurrent furunculosis by vitamin C: improvement of clinical course and of impaired neutrophil functions" *International Journal of Dermatology* 1993 32(11):832-834.

22. Levy R, et al, "Vitamin C for the treatment of recurrent furunculosis in patients with impaired neutrophil functions" *The Journal of Infectious Diseases* 1996 173(6):1502-1505.

23. Ciocoiu M, et al, "The involvement of vitamins C and E in changing the immune response" [Article in Romanian] *Revista Medico-Chirurgicala a Societatii de Medici si Naturalisti din Iasi* 1998 102(1-2):93-96.

24. De la Fuente M, et al, "Immune function in aged women is improved by ingestion of vitamins C and E" *Canadian Journal of Physiology and Pharmacology* 1998 76(4):373-380.

25. Glick D, Hosoda S, "Histochemistry. LXXViii. Ascorbic acid in normal mast cells and macrophages and neoplastic mast cells" *Proceedings of the Society for Experimental Biology and Medicine* 1965 119:52-56.

26. Thomas W, Holt P, "Vitamin C and immunity: an assessment of the evidence" *Clinical and Experimental Immunology* 1978 32(2):370-379.

27. Evans R, Currie L, Campbell A, "The distribution of ascorbic acid between various cellular components of blood, in normal individuals, and its relation to the plasma concentration" *The British Journal of Nutrition* 1982 47(3):473-482.

28. Goldschmidt M, "Reduced bactericidal activity in neutrophils from scorbutic animals and the effect of ascorbic acid on these target bacteria *in vivo* and *in vitro*" *The American Journal of Clinical Nutrition* 1991 54(6 Suppl):1214S-1220S.

29. Washko P, Wang Y, Levine M, "Ascorbic acid recycling in human neutrophils" *The Journal of Biological Chemistry* 1993 268(21):15531-15535.

30. Siegel B, Morton J, "Vitamin C and the immune response" *Experientia* 1977 33(3):393-395.

31. Jeng K, et al, "Supplementation with vitamins C and E enhances cytokine production by peripheral blood mononuclear cells in healthy adults" *The American Journal of Clinical Nutrition* 1996 64(6):960-965.

32. Campbell J, et al, "Ascorbic acid is a potent inhibitor of various forms of T cell apoptosis" *Cellular Immunology* 1999 194(1):1-5.

33. Mizutani A, et al, "Ascorbate-dependent enhancement of nitric oxide formation in activated macrophages. *Nitric Oxide: Biology and Chemistry* 1998 2(4):235-241.

34. Mizutani A. Tsukagoshi N, "Molecular role of ascorbate in enhancement of NO production in activated macrophage-like cell line, J774.1" *Journal of Nutritional Science and Vitaminology* 1999 45(4):423-435.

35. Fraser R, et al, "The effect of variations in vitamin C intake on the cellular immune response of guinea pigs" *The American Journal of Clinical Nutrition* 1980 33(4):839-847.

36. Kennes B, et al, "Effect of vitamin C supplements on cell-mediated immunity in old people" *Gerontology* 1983 29(5):305-310.

37. Wu C, Dorairajan T, Lin T, "Effect of ascorbic acid supplementation on the immune response of chickens vaccinated and challenged with infectious bursal disease virus" *Veterinary Immunology and Immunopathology* 2000 74(1-2):145-152.

38. Schwager J, Schulze J, "Influence of ascorbic acid on the response to mitogens and interleukin production of porcine lymphocytes" *International Journal for Vitamin and Nutrition* Research 1997 67(1):10-16.

39. Rotman D, "Sialoresponsin and an antiviral action of ascorbic acid" *Medical Hypotheses* 1978 4(1):40-43.

40. Ecker E, Pillemer L, "Vitamin C requirement of the guinea pig" *Proceedings of the Society for Experimental Biology and Medicine* 1940 44:262.

41. Bourne G, "Vitamin C and immunity" *The British Journal of Nutrition* 1949 2:342.

42. Prinz W, et al, "The effect of ascorbic acid supplementation on some parameters of the human immunological defence system" *International Journal for Vitamin and Nutrition Research* 1977 47(3):248-257.

43. Vallance S, "Relationships between ascorbic acid and serum proteins of the immune system" *British Medical Journal* 1977 2(6084):437-438.

44. Sakamoto M, et al, "The effect of vitamin C deficiency on complement systems and complement components" *Journal of Nutritional Science and Vitaminology* 1981 27(4):367-378.

45. Feigen G, et al, "Enhancement of antibody production and protection against systemic anaphylaxis by large doses of vitamin C" *Research Communications in Chemical Pathology and Pharmacology* 1982 38(2):313-333.

46. Li Y, Lovell T, "Elevated levels of dietary ascorbic acid increase immune responses in channel catfish" *The Journal of Nutrition* 1985 115(1):123-131.

47. Wahli T, Meier W, Pfister K, "Ascorbic acid induced immune-mediated decrease in mortality in *Ichthyophthirius multifiliis* infected rainbow-trout (*Salmo gairdneri*)" *Acta Tropica* 1986 43(3):287-289.

48. Johnston C, Kolb W, Haskell B, "The effect of vitamin C nutriture on complement component C1q concentrations in guinea pig plasma" *The Journal of Nutrition* 1987 117(4):764-768.

49. Haskell B, Johnston C, "Complement component C1q activity and ascorbic acid nutriture in guinea pigs" *The American Journal of Clinical Nutrition* 1991 54(6 Suppl):1228S-1230S.

50. Wu C, Dorairajan T, Lin T, "Effect of ascorbic acid supplementation on the immune response of chickens vaccinated and challenged with infectious bursal disease virus" *Veterinary Immunology and Immunopathology* 2000 74(1-2):145-152.

51. Heuser G, Vojdani A, "Enhancement of natural killer cell activity and T and B cell function by buffered vitamin C in patients exposed to toxic chemicals: the role of protein kinase-C" *Immunopharmacology and Immunotoxicology* 1997 19(3):291-312.

52. Horrobin D, et al, "The nutritional regulation of T lymphocyte function" *Medical Hypotheses* 1979 5(9):969-985.

53. Scott J, "On the biochemical similarities of ascorbic acid and interferon" *Journal of Theoretical Biology* 1982 98(2):235-238.

54. Siegel B, Morton J, "Vitamin C and immunity: influence of ascorbate on prostaglandin E2 synthesis and implications for natural killer cell activity" *International Journal for Vitamin and Nutrition Research* 1984 54(4):339-342.

55. Atkinson J, et al, "Effects of ascorbic acid and sodium ascorbate on cyclic nucleotide metabolism in human lymphocytes" *Journal of Cyclic Nucleotide Research* 1979 5(2):107-123.

56. Panush R, et al, "Modulation of certain immunologic responses by vitamin C. III. Potentiation of *in vitro* and *in vivo* lymphocyte responses" *International Journal for Vitamin and Nutrition Research. Supplement* 1982 23:35-47.

57. Strangeways W, "Observations on the trypanocidal action *in vitro* of solutions of glutathione and ascorbic acid" *Annals of Tropical Medicine and Parasitology* 1937 31:405-416.

58. Miller T, "Killing and lysis of gram-negative bacteria through the synergistic effect of hydrogen peroxide, ascorbic acid, and lysozyme" *Journal of Bacteriology* 1969 98(3):949-955.

59. Tappel A, "Lipid peroxidation damage to cell components" *Federation Proceedings* 1973 32(8):1870-1874.

60. Kraut E, Metz E, Sagone A, "*In vitro* effects of ascorbate on white cell metabolism and the chemiluminescence response" *Journal of the Reticuloendothelial Society* 1980 27(4):359-366.

61. Robertson W, Ropes M, Bauer W, "The degradation of mucins and polysaccharides by ascorbic acid and hydrogen peroxide" *The Biochemical Journal* 1941 35:903.

62. Nandi B, et al, "Effect of ascorbic acid on detoxification of histamine under stress conditions" *Biochemical Pharmacology* 1974 23(3):643-647.

63. Johnston C, Martin L, Cai X, "Antihistamine effect of supplemental ascorbic acid and neutrophil chemotaxis" *Journal of the American College of Nutrition* 1992 11(2):172-176.

64. Kastenbauer S, et al, "Oxidative stress in bacterial meningitis in humans" *Neurology* 2002 58(2):186-191.

65. Versteeg J, "Investigations on the effect of ascorbic acid on antibody production in rabbits after injection of bacterial and viral antigens by different routes. Proceedings of the Koninklijke Nederlandse Akademie van Wetenschappen. Series C" *Biological and Medical Sciences* 1970 73(5):494-501.

66. Banic S, "Immunostimulation by vitamin C" *International Journal for Vitamin and Nutrition Research. Supplement* 1982 23:49-52.
67. Wu C, Dorairajan T, Lin T, "Effect of ascorbic acid supplementation on the immune response of chickens vaccinated and challenged with infectious bursal disease virus" *Veterinary Immunology and Immunopathology* 2000 74(1-2):145-152.
68. Ericsson Y, "The effect of ascorbic acid oxidation on mucoids and bacteria in body secretions" *Acta Pathologica et Microbiologica Scandinavica* 1954 35:573-583.
69. Rawal B, "Bactericidal action of ascorbic acid on *Pseudomonas aeruginosa*: alteration of cell surface as a possible mechanism" *Chemotherapy* 1978 24(3):166-171.

## Resource C

1. Smith VH, "Vitamin C deficiency is an under-diagnosed contributor to degenerative disc disease in the elderly" *Med Hypotheses* 2010 Apr 74(4):695-7.
2. Duarte TL, Cooke MS, Jones GD, "Gene expression profiling reveals new protective roles for vitamin C in human skin cells" *Free Radic Biol Med* 2009 Jan 1 46(1):78-87.
3. Hashem MA, et al, "A rapid and sensitive screening system for human type I collagen with the aim of discovering potent anti-aging or anti-fibrotic compounds" *Mol Cells* 2008 Dec 31 26(6):625-30.
4. Qiao H, et al, "Ascorbic acid uptake and regulation of type I collagen synthesis in cultured vascular smooth muscle cells" *J Vasc Res* 2009 46(1):15-24.
5. Boyera N, Galey I, Bernard BA, "Effect of vitamin C and its derivatives on collagen synthesis and cross-linking by normal human fibroblasts" *Int J Cosmet Sci* 1998 Jun 20(3):151-8.
6. May JM, Qu ZC, "Transport and intracellular accumulation of vitamin C in endothelial cells: relevance to collagen synthesis" *Arch Biochem Biophys* 2005 Feb 1 434(1):178-86.
7. Saitoh Y, Nagai Y, Miwa N, "Fucoidan-Vitamin C complex suppresses tumor invasion through the basement membrane, with scarce injuries to normal or tumor cells, via decreases in oxidative stress and matrix metalloproteinases" *Int J Oncol* 2009 Nov 35(5):1183-9.
8. Mahmoodian F, Peterkofsky B, "Vitamin C deficiency in guinea pigs differentially affects the expression of type IV collagen, laminin, and elastin in blood vessels" *J Nutr* 1999 Jan 129(1):83-91.
9. Marionnet C, et al, "Morphogenesis of dermal-epidermal junction in a model of reconstructed skin: beneficial effects of vitamin C" *Exp Dermatol* 2006 Aug 15(8):625-33.
10. Boyce ST, et al, "Vitamin C regulates keratinocyte viability, epidermal barrier, and basement membrane *in vitro*, and reduces wound contraction after grafting of cultured skin substitutes" *J Invest Dermatol* 2002 Apr 118(4):565-72.
11. Heyman H, "Benefits of an oral nutritional supplement on pressure ulcer healing in long-term care residents" *J Wound Care* 2008 Nov 17(11):476-8, 480.
12. Otsuka M, et al, "Contribution of a high dose of L-ascorbic acid to carnitine synthesis in guinea pigs fed high-fat diets" *J Nutr Sci Vitaminol* (Tokyo). 1999 Apr 45(2):163-71.
13. Rebouche CJ, "Ascorbic acid and carnitine biosynthesis" *Am J Clin Nutr* 1991 Dec 54(6 Suppl):1147S-1152S.
14. Naidu KA, "Vitamin C in human health and disease is still a mystery? An overview" *Nutr J* 2003 Aug 21 2:7.
15. Gabbay KH, et al, "Ascorbate synthesis pathway: dual role of ascorbate in bone homeostasis" *J Biol Chem* 2010 Jun 18 285(25):19510-20.

16. Yalin S, et al, "Is there a role of free oxygen radicals in primary male osteoporosis?" *Clin Exp Rheumatol* 2005 Sep-Oct 23(5):689-92.

17. Park JB, "The Effects of Dexamethasone, Ascorbic Acid, and β-Glycerophosphate on Osteoblastic Differentiation by Regulating Estrogen Receptor and Osteopontin Expression" *J Surg Res* 2010 Oct 8.

18. Hie M, Tsukamoto I, "Vitamin C-deficiency stimulates osteoclastogenesis with an increase in RANK expression" *J Nutr Biochem* 2011 Feb 22(2):164-71.

19. Sheweita SA, Khoshhal KI, "Calcium metabolism and oxidative stress in bone fractures: role of antioxidants" *Curr Drug Metab* 2007 Jun 8(5):519-25.

20. Saito M, "Nutrition and bone health. Roles of vitamin C and vitamin B as regulators of bone mass and quality" *Clin Calcium* 2009 Aug 19(8):1192-9.

21. Maehata Y, et al, "Type III collagen is essential for growth acceleration of human osteoblastic cells by ascorbic acid 2-phosphate, a long-acting vitamin C derivative" *Matrix Biol* 2007 Jun 26(5):371-81.

22. Hie M, Tsukamoto I, "Vitamin C-deficiency stimulates osteoclastogenesis with an increase in RANK expression" *J Nutr Biochem* 2011 Feb 22(2):164-71. Epub 2010 May 4.

23. Chuin A, et al, "Effect of antioxidants combined to resistance training on BMD in elderly women: a pilot study" *Osteoporos Int* 2009 Jul 20(7):1253-8.

24. Sahni S, et al, "High vitamin C intake is associated with lower 4-year bone loss in elderly men" *J Nutr* 2008 Oct 138(10):1931-8.

25. Pasco JA, et al, "Antioxidant vitamin supplements and markers of bone turnover in a community sample of nonsmoking women" *J Womens Health (Larchmt)* 2006 Apr 15(3):295-300.

26. Sugiura M, et al, "Dietary patterns of antioxidant vitamin and carotenoid intake associated with bone mineral density: findings from post-menopausal Japanese female subjects" *Osteoporos Int* 2011 Jan 22(1):143-52

27. Ruiz-Ramos M, et al, "Supplementation of ascorbic acid and alpha-tocopherol is useful to preventing bone loss linked to oxidative stress in elderly" *J Nutr Health Aging* 2010 Jun 14(6):467-72.

28. Zinnuroglu M, et al, "Prospective evaluation of free radicals and antioxidant activity following 6-month risedronate treatment in patients with postmenopausal osteoporosis" *Rheumatol Int* 2011 Jan 8.

29. Sahni S, et al, "Protective effect of total and supplemental vitamin C intake on the risk of hip fracture — a 17-year follow-up from the Framingham Osteoporosis Study" *Osteoporos Int* 2009 Nov 20(11):1853-61.

30. Falch JA, Mowé M, Bøhmer T, "Low levels of serum ascorbic acid in elderly patients with hip fracture" *Scand J Clin Lab Invest* 1998 May 58(3):225-8.

31. Subramanian N, et al, "Effect of ascorbic acid on detoxification of histamine in rats and guinea pigs under drug treated conditions" *Pharmacol* 1974 Feb 1 23(3):637-41.

32. Johnston C, Martin L, Cai X, "Antihistamine effect of supplemental ascorbic acid and neutrophil chemotaxis" *Journal of the American College of Nutrition* 1992 11(2):172-176.

33. Johnston CS, Huang SN, "Effect of ascorbic acid nutriture on blood histamine and neutrophil chemotaxis in guinea pigs" *J Nutr* 1991 Jan 121(1):126-30.

34. Cathcart RF 3rd, "The vitamin C treatment of allergy and the normally unprimed state of antibodies" *Med Hypotheses* 1986 Nov 21(3):307-21.

### *Resource D*

1. Blanck T, Peterkofsky B, "The stimulation of collagen secretion by ascorbate as a result of increased proline hydroxylation in chick embryo fibroblasts" *Archives of Biochemistry and Biophysics* 1975 171(1):259-267.

2. Wendt M, et al, "Ascorbate stimulates type I and type III collagen in human Tenon's fibroblasts" *Journal of Glaucoma* 1997 6(6):402-407.

3. May J, Qu Z, "Transport and intracellular accumulation of vitamin C in endothelial cells: relevance to collagen synthesis" *Archives of Biochemistry and Biophysics* 2005 434(1):178-186.

4. Galley H, et al, "Combination oral antioxidant supplementation reduces blood pressure" *Clinical Science* 1997 92(4):361-365.

5. Duffy S, et al, "Treatment of hypertension with ascorbic acid" *Lancet* 1999 354(9195):2048-2049.

6. Moran J, et al, "Plasma ascorbic acid concentrations relate inversely to blood pressure in human subjects" *The American Journal of Clinical Nutrition* 1993 57(2):213-217.

7. Ness A, "Vitamin C status and blood pressure" *Journal of Hypertension* 1996 14(4):503-508.

8. Ness A, Chee D, Elliott P, "Vitamin C and blood pressure—an overview" *Journal of Human Hypertension* 1997 11(6):343-350.

9. Sakai, N, et al, "An inverse relationship between serum vitamin C and blood pressure in a Japanese community" *Journal of Nutritional Science and Vitaminology* 1998 44(6):853-867.

10. Lanman T, Ingalls T, "Vitamin C deficiency and wound healing: an experimental and clinical study" *Annals of Surgery* 1937 105(4):616-625.

11. Stolman J, Goldman H, Gould B, "Ascorbic acid and blood vessels" *Archives of Pathology* 1961 72:535-545.

12. Abt A, von Schuching S, Roe J, "Connective tissue studies. II. The effect of vitamin C deficiency on healed wounds" *Bulletin of the Johns Hopkins Hospital* 1959 105:67-76.

13. Pirani C, Levenson S, "Effect of vitamin C deficiency on healed wounds" *Proceedings of the Society for Experimental Biology and Medicine* 1953 82:95-99.

14. Bates C, et al, "Does vitamin C reduce blood pressure? Results of a large study of people aged 65 or older" *Journal of Hypertension* 1998 16(7):925-932.

15. Fotherby M, et al, "Effect of vitamin C on ambulatory blood pressure and plasma lipids in older persons" *Journal of Hypertension* 2000 18(4):411-415.

16. May J, "How does ascorbic acid prevent endothelial dysfunction?" *Free Radical Biology & Medicine* 2000 28(9):1421-1429.

17. Figueiredo P, et al, "Serum high-density lipoprotein (HDL) inhibits *in vitro* enterohemolysin (EHly) activity produced by enteropathogenic *Escherichia coli*" *FEMS Immunology and Medical Microbiology* 2003 38(1):53-57.

18. Park, K., et al, "Low density lipoprotein inactivates *Vibrio vulnificus* cytolysin through the oligomerization of toxin monomer" *Medical Microbiology and Immunology* 2005 194(3):137-141.

19. Carlson L, Bottiger L, "Risk factors for ischaemic heart disease in men and women. Results of the 19-year follow-up of the Stockholm Prospective Study" *Acta Medica Scandinavica* 1985 218(2):207-211.

20. Alouf J, "Thiol-dependent cytolytic bacterial toxins: streptolysin O and prominent toxins" [French] *Archives de l'Institut Pasteur de Tunis* 1981 58(3):355-373.

21. Alouf J, "Cholesterol-binding cytolytic protein toxins" *International Journal of Medical Microbiology* 2000 290(4-5):351-356.

22. Chi M, et al, "Effects of T-2 toxin on brain catecholamines and selected blood components in growing chickens" *Poultry Science* 1981 60(1):137-141.

23. Watson K, Kerr E, "Functional role of cholesterol in infection and autoimmunity" *Lancet* 1975 1(7902):308-310.

24. Bloomer A, et al, "A study of pesticide residues in Michigan's general population, 1968-70" *Pesticides Monitoring Journal* 1977 11(3):111-115.

25. Tarugi P, et al "Heavy metals and experimental atherosclerosis. Effect of lead intoxication on rabbit plasma lipoproteins" *Atherosclerosis* 1982 45(2):221-234.

26. Yousef M, et al, "Influence of ascorbic acid supplementation on the haematological and clinical biochemistry parameters of male rabbits exposed to aflatoxin B1" *Journal of Environmental Science and Health. Part B. Pesticides, Food Contaminants, and Agricultural Wastes* 2003 38(2):193-209.

27. Ginter E, "Marginal vitamin C deficiency, lipid metabolism, and atherogenesis" *Advances in Lipid Research* 1978 16:167-220.

28. Willis G, "An experimental study of the intimal ground substance in atherosclerosis" *Canadian Medical Association Journal* 1953 69:17-22.

29. Datey K, et al, "Ascorbic acid and experimental atherosclerosis" *Journal of the Association of Physicians of India* 1968 16(9):567-570.

30. Duff G, "Experimental cholesterol arteriosclerosis and its relationship to human arteriosclerosis" *Archives of Pathology* 1935 20:81-123, 259-304.

31. Willis G, Fishman S, "Ascorbic acid content of human arterial tissue" *Canadian Medical Association Journal* 1955 72:500-503.

32. Zaitsv V, et al, "The effect of ascorbic acid on experimental atherosclerosis" *Cor et Vasa* 1964 6(1):19-25.

33. Beetens, et al, "Influence of vitamin C on the metabolism of arachidonic acid and the development of aortic lesions during experimental atherosclerosis in rabbits" *Biomedica Biochimica Acta* 1984 43(8-9):S273-S276.

34. Ginter E, *The Role of Vitamin C in Cholesterol Catabolism and Atherogenesis* 1975 Bratislava, Czechoslovakia: Veda, Vydavatelstvo Slovenskej Akademie Vied.

35. Dent F, Hayes R, Booker W, "Further evidence of cholesterol-ascorbic acid antagonism in blood; role of adrenocortical hormones" *Federation Proceedings* 1951 18:291.

36. Booker W, et al "Cholesterol-ascorbic acid relationship; changes in plasma and cell ascorbic acid and plasma cholesterol following administration of ascorbic acid and cholesterol" *American Journal of Physiology* 1957 189:75-77.

37. Turley S, West C, Horton B, "The role of ascorbic acid in the regulation of cholesterol metabolism and in the pathogenesis of atherosclerosis" *Atherosclerosis* 1976 24(1-2):1-18.

38. Banerjee S, Singh H, "Cholesterol metabolism in scorbutic guinea pigs" *Journal of Biological Chemistry* 1958 233(1):336-339.

39. Maeda N, et al, "Aortic wall damage in mice unable to synthesize ascorbic acid" *Proceedings of the National Academy of Sciences of the United States of America* 2000 97(2):841-846.

40. Ginter E, "Cholesterol: vitamin C controls its transformation to bile acids" *Science* 1973 179(74):702-704.

41. Sitaramayya C, Ali T, "Studies on experimental hypercholesterolemia and atherosclerosis" *Journal of Physiology and Pharmacology* 1962 6:192-204.

42. Sadava D, et al, "The effect of vitamin C on the rapid induction of aortic changes in rabbits" *Journal of Nutritional Science and Vitaminology* 1982 28(2):85-92.

43. Ginter E, "Ascorbic acid in cholesterol and bile acid metabolism" *Annals of the New York Academy of Sciences* 1975 258:410-421.

44. Ginter E, et al, "Lowered cholesterol catabolism in guinea pigs with chronic ascorbic acid deficiency" *American Journal of Clinical Nutrition* 1971 24(10):1238-1245.

45. Ginter E, Kajaba T, Nizner O, "The effect of ascorbic acid on cholesterolemia in healthy subjects with seasonal deficit of vitamin C" *Nutrition and Metabolism* 1970 2(2):76-86.

46. Ginter E, et al, "Effect of ascorbic acid on plasma cholesterol in humans in a long-term experiment. *International Journal for Vitamin and Nutrition Research* 1977 47(2):123-134.

47. Sokoloff B, et al, "Aging, atherosclerosis and ascorbic acid metabolism" *Journal of the American Geriatrics Society* 1966 14(12):1239-1260.

48. Erden F, et al, "Ascorbic acid effect on some lipid fractions in human beings" *Acta Vitaminologica et Enzymologica* 1985 7(1-2):131-137.

49. Bishop N, Schorah C, Wales J, "The effect of vitamin C supplementation on diabetic hyperlipidaemia: a double blind, crossover study" *Diabetic Medicine: A Journal of the British Diabetic Association* 1985 2(2):121-124.

50. Ness A, et al, "Vitamin C status and serum lipids" *European Journal of Clinical Nutrition* 1996 50(11):724-729.

51. Bobek P, et al, "The effect of chronic marginal vitamin C deficiency on the rate of secretion and the removal of plasma triglycerides in guinea-pigs" *Physiologia Bohemoslovaca* 1980 29(4):337-343.

52. Ha T, Otsuka M, Arakawa N, "The effect of graded doses of ascorbic acid on the tissue carnitine and plasma lipid concentrations" *Journal of Nutritional Science and Vitaminology* 1990 36(3):227-234.

53. Adams C, et al, "Modification of aortic atheroma and fatty liver in saturated and polyunsaturated lecithins" *Journal of Pathology and Bacteriology* 1967 94(1):77-87.

54. Wilson T, Meservey C, Nicolosi R, "Soy lecithin reduces plasma lipoprotein cholesterol and early atherogenesis in hypercholesterolemic monkeys and hamsters: beyond lineoleate" *Atherosclerosis* 1998 140(1):147-153.

55. Mastellone I, et al, "Dietary soybean phosphatidylcholines lower lipidemia: Mechanisms at the levels of intestine, endothelial cell, and hepato-biliary axis" *Journal of Nutritional Biochemistry* 2000 11(9):461-466.

56. Polichetti E, et al, "Cholesterol-lowering effect of soyabean lecithin in normolipidaemic rats by stimulation of biliary lipid secretion" *British Journal of Nutrition* 1996 75(3):471-478.

57. Polichetti E, et al, "Dietary polyenylphosphatidylcholine decreases cholesterolemia in hypercholesterolemic rabbits: role of the hepato-biliary axis" *Life Sciences* 2000 67(21):2563-2576.

58. Altman R, et al, "Phospholipids associated with vitamin C in experimental atherosclerosis. *Arzneimittelforschung* 1980 30(4):627-630.

59. Pleiner J, et al, "Inflammation-induced vasoconstrictor hyporeactivity is caused by oxidative stress" *Journal of the American College of Cardiology* 2003 42(9):1656-1662.

60. Willis G, Fishman S, "Ascorbic acid content of human arterial tissue" *Canadian Medical Association Journal* 1955 72:500-503.

61. Yu H, Rifai N, "High-sensitivity C-reactive protein and atherosclerosis: from theory to therapy" *Clinical Biochemistry* 2000 33(8):601-610.

62. MacCallum P, "Markers of hemostasis and systemic inflammation in heart disease and atherosclerosis in smokers" *Proceedings of the American Thoracic Society* 2005 2(1):34-43.

63. Boos C, Lip G, "Blood clotting, inflammation, and thrombosis in cardiovascular events: perspectives" *Frontiers in Bioscience: a Journal and Virtual Library* 2006 11:328-336.

64. Becker A, de Boer O, van der Wal A, "The role of inflammation and infection in coronary heart disease" *Annual Review of Medicine* 2001 52:289-297.

65. Corti R, et al, "Evolving concepts in the triad of atherosclerosis, inflammation and thrombosis" *Journal of Thrombosis and Thrombolysis* 2004 17(1):35-44.

66. Licastro F, et al, "Innate immunity and inflammation in ageing: a key for understanding age-related diseases" *Immunity & Ageing* 2005 2:8.

67. Langlois M, et al, "Serum vitamin C concentration is low in peripheral arterial disease and is associated with inflammation and severity of atherosclerosis" *Circulation* 2001 103(14):1863-1868.

68. Beck J, et al, "Dental infections and atherosclerosis" *American Heart Journal* 1999 138(5 Pt 2):S528-533.

69. Muhlestein J, "Infectious agents, antibiotics, and coronary artery disease" *Current Interventional Cardiology Reports* 2000 2(4):342-348.

70. Emingil G, et al, "Association between periodontal disease and acute myocardial infarction" *Journal of Periodontology* 2000 71(12):1882-1886.

71. Hajishengallis G, et al, "Interactions of oral pathogens with toll-like receptors: possible role in atherosclerosis" *Annals of Periodontology* 2002 7(1):72-78.

72. Soder P, et al, "Early carotid atherosclerosis in subjects with periodontal diseases" *Stroke: A Journal of Cerebral Circulation* 2005 36(6):1195-1200.

73. Willis G, Fishman S, "Ascorbic acid content of human arterial tissue" *Canadian Medical Association Journal* 1955 72:500-503.

74. Becker A, de Boer O, van der Wal A, "The role of inflammation and infection in coronary heart disease" *Annual Review of Medicine* 2001 52:289-297.

75. Klotz O, "A discussion of the classification and experimental production of arteriosclerosis" *British Medical Journal* 1906 2:1767.

76. Klotz O, "The relation of experimental arterial disease in animals to arteriosclerosis in man" *Journal of Experimental Medicine, N.Y.* 1906 8:504.

77. Kiechl S, et al, "Chronic infections and the risk of carotid atherosclerosis. Prospective results from a large population study" *Circulation* 2001 103(8):1064-1070.

78. Leskov V, Zatevakhin I, "The role of the immune system in the pathogenesis of atherosclerosis [article in Russian] *Angiologiia i Sosudistaia Khirurgiia* 2005 11(2):9-14.

79. Wick G, et al, "Atherosclerosis, autoimmunity, and vascular-associated lymphoid tissue" *Federation of American Societies for Experimental Biology Journal* 1997 11(13):1199-1207.

80. Mayr M, et al, "Endothelial cytotoxicity mediated by serum antibodies to heat shock proteins of *Escherichia coli* and *Chlamydia pneumoniae*: immune reactions to heat shock proteins as a possible link between infection and atherosclerosis" *Circulation* 1999 99(12):1560-1566.

81. Xu Q, et al, "Association of serum antibodies to heat-shock protein 65 with carotid atherosclerosis: clinical significance determined in a follow-up study" *Circulation* 1999 100(11):1169-1174.

82. Xu Q, et al, "Serum soluble heat shock protein 60 is elevated in subjects with atherosclerosis in a general population" *Circulation* 2000 102(1):14-20.

83. de Leeuw K, Kallenberg C, Bijl M, "Accelerated atherosclerosis in patients with systemic autoimmune diseases" *Annals of the New York Academy of Sciences* 2005 1051:362-371.

84. Doria A, et al, "Inflammation and accelerated atherosclerosis: basic mechanisms" *Rheumatic Diseases Clinics of North America* 2005 31(2):355-362, viii.

85. Frostegard J, "Atherosclerosis in patients with autoimmune disorders" *Arteriosclerosis, Thrombosis, and Vascular Biology* 2005 25(9):1776-1785.

86. Kleindienst R, et al, "Atherosclerosis as an autoimmune condition" *Israel Journal of Medical Sciences* 1995 31(10):596-599.

87. Kodama M, et al, "Diabetes mellitus is controlled by vitamin C treatment" *In Vivo* 1993 7(6A):535-542.

88. Adam E, et al, "High levels of cytomegalovirus antibody in patients requiring vascular surgery for atherosclerosis" *Lancet* 1987 2(8554):291-293.

89. Cunningham M, Pasternak R, "The potential role of viruses in the pathogenesis of atherosclerosis" *Circulation* 1988 77(5):964-966.

90. Melnick J, Adam E, DeBakey M, "Cytomegalovirus and atherosclerosis" *Bioessays* 1995 17(10):899-903.

91. Eryol N, et al, "Are the high levels of cytomegalovirus antibodies a determinant in the development of coronary artery disease?" *International Heart Journal* 2005 46(2):205-209.

92. Fabricant C, et al, "Virus-induced atherosclerosis" *Journal of Experimental Medicine* 1978 148(1):335-340.

93. Minick C, et al, "Atheroarteriosclerosis induced by infection with a herpesvirus" *American Journal of Pathology* 1979 96(3):673-706.

94. Fabricant C,et al, "Herpesvirus-induced atherosclerosis in chickens" *Federation Proceedings* 1983 42(8):2476-2479.

95. Blum A, et al, "Viral load of the human immunodeficiency virus could be an independent risk factor for endothelial dysfunction" *Clinical Cardiology* 2005 28(3):149-153.

96. Nicholson A, Hajjar D, "Herpesviruses and thrombosis: activation of coagulation on the endothelium" *Clinica Chimica Acta (International Journal of Clinical Chemistry)* 1999 286(1-2):23-29.

97. Morrow D, Ridker P, "C-reactive protein, inflammation, and coronary risk" *Medical Clinics of North America* 2000 84(1):149-161, ix.

98. Ilhan F, et al, "Procalcitonin, C-reactive protein, and neopterin levels in patients with coronary atherosclerosis" *Acta Cardiologica* 2005 60(4):361-365.

99. Makita S, Nakamura M, Hiramori K, "The association of C-reactive protein levels with carotid intima-media complex thickness and plaque formation in the general population" *Stroke: a Journal of Cerebral Circulation* 2005 36(10):2138-2142.

100. Sun H, et al, "C-reactive protein in atherosclerotic lesions: its origin and pathophysiological significance" *The American Journal of Pathology* 2005 167(4):1139-1148.

101. von Eckardstein A, et al, "Lipoprotein(a) further increases the risk of coronary events in men with high global cardiovascular risk" *Journal of the American College of Cardiology* 2001 37(2):434-439.

102. Stubbs P, et al, "A prospective study of the role of lipoprotein(a) in the pathogenesis of unstable angina" *European Heart Journal* 1997 18(4):603-607.

103. Rath M, Pauling L, "Hypothesis: lipoprotein(a) is a surrogate for ascorbate" *Proceedings of the National Academy of Science USA* 1990 87(16):6204-6207.

104. Rath M, et al, "Detection and quantification of lipoprotein(a) in the arterial wall of 107 coronary bypass patients" *Arteriosclerosis* 1989 9(5):579-592.

105. Rath M, Pauling L, "Solution to the puzzle of human cardiovascular disease: its primary cause is ascorbate deficiency leading to the deposition of lipoprotein(a) and fibrinogen/fibrin in the vascular wall" *Journal of Orthomolecular Medicine* 1991 6(3&4):125-134.

106. Niendorf A, et al, "Morphological detection and quantification of lipoprotein(a) deposition in atheromatous lesions of human aorta and coronary arteries" *Virchows Arch A, Pathological Anatomy and Histopathology* 1990 417(2):105-111.

107. Cushing G, et al, "Quantitation and localization of apolipoproteins(a) and B in coronary artery bypass vein grafts resected at re-operation" *Arteriosclerosis* 1989 9(5):593-603.

108. Pauling L, "Case report: lysine/ascorbate-related amelioration of angina pectoris" *Journal of Orthomolecular Medicine* 1991 6(3&4):144-146.

109. Pauling L, "Third case report on lysine-ascorbate amelioration of angina pectoris" *Journal of Orthomolecular Medicine* 1993 8(3):137-138.

110. McBeath M, Pauling L, "A case history: lysine/ascorbate-related amelioration of angina pectoris" *Journal of Orthomolecular Medicine* 1993 8(2):77-78.

111. Kaufmann P, et al, "Coronary heart disease in smokers: vitamin C restores coronary microcirculatory function" *Circulation* 2000 102(11):1233-1238.

112. Rath M, "Reducing the risk for cardiovascular disease with nutritional supplements" *Journal of Orthomolecular Medicine* 1992 7(3):153-162.

113. Katz E, "Reduction of cholesterol and Lp(a) and regression of coronary artery disease: a case study" *Journal of Orthomolecular Medicine* 1996 11(3):173-179.

114. Dahl-Jorgensen K, Larsen J, Hanssen K, "Atherosclerosis in childhood and adolescent type I diabetes: early disease, early treatment?" *Diabetologia* 2005 48(8):1445-1453.

115. Haffner S, "Rationale for new American Diabetes Association Guidelines: are national cholesterol education program goals adequate for the patient with diabetes mellitus?" *The American Journal of Cardiology* 2005 96(4A):33E-36E.

116. Ginter E, "Marginal vitamin C deficiency, lipid metabolism, and atherogenesis" *Advances in Lipid Research* 1978 16:167-220.

117. Hunt J, Bottoms M, Mitchinson M, "Ascorbic acid oxidation: a potential cause of the elevated severity of atherosclerosis in diabetes mellitus?" *FEBS Letters* 1992 311(2):161-164.

118. Gupta M, Chari S "Lipid peroxidation and antioxidant status in patients with diabetic retinopathy" *Indian Journal of Physiology and Pharmacology* 2005 49(2):187-192.

119. Wolff S, Jiang Z, Hunt J, "Protein glycation and oxidative stress in diabetes mellitus and ageing" *Free Radical Biology & Medicine* 1991 10(5):339-352.

120. Baynes J, "Role of oxidative stress in development of complications in diabetes" *Diabetes* 1991 40(4):405-412.

121. Sato Y, et al, "Lipid peroxide level in plasma of diabetic patients" *Biochemical Medicine* 1979 21(1):104-107.

122. Ginter E, "Marginal vitamin C deficiency, lipid metabolism, and atherogenesis" *Advances in Lipid Research* 1978 16:167-220.

123. Som S, et al, "Ascorbic acid metabolism in diabetes mellitus" *Metabolism: Clinical and Experimental* 1981 30(6):572-577.

124. Stankova L, et al, "Plasma ascorbate concentrations and blood cell dehydroascorbate transport in patients with diabetes mellitus" *Metabolism: Clinical and Experimental* 1984 33(4):347-353.

125. Mooradian A, Morley J, "Micronutrient status in diabetes mellitus "*The American Journal of Clinical Nutrition* 1987 45(5):877-895.

126. Simon J, "Vitamin C and cardiovascular disease: a review" *Journal of the American College of Nutrition* 1992 11(2):107-125.

127. Price K, Price C, Reynolds R, "Hyperglycemia-induced latent scurvy and atherosclerosis: the scorbutic-metaplasia hypothesis" *Medical Hypotheses* 1996 46(2):119-129.

128. Bigley R, et al, "Interaction between glucose and dehydroascorbate transport in human neutrophils and fibroblasts" *Diabetes* 1983 32(6):545-548.

129. Kapeghian J, Verlangieri A, "The effects of glucose on ascorbic acid uptake in heart endothelial cells: possible pathogenesis of diabetic angiopathies" *Life Sciences* 1984 34(6):577-584.

130. Khatami M, Li W, Rockey J, "Kinetics of ascorbate transport by cultured retinal capillary pericytes. Inhibition by glucose" *Investigative Ophthalmology & Visual Science* 1986 27(11):1665-1671.

131. Sagun K, Carcamo J, Golde D, "Vitamin C enters mitochondria via facilitative glucose transporter 1 (Glut1) and confers mitochondrial protection against oxidative injury" *The FASEB Journal: Official Publication of the Federation of American Societies for Experimental Biology* 2005 19(12):1657-1667.

132. Wilson J, "Regulation of vitamin C transport" *Annual Review of Nutrition* 2005 25:105-125.

133. Cunningham J, "The glucose/insulin system and vitamin C: implications in insulin-dependent diabetes mellitus" *Journal of the American College of Nutrition* 1998 17(2):105-108.

134. Sherry S, Ralli E, "Further studies of the effects of insulin on the metabolism of vitamin C" *Journal of Clinical Investigation* 1948 27:217-225.

135. Will J, Byers T, "Does diabetes mellitus increase the requirement for vitamin C? *Nutrition Reviews* 1996 54(7):193-202.

136. Fisher E, et al, "Interaction of ascorbic acid and glucose on production of collagen and proteoglycan by fibroblasts" *Diabetes* 1991 40(3):371-376.

137. Chen M, et al, "Hyperglycemia-induced intracellular depletion of ascorbic acid in human mononuclear leukocytes" *Diabetes* 1983 32(11):1078-1081.

138. Karpen C, et al, "Interrelation of platelet vitamin E and thromboxane synthesis in type I diabetes mellitus" *Diabetes* 1984 33(3):239-243.

139. Sarji K, et al, "Decreased platelet vitamin C in diabetes mellitus: possible role in hyperaggregation" *Thrombosis Research* 1979 15(5/6):639-650.

140. Ibid.

141. Will J, Ford E, Bowman B, "Serum vitamin C concentrations and diabetes: findings from the Third National Health and Nutrition Examination Survey, 1988-1994" *American Journal of Clinical Nutrition* 1999 70(1):49-52.

142. Spittle C, "Vitamin C and deep-vein thrombosis" *Lancet* 1973 2(7822):199-201 & "The action of vitamin C on blood vessels" *American Heart Journal* 1974 88(3):387-388.

143. Dou C, Xu D, Wells W, "Studies on the essential role of ascorbic acid in the energy dependent release of insulin from pancreatic islets" *Biochemical and Biophysical Research Communications* 1997 231(3):820-822.

144. Kodama M, et al, "Diabetes mellitus is controlled by vitamin C treatment" *In Vivo* 1993 7(6A):535-542.

145. Belting C, Hinkler J, Dummett C, "Influence of diabetes mellitus on the severity of periodontal disease" *Journal of Periodontology* 1964 35:476.

146. Aleo J, "Diabetes and periodontal disease. Possible role of vitamin C deficiency: an hypothesis" *Journal of Periodontology* 1981 52(5):251-254.

147. Frank E, "Benefits of stopping smoking" *The Western Journal of Medicine* 1993 159(1):83-86.

148. Mennoti A, et al, "Forty-year mortality from cardiovascular diseases and all causes of death in the US Railroad cohort of the Seven Countries Study" *European Journal of Epidemiology* 2004 19(5):417-424.

149. Bourquin A, Musmanno E, "Preliminary report on the effect of smoking on the ascorbic acid content of whole blood" *American Journal of Digestive Diseases* 1953 20:75-77.

150. Strauss I, Scheer P, "Effect of nicotine on vitamin C metabolism" *Internationale Zeitschrift fur Vitaminforschung* 1939 9:39-49.

151. McCormick W, "Coronary thrombosis: a new concept of mechanism and etiology" *Clinical Medicine* 1957)July, pp. 839-845.

152. Durand C, Audinot M, Frajdenrajch S, "Hypovitaminose C latente et tabac" *Concours Medical* 1962 84:4801.

153. Strauss R, "Environmental tobacco smoke and serum vitamin C levels in children" *Pediatrics* 2001 107(3):540-542.

154. Preston A, et al, "Influence of environmental tobacco smoke on vitamin C status in children" *The American Journal of Clinical Nutrition* 2003 77(1):167-172.

155. Pelletier O, "Vitamin C and cigarette smokers" *Annals of the New York Academy of Sciences* 1975 258:156-167.

156. Pelletier O, "Vitamin C and tobacco" *International Journal for Vitamin and Nutrition Research. Supplement* 1977 16:147.

157. Maritz G, "Ascorbic acid. Protection of lung tissue against damage" *Subcellular Biochemistry* 1996 25:265-291.

158. McCormick W, "Coronary thrombosis: a new concept of mechanism and etiology" *Clinical Medicine* 1957 July, pp. 839-845.

159. Solomon H, Priore R, Bross I, "Cigarette smoking and periodontal disease" *Journal of the American Dental Association* 1968 77(5):1081-1084.

160. Shannon I, "Significant correlations between gingival scores and ascorbic acid status" *Journal of Dental Research* 1973 52(2):394.

161. Cohen M, "The effect of large doses of ascorbic acid on gingival tissue at puberty" *Journal of Dental Research* 1955 34(Abstract):750.

162. Teramoto K, et al, "Acute effect of oral vitamin C on coronary circulation in young healthy smokers" *American Heart Journal* 2005 148(2):300-305.

163. Gamble J, Grewal P, Gartside I, "Vitamin C modifies the cardiovascular and microvascular responses to cigarette smoke inhalation in man" *Clinical Science* 2000 98(4):455-460.

164. Janoff A, "Elastases and emphysema. Current assessment of the protease-antiprotease hypothesis" *The American Review of Respiratory Disease* 1985 132(2):417-433.

165. Ross R, "Rous-Whipple Award Lecture. Atherosclerosis: a defense mechanism gone awry" *American Journal of Pathology* 1993 143(4):987-1002.

166. Weiss S, "Tissue destruction by neutrophils" *The New England Journal of Medicine* 1989 320(6):365-376.

167. Lehr H, Arfors K, "Mechanisms of tissue damage by leukocytes" *Current Opinion in Hematology* 1994 1(1):92-99.

168. Lehr H, Frei B, Arfors K, "Vitamin C prevents cigarette smoke-induced leukocyte aggregation and adhesion to endothelium *in vivo*" *Proceedings of the National Academy of Sciences of the United States of America* 1994 91(16):7688-7692.

169. Kannel W, et al, "Fibrinogen and risk of cardiovascular disease. The Framingham Study" *The Journal of the American Medical Association* 1987 258(9):1183-1186.

170. Tunstall-Pedoe H, et al, "Comparison of the prediction by 27 different factors of coronary heart disease and death in men and women of the Scottish heart health study: cohort study" *BMJ* 1997 315(7110):722-729.

171. Nyyssonen K, et al, "Vitamin C deficiency and risk of myocardial infarction: prospective population study of men from eastern Finland" *BMJ* 1997 314(7081):634-638.

172. Bielak L, et al, "Association of fibrinogen with quantity of coronary artery calcification measured by electron beam computed tomography" *Arteriosclerosis, Thrombosis, and Vascular Biology* 2000 20(9):2167-2171.

173. Paramo J, et al, "Validation of plasma fibrinogen as a marker of carotid atherosclerosis in subjects free of clinical cardiovascular disease" *Haematologica* 2004 89(10):1226-1231.

174. Khaw K, Woodhouse P, "Interrelation of vitamin C, infection, haemostatic factors, and cardiovascular disease" *BMJ (Clinical Research ed)* 1995 310(6994):1559-1563.

175. Hume R, Vallance B, Muir M, "Ascorbate status and fibrinogen concentrations after cerebrovascular accident" *Journal of Clinical Pathology* 1982 35(2):195-199.

176. Bordia A, et al, "Acute effect of ascorbic acid on fibrinolytic activity" *Atherosclerosis* 1978 30(4):351-354.

177. Shimizu M, et al, "Effect of ascorbic acid on fibrinolysis" *Acta Haemotologica Japonica* 1970 33(1):137-148.

## Resource E

1. Hagler L, Herman R, "Oxalate metabolism. III" *The American Journal of Clinical Nutrition* 1973 26(9):1006-1010.

2. Ogawa Y, Miyazato T, Hatano T, "Oxalate and urinary stones" *World Journal of Surgery* 2000 24(10):1154-1159.

3. Oke O, "Oxalic acid in plants and in nutrition" *World Review of Nutrition and Dietetics* 1969 10:262-303.

4. Lawton J, et al, "Acute oxalate nephropathy after massive ascorbic acid administration" *Archives of Internal Medicine* 1985 145(5):950-951.

5. Noe H, "Hypercalciuria and pediatric stone recurrences with and without structural abnormalities" *The Journal of Urology* 2000 164(3 Pt 2):1094-1096.

6. Kinder J, et al, "Urinary stone risk factors in the siblings of patients with calcium renal stones" *The Journal of Urology* 2002 167(5):1965-1967.

7. Bushinsky D, et al, "Calcium oxalate stone formation in genetic hypercalciuric stone-forming rats" *Kidney International* 2002 61(3):975-987.

8. Borghi L, et al, "Comparison of two diets for the prevention of recurrent stones in idiopathic hypercalciuria" *The New England Journal of Medicine* 2002 346(2):77-84.

9. Swartz R, et al, "Hyperoxaluria and renal insufficiency due to ascorbic acid administration during total parenteral nutrition" *Annals of Internal Medicine* 1984 100(4):530-531.

10. Alvarez M, Traba M, Rapado A, "Hypocitraturia as a pathogenic risk factor in the mixed (calcium oxalate/uric acid) renal stones" *Urologia Internationalis* 1992 48(3):342-346.

11. Tekin A, et al, "A study of the etiology of idiopathic calcium urolithiasis in children: hypocitruria is the most important risk factor" *The Journal of Urology* 2000 164(1):162-165.

12. Yagisawa T, et al, "Contributory metabolic factors in the development of nephrolithiasis in patients with medullary sponge kidney" *American Journal of Kidney Diseases* 2001 37(6):1140-1143.

13. Martins M, et al, "Cystine: a promoter of the growth and aggregation of calcium oxalate crystals in normal undiluted human urine" *The Journal of Urology* 2002 167(1):317-321.

14. Prie D, et al, "Frequency of renal phosphate leak among patients with calcium nephrolithiasis" *Kidney International* 2001 60(1):272-276.

15. Koide T, "Hyperuricosuria and urolithiasis" [Article in Japanese] *Nippon Rinsho* 1996 54(12):3273-3276.

16. Yagisawa T, et al, "Metabolic characteristics of the elderly with recurrent calcium oxalate stones" *BJU International* 1999 83(9):924-928.

17. Khan S, Shevock P, Hackett R, "Presence of lipids in urinary stones: results of preliminary studies" *Calcified Tissue International* 1988 42(2):91-96.

18. Khan S, Glenton P, "Increased urinary excretion of lipids by patients with kidney stones" 1996 *British Journal of Urology* 77(4):506-511.

19. Mousson C, et al, "Piridoxilate-induced oxalate nephropathy can lead to end-stage renal failure" *Nephron* 1993 63(1):104-106.

20. Bellizzi V, et al, "Effects of water hardness on urinary risk factors for kidney stones in patients with idiopathic nephrolithiasis" *Nephron* 1999 81(Suppl 1):66-70.

21. Sakhaee K, et al, "Assessment of the pathogenetic role of physical exercise in renal stone formation" *The Journal of Clinical Endocrinology and Metabolism* 1987 65(5):974-979.

22. Borghi L, et al, "Urinary volume, water and recurrences in idiopathic calcium nephrolithiasis: a 5-year randomized prospective study" *The Journal of Urology* 1996 155(3):839-843.

23. Riobo P, et al, "Update on the role of diet in recurrent nephrolithiasis" [Article in Spanish] *Nutricion Hospitalaria* 1998 13(4):167-171.

24. Borghi L, et al, "Urine volume: stone risk factor and preventive measure" *Nephron* 1999a 81(Suppl 1):31-37.

25. Wall I, Tiselius H, "Long-term acidification of urine in patients treated for infected renal stones" *Urologia Internationalis* 1990 45(6):336-341.

26. Hokama S, et al, "Ascorbate conversion to oxalate in alkaline milieu and *Proteus mirabilis* culture" *Molecular Urology* 2000 4(4):321-328.

27. Murayama T, et al, "Role of the diurnal variation of urinary pH and urinary calcium in urolithiasis: a study in outpatients" *International Journal of Urology* 2001 8(10):525-531.

28. Hsu T, et al, "Association of changes in the pattern of urinary calculi in Taiwanese with diet habit change between 1956 and 1999" *Journal of the Formosan Medical Association* 2002 101(1):5-10.

29. Curhan G, et al, "Comparison of dietary calcium with supplemental calcium and other nutrients as factors affecting the risk for kidney stones in women" *Annals of Internal Medicine* 1997 126(7):497-504.

30. Powell R, "Pure calcium carbonate gallstones in a two year old in association with prenatal calcium supplementation" *Journal of Pediatric Surgery* 1985 20(2):143-144.

31. Black J, "Oxaluria in British troops in India" *British Medical Journal* 1945 1:590.

32. Hodgkinson A, Zarembski P, "Oxalic acid metabolism in man: a review" *Calcified Tissue Research* 1968 2(2):115-132.

33. Broadus A, et al, "The importance of circulating 1,25-dihydroxyvitamin D in the pathogenesis of hypercalciuria and renal-stone formation in primary hyperparathyroidism" *The New England Journal of Medicine* 1980 302(8):421-426.

34. Ichioka K, et al, "A case of urolithiasis due to vitamin D intoxication in a patient with idiopathic hypoparathyroidism" [Article in Japanese] *Hinyokika Kiyo. Acta Urologica Japonica* 2002 48(4):231-234.

35. Williams H, Smith L, "Disorders of oxalate metabolism" *The American Journal of Medicine* 1968 45(5):715-735.

36. Oren A, et al, "Calcium oxalate kidney stones in patients on continuous ambulatory peritoneal dialysis" *Kidney International* 1984 25(3):534-538.

37. Chen S, et al, "Renal excretion of oxalate in patients with chronic renal failure or nephrolithiasis" *Journal of the Formosan Medical Association* 1990 89(8):651-656.

38. Daudon M, et al, "Urolithiasis in patients with end stage renal failure" *The Journal of Urology* 1992 147(4):977-980.

39. Khan S, Thamilselvan S, "Nephrolithiasis: a consequence of renal epithelial cell exposure to oxalate and calcium oxalate crystals" *Molecular Urology* 2000 4(4):305-312.

40. Bakane B, Nagtilak S, Patil B, "Urolithiasis: a tribal scenario" *Indian Journal of Pediatrics* 1999 66(6):863-865.

41. Massey L, Palmer R, Horner H, "Oxalate content of soybean seeds (Glycine max: Leguminosae), soyfoods, and other edible legumes" *Journal of Agricultural and Food Chemistry* 2001 49(9):4262-4266.

42. McKay D, et al, "Herbal tea: an alternative to regular tea for those who form calcium oxalate stones" *Journal of the American Dietetic Association* 1995 95(3):360-361.

43. Curhan G, et al, "Prospective study of beverage use and the risk of kidney stones" *American Journal of Epidemiology* 1996 143(3):240-247.

44. Terris M, Issa M, Tacker J, "Dietary supplementation with cranberry concentrate tablets may increase the risk of nephrolithiasis" *Urology* 2001 57(1):26-29.

45. Shields M, Simmons R, "Urinary calculus during methazolamide therap". *American Journal of Ophthalmology* 1976 81(5):622-624.

46. Fleisch H, "Inhibitors and promoters of stone formation" *Kidney International* 1978 13(5):361-371.

47. Ettinger B, Oldroyd N, Sorgel F, "Triamterene nephrolithiasis" *The Journal of the American Medical Association* 1980 244(21):2443-2445.

48. Wolf C, et al, "Calcium oxalate stones and hyperoxaluria secondary to treatment with pyridoxilate" [Article in French] *Annales d'urologie* 1985 19(5):313-317.

49. Ahlstrand C, Tiselius H, "Urine composition and stone formation during treatment with acetazolamide" *Scandinavian Journal of Urology and Nephrology* 1987 21(3):225-228.

50. Daudon M, et al, "Piridoxilate-induced calcium oxalate calculi: a new drug-induced metabolic nephrolithiasis" *The Journal of Urology* 1987 138(2):258-261.

51. Michelacci Y, et al, "Possible role for chondroitin sulfate in urolithiasis: *in vivo* studies in an experimental model" *Clinica Chimica Acta* 1992 208(1-2):1-8.

52. Kohan A, Armenakas N, Fracchia J, "Indinavir urolithiasis: an emerging cause of renal colic in patients with human immunodeficiency virus" *The Journal of Urology* 1999 161(6):1765-1768.

53. Sundaram C, Saltzman B, "Urolithiasis associated with protease inhibitors" *Journal of Endourology* 1999 13(4):309-312.

54. Gonzalez C, et al, "Renal colic and lithiasis in HIV(+)-patients treated with protease inhibitors" [Article in Spanish] *Actas Urologicas Espanolas* 2000 24(3):212-218.

55. Wu D, Stoller M, "Indinavir urolithiasis" *Current Opinion in Urology* 2000 10(6):557-561.

56. Conyers R, Bais R, Rofe A, "The relation of clinical catastrophes, endogenous oxalate production, and urolithiasis" *Clinical Chemistry* 1990 36(10):1717-1730.

57. Muthukumar A, Selvam R, "Role of glutathione on renal mitochondrial status in hyperoxaluria" *Molecular and Cellular Biochemistry* 1998 185(1-2):77-84.

58. Friedman A, et al, "Secondary oxalosis as a complication of parenteral alimentation in acute renal failure" *American Journal of Nephrology* 1983 3(5):248-252.

59. Swartz R, et al, "Hyperoxaluria and renal insufficiency due to ascorbic acid administration during total parenteral nutrition" *Annals of Internal Medicine* 1984 100(4):530-531.

60. Gershoff S, et al, "Vitamin B6 deficiency and oxalate nephrocalcinosis in the cat" *The American Journal of Medicine* 1959 27:72.

61. Faber S, et al, "The effects of an induced pyridoxine and pantothenic acid deficiency on excretions of oxalic and xanthurenic acids in the urine" *The American Journal of Clinical Nutrition* 1963 12:406.

62. Gershoff S, "Vitamin B6 and oxalate metabolism" *Vitamins and Hormones* 1964 22:581.

63. Mitwalli A, et al, "Control of hyperoxaluria with large doses of pyridoxine in patients with kidney stones" *International Urology and Nephrology* 1988 20(4):353-359.

64. Alkhunaizi A, Chan L, "Secondary oxalosis: a cause of delayed recovery of renal function in the setting of acute renal failure" *Journal of the American Society of Nephrology* 1996 7(11):2320-2326.

65. Curhan G, et al, "Intake of vitamins B6 and C and the risk of kidney stones in women" *Journal of the American Society of Nephrology* 1999 10(4):840-845.

66. Buckle R, "The glyoxylic acid content of human blood and its relationship to thiamine deficiency" *Clinical Science* 1963 25:207.

67. Gregory J, Park K, Schoenberg H, "Oxalate stone disease after intestinal resection" *The Journal of Urology* 1977 117(5):631-634.
68. Drenick E, et al, "Renal damage with intestinal bypass" *Annals of Internal Medicine* 1978 89(5):594-599.
69. Nightingale J, "Management of patients with a short bowel" *Nutrition* 1999 15(7-8):633-637.
70. Nightingale J, "Management of patients with a short bowel" *World Journal of Gastroenterology* 2001 7(6):741-751.
71. Trinchieri A, et al, "Clinical observations on 2086 patients with upper urinary tract stone" *Archivio Italiano di Urologia, Andrologia* 1996 68(4):251-262.
72. Dewan B, et al, "Upper urinary tract stones & *Ureaplasma urealyticum*" *The Indian Journal of Medical Research* 1997 105:15-21.
73. Daskalova S, et al, "Are bacterial proteins part of the matrix of kidney stones?" *Microbial Pathogenesis* 1998 25(4):197-201.
74. Hokama S, et al, "Ascorbate conversion to oxalate in alkaline milieu and *Proteus mirabilis* culture" *Molecular Urology* 2000 4(4):321-328.
75. Sohshang H, et al, "Biochemical and bacteriological study of urinary calculi" *The Journal of Communicable Diseases* 2000 32(3):216-221.
76. Kim H, Cheigh J, Ham H, "Urinary stones following renal transplantation" *The Korean Journal of Internal Medicine* 2001 16(2):118-122.
77. Scheid C, et al, "Oxalate toxicity in LLC-PK1 cells: role of free radicals" *Kidney International* 1996 49(2):413-419.
78. Muthukumar A, Selvam R, "Role of glutathione on renal mitochondrial status in hyperoxaluria" *Molecular and Cellular Biochemistry* 1998 185(1-2):77-84.
79. Daudon M, et al, "Unusual morphology of calcium oxalate calculi in primary hyperoxaluria" *Journal of Nephrology* 1998 11(Suppl 1):51-55.
80. Ralph-Edwards A, et al, "A jejuno-ileal bypass patient presenting with recurrent renal stones due to primary hyperparathyroidism" *Obesity Surgery* 1992 2(3):265-268.
81. Yamaguchi S, et al, "Early stage of urolithiasis formation in experimental hyperparathyroidism" *The Journal of Urology* 2001 165(4):1268-1273.
82. Nikakhtar B, et al, "Urolithiasis in patients with spinal cord injury" *Paraplegia* 1981 19(6):363-366.
83. Sarkissian A, et al, "Pediatric urolithiasis in Armenia: a study of 198 patients observed from 1991 to 1999" *Pediatric Nephrology* 2001 16(9):728-732.
84. Torres V, et al, "The association of nephrolithiasis and autosomal dominant polycystic kidney disease" *American Journal of Kidney Diseases* 1988 11(4):318-325.
85. Torres V, et al, "Renal stone disease in autosomal dominant polycystic kidney disease" *American Journal of Kidney Diseases* 1993 22(4):513-519.
86. Shiraishi K, et al, "Urolithiasis associated with Crohn's disease: a case report" [Article in Japanese] *Hinyokika Kiyo. Acta Urologica Japonica.* 1998 44(10):719-723.
87. Buno A, et al, "Lithogenic risk factors for renal stones in patients with Crohn's disease" *Archivos Espanoles de Urologia* 2001 54(3):282-292.
88. McConnell N, et al, "Risk factors for developing renal stones in inflammatory bowel disease" *BJU International* 2002 89(9):835-841.
89. Turner M, Goldwater D, David T, "Oxalate and calcium excretion in cystic fibrosis" *Archives of Disease in Childhood* 2000 83(3):244-247.
90. Perez-Brayfield M, et al, "Metabolic risk factors for stone formation in patients with cystic fibrosis" *The Journal of Urology* 2002 167(2 Pt 1):480-484.
91. Sharma O, "Vitamin D, calcium, and sarcoidosis" *Chest* 1996 109(2):535-539.

92. Rodman J, Mahler R, "Kidney stones as a manifestation of hypercalcemic disorders. Hyperparathyroidism and sarcoidosis" *The Urologic Clinics of North America* 2000 27(2):275-285, viii.

93. Bohles H, et al, "Antibiotic treatment-induced tubular dysfunction as a risk factor for renal stone formation in cystic fibrosis" *Journal of Pediatrics* 2002 140(1):103-109.

94. Singh P, et al, "Evidence suggesting that high intake of fluoride provokes nephrolithiasis in tribal populations" *Urological Research* 2001 29(4):238-244.

95. Hwang T, et al, "Effect of prolonged bedrest on the propensity for renal stone formation" *The Journal of Clinical Endocrinology and Metabolism* 1988 66(1):109-112.

96. Torrecilla C, et al, "Incidence and treatment of urinary lithiasis in renal transplantation" [Article in Spanish] *Actas Urologicas Espanolas* 2001 25(5):357-363.

97. Borghi L, et al, "Essential arterial hypertension and stone disease" *Kidney International* 1999 55(6):2397-2406.

98. Hall W, et al, "Risk factors for kidney stones in older women in the southern United States" *The American Journal of the Medical Sciences* 2001 322(1):12-18.

99. Hughes J, Norman R, "Diet and calcium stones. *Canadian Medical Association Journal* 1992 146(2):137-143.

100. Burns J, Burch H, King C, "The metabolism of 1-C14-L-ascorbic acid in guinea pigs" *The Journal of Biological Chemistry* 1951 191:501.

101. Nguyen N, et al, "Urinary calcium and oxalate excretion during oral fructose or glucose load in man" *Hormone and Metabolic Research* 1989 21(2):96-99.

102. Hildebrandt R, Shanklin D, "Oxalosis and pregnancy" *American Journal of Obstetrics and Gynecology* 1962 84:65.

103. Maikranz P, et al, "Gestational hypercalciuria causes pathological urine calcium oxalate supersaturations" *Kidney International* 1989 36(1):108-113.

104. Mazze R, Shue G, Jackson S, "Renal dysfunction associated with methoxyflurane anesthesia. A randomized, prospective clinical evaluation" *The Journal of the American Medical Association* 1971 216(2):278-288.

105. Mazze R, Trudell J, Cousins M "Methoxyflurane metabolism and renal dysfunction: clinical correlation in man" *Anesthesiology* 1971 35(3):247-252.

106. Silverberg D, et al, "Oxalic acid excretion after methoxyflurane and halothane anaesthesia" *Canadian Anaesthetists' Society Journal* 1971 18(5):496-504.

107. Furth S, et al, "Risk factors for urolithiasis in children on the ketogenic diet" *Pediatric Nephrology* 2000 15(1-2):125-128.

108. Whitson P, Pietrzyk R, Pak C, "Renal stone risk assessment during Space Shuttle flights" *The Journal of Urology* 1997 158(6):2305-2310.

109. Whitson P, Pietrzyk R, Pak C, "Space flight and the risk of renal stones" *Journal of Gravitational Physiology* 1999 6(1):P87-P88.

110. Pru C, Eaton J, Kjellstrand C, "Vitamin C intoxication and hyperoxalemia in chronic hemodialysis patients" *Nephron* 1985 39(2):112-116.

111. Urivetzky M, Kessaris D, Smith A, "Ascorbic acid overdosing: a risk factor for calcium oxalate nephrolithiasis" *The Journal of Urology* 1992 147(5):1215-1218.

112. Auer B, Auer D, Rodgers A, "Relative hyperoxaluria, crystalluria and haematuria after megadose ingestion of vitamin C" *European Journal of Clinical Investigation* 1998 28(9):695-700.

113. Kalokerinos A, Dettman I, Dettman G, "Vitamin C. The dangers of calcium and safety of sodium ascorbate" *The Australasian Nurses Journal* 1981 10(3):22.

114. Tsugawa N, et al, "Intestinal absorption of calcium from calcium ascorbate in rats" *Journal of Bone and Mineral Metabolism* 1999 17(1):30-36.

## Resource H

### Aflatoxin

1. *Cecil Medicine, 23rd Edition*, Saunders, an imprint of Elsevier Inc., 2008, Chap. 206.
2. Online article at: http://en.wikipedia.org/wiki/Aflatoxin
3. Netke S, et al, "Ascorbic acid protects guinea pigs from acute aflatoxin toxicity" *Toxicology and Applied Pharmacology* 1997 143(2):429-435.
4. Salem M, et al, "Protective role of ascorbic acid to enhance semen quality of rabbits treated with sublethal doses of aflatoxin B(1)" *Toxicology* 2001 162(3):209-218.
5. Verma R, Shukla R, Mehta D, "Interaction of aflatoxin with L-ascorbic acid: a kinetic and mechanistic approach" *Natural Toxins* 1999 7(1):25-29.
6. Bose S, Sinha S, "Aflatoxin-induced structural chromosomal changes and mitotic disruption in mouse bone marrow" 1991 *Mutation Research* 261(1):15-19.
7. Raina V, Gurtoo H, "Effects of vitamins A, C, and E on aflatoxin B1-induced mutagenesis in *Salmonella typhimurium* TA-98 and TA-100" 1985 *Teratogenesis, Carcinogenesis, and Mutagenesis* 5(1):29-40.
8. Bhattacharya R, Francis A, Shetty T, "Modifying role of dietary factors on the mutagenicity of aflatoxin B1: *in vitro* effect of vitamins" 1987 *Mutation Research* 188(2):121-128.

### AIDS

1. *Cecil Medicine, 23rd Edition*, "History," Saunders, an imprint of Elsevier Inc., 2008, Chap. 412.
2. *Cecil Medicine*, 23rd Edition, "Treatment," Saunders, an imprint of Elsevier Inc., 2008, Chap. 412.
3. Cathcart R, "Vitamin C in the treatment of acquired immune deficiency syndrome (AIDS)" *Medical Hypotheses* 1984 14(4):423-433.
4. Cathcart R, "Letter to the Editor" *Lancet* 1990 335:235.
5. Everall I, Hudson L, Kerwin R, "Decreased absolute levels of ascorbic acid and unaltered vasoactive intestinal polypeptide receptor binding in the frontal cortex in acquired immunodeficiency syndrome" *Neuroscience Letters* 1997 224(2):119-122.
6. Allard J, et al, "Effects of vitamin E and C supplementation on oxidative stress and viral load in HIV infected subjects" *AIDS* 1998 12(13):1653-1659.
7. Kotler D, "Antioxidant therapy and HIV infection: 1998 [editorial]" *The American Journal of Clinical Nutrition* 1998 67:7-9.
8. Cathcart R, "Letter to the Editor" *Lancet* 1990 335:235.
9. Harakeh S, Jariwalla R, "Comparative study of the anti-HIV activities of ascorbate and thiol-containing reducing agents in chronically HIV-infected cells" *The American Journal of Clinical Nutrition* 1991 54(6 Suppl):1231S-1235S.
10. Harakeh S, Jariwalla R, Pauling L, "Suppression of human immunodeficiency virus replication by ascorbate in chronically and acutely infected cells" *Proceedings of the National Academy of Sciences of the United States of America* (1990) 87(18):7245-7249.
11. Muller R, et al, "Virological and immunological effects of antioxidant treatment in patients with HIV infection" *European Journal of Clinical Investigation* 2000 30(10):905-914.
12. Tang A, et al, "Dietary micronutrient intake and risk of progression to acquired immunodeficiency syndrome (AIDS) in human immunodeficiency virus type 1 (HIV-1)-infected homosexual men" *American Journal of Epidemiology* 1993 138(11):937-951.

13. Treitinger A, et al, "Decreased antioxidant defence in individuals infected by the human immunodeficiency virus" *European Journal of Clinical Investigation* 2000 30(5):454-459.

14. Kataoka A, et al, "Intermittent high-dose vitamin C therapy in patients with HTLV-1 associated myelopathy" *Journal of Neurology, Neurosurgery, and Psychiatry* 1993 56(11):1213-1216.

15. Kataoka A, et al, "Intermittent high-dose vitamin C therapy in patients with HTLV-1-associated myelopathy" [Article in Japanese] *Rinsho Shinkeigaku. Clinical Neurology* 1993 33(3):282-288.

16. De la Asuncion J, et al, "AZT treatment induces molecular and ultrastructural oxidative damage to muscle mitochondria. Prevention by antioxidant vitamins" *The Journal of Clinical Investigation* 1998 102(1):4-9.

## Alcohol

1. Miquel M, Aguilar M, Aragon C, "Ascorbic acid antagonizes ethanol-induced locomotor activity in the open-field" *Pharmacology, Biochemistry, and Behavior* 1999 62(2):361-366.

2. Susick Jr R, Zannoni V, "Effect of ascorbic acid on the consequences of acute alcohol consumption in humans" *Clinical Pharmacology and Therapeutics* 1987 41(5):502-509.

3. Busnel R, Lehmann A, "Antagonistic effect of sodium ascorbate on ethanol-induced changes in swimming of mice" *Behavioural Brain Research* 1980 1(4):351-356.

4. Klenner F, "Observations on the dose and administration of ascorbic acid when employed beyond the range of a vitamin in human pathology" *Journal of Applied Nutrition* 1971 23(3&4):61-88.

5. Meagher E, et al, "Alcohol-induced generation of lipid peroxidation products in humans" *The Journal of Clinical Investigation* 1999 104(6):805-813.

6. Zhou J, Chen P, "Studies on the oxidative stress in alcohol abusers in China" *Biomedical and Environmental Sciences* 2001 14(3):180-188.

7. Faizallah R, ET AL, "Alcohol enhances vitamin C excretion in the urine" *Alcohol and Alcoholism* 1986 21(1):81-84.

8. van der Gaag M, et al, "Moderate consumption of beer, red wine and spirits has counteracting effects on plasma antioxidants in middle-aged men" *European Journal of Clinical Nutrition* 2000 54(7):586-591.

9. Wickramasinghe S, Hasan R, "*In vivo* effects of vitamin C on the cytotoxicity of post-ethanol serum" *Biochemical Pharmacology* 1994 48(3):621-624.

10. Krasner N, et al, "Ascorbic-acid saturation and ethanol metabolism" Lancet 1974 2(7882):693-695.

11. Moldowan M, Acholonu W, "Effect of ascorbic acid or thiamine on acetaldehyde, disulfiram-ethanol- or disulfiram-acetaldehyde-induced mortality" *Agents and Actions* 1982 12(5-6):731-736.

12. Yunice A, Lindeman R, "Effect of ascorbic acid and zinc sulfate on ethanol toxicity and metabolism" *Proceedings of the Society for Experimental Biology and Medicine* 1977 154(1):146-150.

13. Tamura T, et al, "Studies on the antidotal action of drugs. Part 1. Vitamin C and its antidotal effect against alcoholic and nicotine poisoning" *The Journal of Nihon University School of Dentistry* 1969 11(4):149-151.

14. Navasumrit P, et al, "Ethanol-induced free radicals and hepatic DNA strand breaks are prevented *in vivo* by antioxidants: effects of acute and chronic ethanol exposure" *Carcinogenesis* 2000 21(1):93-99.

15. Suresh M, Menon B, Indira M, "Effects of exogenous vitamin C on ethanol toxicity in rats" *Indian Journal of Physiology and Pharmacology* 2000 44(4):401-410.

16. Ginter E, Zloch Z, "Influence of vitamin C status on the metabolic rate of a single dose of ethanol-1-(14)C in guinea pigs" *Physiological Research* 1999 48(5):369-373.

17. Ginter E, Zloch Z, Ondreicka R, "Influence of vitamin C status on ethanol metabolism in guinea-pigs" *Physiological Research* 1998 47(2):137-141.

18. Suresh M, et al, "Interaction of ethanol and ascorbic acid on lipid metabolism in guinea pigs" *Indian Journal of Experimental Biology* 1997 35(10):1065-1069.

19. Susick Jr R, Zannoni V, "Ascorbic acid and elevated SGOT levels after an acute dose of ethanol in the guinea pig" *Alcoholism, Clinical and Experimental Research* 1987 11(3):265-268.

20. Zannoni V, et al, "Ascorbic acid, alcohol, and environmental chemicals" *Annals of the New York Academy of Sciences* 1987 498:364-388.

## Aluminum

1. *Cecil Medicine, 23rd Edition*, "History," Saunders, an imprint of Elsevier Inc., 2008, Chap. 20.

2. Anane R, Creppy E, "Lipid peroxidation as pathway of aluminium cytotoxicity in human skin fibroblast cultures: prevention by superoxide dismutase+catalase and vitamins E and C" *Human & Experimental Toxicology* 2001 20(9):477-481.

3. Swain C, Chainy G, "*In vitro* stimulation of chick brain lipid peroxidation by aluminium, and effects of Tiron, EDTA and some antioxidants" *Indian Journal of Experimental Biology* 2000 38(12):1231-1235.

4. Fulton B, Jeffery E, "Absorption and retention of aluminum from drinking water. Effect of citric and ascorbic acids on aluminum tissue levels in rabbits" *Fundamental and Applied Toxicology* 1990 14(4):788-796.

5. Dhir H, et al, "Modification of clastogenicity of lead and aluminium in mouse bone marrow cells by dietary ingestion of Phyllanthus emblica fruit extract" *Mutation Research* 1990 241(3):305-312.

6. Roy A, Dhir H, Sharma A, "Modification of metal-induced micronuclei formation in mouse bone marrow erythrocytes by Phyllanthus fruit extract and ascorbic acid" *Toxicology Letters* 1992 62(1):9-17.

## Alzheimer's / Dementia

1. *Cecil Medicine, 23rd Edition*, "Dementia Definition," Saunders, an imprint of Elsevier Inc., 2008, Chap. 425.

2. Bennett S, Grant MM, Aldred S, "Oxidative stress in vascular dementia and Alzheimer's disease: a common pathology," J Alzheimers Dis. 2009;17(2):245-57.

3. Cecil Medicine, 23rd Edition, "Prevention and Treatment," Saunders, an imprint of Elsevier Inc., 2008, Chap. 425.

4. Harrison FE, et al, "Vitamin C deficiency increases basal exploratory activity but decreases scopolamine-induced activity in APP/PSEN1 transgenic mice," *Pharmacol Biochem Behav.* 2010 Feb; 94(4):543-52.

5. Harrison FE, et al, "Antioxidants and cognitive training interact to affect oxidative stress and memory in APP/PSEN1 mice," *Nutr Neurosci.* 2009 Oct;12(5):203-18.

6. Harrison FE, et al, "Ascorbic acid attenuates scopolamine-induced spatial learning deficits in the water maze," *Behav Brain Res.* 2009 Dec 28;205(2):550-8.

7. Fotuhi M, et al. "Better cognitive performance in elderly taking antioxidant vitamins E and C supplements in combination with nonsteroidal anti-inflammatory drugs: the Cache County Study," *Alzheimers Dement.* 2008 May;4(3):223-7.

8. Cornelli U, "Treatment of Alzheimer's disease with a cholinesterase inhibitor combined with antioxidants," *Neurodegener Dis.* 2010;7(1-3):193-202

## Amphetamine Poisoning

1. Online article at http://emedicine.medscape.com/article/812518-treatment#a1126

2. Beyer C, "Rapid recovery from Ecstasy intoxication" *South African Medical Journal* 2001 91(9):708-709.

3. Wagner G, Carelli R, Jarvis M, "Pretreatment with ascorbic acid attenuates the neurotoxic effects of methamphetamine in rats" Research Communications in Chemical Pathology and Pharmacology 1985 47(2):221-228.

4. Miquel M, Aguilar M, Aragon C, "Ascorbic acid antagonizes ethanol-induced locomotor activity in the open-field" *Pharmacology, Biochemistry, and Behavior* 1999 62(2):361-366.

5. De Vito M, Wagner G, "Methamphetamine-induced neuronal damage: a possible role for free radicals" *Neuropharmacology* 1989 28(10):1145-1150.

6. Rebec G, et al, "Ascorbic acid and the behavioral response to haloperidol: implications for the action of antipsychotic drugs" *Science* 1985 227(4685):438-440.

7. White L, et al, "Ascorbate antagonizes the behavioral effects of amphetamine by a central mechanism" *Psychopharmacology* 1988 94(2):284-287.

## Arsenic Poisoning

1. *Cecil Medicine, 23rd Edition*, "Arsenic," Saunders, an imprint of Elsevier Inc., 2008, Chap. 20.

2. *Cecil Medicine, 23rd Edition*, "Arsenic: Treatment," Saunders, an imprint of Elsevier Inc., 2008, Chap. 20.

3. Lahiri K, "Advancement in the treatment of arsenical intolerance" *Indian Journal of Venereal Diseases and Dermatology* 1943 9(1):115-117.

4. Chattopadhyay S, et al, "Protection of sodium arsenite-induced ovarian toxicity by coadministration of L-ascorbate (vitamin C) in mature Wistar strain rat" *Archives of Environmental Contamination and Toxicology* 2001 41(1):83-89.

5. Grad J, et al, "Ascorbic acid enhances arsenic trioxide-induced cytotoxicity in multiple myeloma cells" *Blood* 2001 98(3):805-813.

6. Gao F, et al, "Ascorbic acid enhances the apoptosis of U937 cells induced by arsenic trioxide in combination with DMNQ and its mechanism" [Article in Chinese] *Zhonghua Xueyexue Zazhi* 2002 23(1):9-11.

7. Bachleitner-Hofmann T, et al, "Arsenic trioxide and ascorbic acid: synergy with potential implications for the treatment of acute myeloid leukaemia?" *British Journal of Haematology* 2001 112(3):783-786.

## Arthritis

1. Yudoh K, et al, "Potential involvement of oxidative stress in cartilage senescence and development of osteoarthritis: oxidative stress induces chondrocyte telomere instability and downregulation of chondrocyte function" *Arthritis Res Ther.* 2005;7(2):R380-91.

2. Jaswal S, et al, "Antioxidant status in rheumatoid arthritis and role of antioxidant therapy" Clin Chim Acta. 2003 Dec;338(1-2):123-9.

3. *Cecil Medicine, 23rd Edition*, "Medical Therapy" Saunders, an imprint of Elsevier Inc., 2008, Chap. 285.

4. *Cecil Medicine, 23rd Edition*, "Medical Therapy" Saunders, an imprint of Elsevier Inc., 2008, Chap. 286.

5. Khodyrev VN, et al, "The influence of the vitamin-mineral complex upon the blood vitamin, calcium and phosphorus of patients with ostreoarthrosis" *Vopr Pitan.* 2006;75(2):44-7.

6. Lau H, Massasso D, Joshua F, "Skin, muscle and joint disease from the 17th century: scurvy" *Int J Rheum Dis.* 2009 Dec;12(4):361-5.

7. Kumar V, Choudhury P, "Scurvy — a forgotten disease with an unusual presentation" *Trop Doct.* 2009 Jul;39(3):190-2.

8. Vitale A, et al, "Arthritis and gum bleeding in two children" J Paediatr Child Health. 2009 Mar;45(3):158-60. Regan EA, Bowler RP, Crapo JD, "oint fluid antioxidants are decreased in osteoarthritic joints compared to joints with macroscopically intact cartilage and subacute injury" Osteoarthritis Cartilage 2008 Apr;16(4):515-21.

9. Choi HK, et al, "Dietary risk factors for rheumatic diseases," Curr Opin Rheumatol. 2005 Mar;17(2):141-6.

10. Pattison DJ, et al, "Vitamin C and the risk of developing inflammatory polyarthritis: prospective nested case-control study" Ann Rheum Dis. 2004 Jul;63(7):843-7.

11. Wang Y, et al, "Effect of antioxidants on knee cartilage and bone in healthy, middle-aged subjects: a cross-sectional study" Arthritis Res Ther. 2007;9(4):R66.

12. Sakai A, at al, "Large-dose ascorbic acid administration suppresses the development of arthritis in adjuvant-infected rats" Arch Orthop Trauma Surg. 1999;119(3-4):121-6.

## Barbiturate Overdose

1. Article online at: http://en.wikipedia.org/wiki/Barbiturate_overdose

2. Article online at: http://emedicine.medscape.com/article/813155-treatment#a1126

3. Klenner F, "Observations on the dose and administration of ascorbic acid when employed beyond the range of a vitamin in human pathology" Journal of Applied Nutrition 1971 23(3&4):61-88.

4. Kao H, Jai S, Young Y, "A study of the therapeutic effect of large dosage of injection ascorbici acidi on the depression of the central nervous system as in acute poisoning due to barbiturates" [Article in Chinese] Acta Pharmaceutica Sinica 1965 12(11):764-765.

## Benzanthrone Poisoning

1. Article onlline at: http://en.wikipedia.org/wiki/Benzanthrone

2. Article online at: http://toxnet.nlm.nih.gov/cgi-bin/sis/search/a?dbs+hsdb:@term+@DOCNO+5245

3. Dwivedi N, Das M, Khanna S, "Role of biological antioxidants in benzanthrone toxicity" Archives of Toxicology 2001 75(4):221-226.

4. Pandya K, SinghG, Joshi N, "Effect of benzanthrone on the body level of ascorbic acid in guinea pigs" Acta Pharmacologica et Toxicologica 1970 28(6):499-506.

5. Das M, et al, "Attenuation of benzanthrone toxicity by ascorbic acid in guinea pigs" Fundamental and Applied Toxicology 1994 22(3):447-456.

6. Dwivedi N, et al, "Modulation by ascorbic acid of the cutaneous and hepatic biochemical effects induced by topically applied benzanthrone in mice" Food and Chemical Toxicology 1993 31(7):503-508.

7. Garg K, et al, "Effect of extraneous supplementation of ascorbic acid on the bio-disposition of benzanthrone in guinea pigs" Food and Chemical Toxicology 1992 30(11):967-971.

8. Das M, et al, "Bio-elimination and organ retention profile of benzanthrone in scorbutic and non-scorbutic guinea pigs" Biochemical and Biophysical Research Communications 1991 178(3):1405-1412.

## Benzene Poisoning

1. Online article at: http://www.nlm.nih.gov/medlineplus/ency/article/002720.htm

2. Online article at: http://www.atsdr.cdc.gov/csem/benzene/treatment_management.html

3. Meyer A, "Benzene poisoning" The Journal of the American Medical Association 1937 108(11):911.

4. Cathala J, Bolgert M, Grenet P, "Scorbut chez un sujet soumis a une intoxication benzolique professionelle" *Bull et Mem Soc d Hop de Paris* 1936 52:1648.

5. Lurie J, "Benzene intoxication and vitamin C" *The Transactions of the Association of Industrial Medical Officers* 1965 15:78-79.

6. Wu J, Karlsson K, Danielsson A, "Protective effects of trolox C, vitamin C, and catalase on bromobenzene-induced damage to rat hepatocytes" *Scandinavian Journal of Gastroenterology* 1996 31(8):797-803.

7. Gontea I, et al, "Influence of chronic benzene intoxication on vitamin C in the guinea pig and rat" *Igiena* 1969 18:1-11.

## Brucellosis

1. *Cecil Medicine, 23rd Edition*, Chap. 331, Saunders, an imprint of Elsevier Inc., 2008.

2. Boura P, et al, "Monocyte locomotion in anergic chronic brucellosis patients: the *in vivo* effect of ascorbic acid" *Immunopharmacology and Immunotoxicology* 1989 11(1):119-129.

3. Mick E, "Brucellosis and its treatment. Observations preliminary report" *Archives of Pediatrics* 1955 72:119-125.

## Cadmium Poisoning

1. Online article at: http://en.wikipedia.org/wiki/Cadmium_poisoning

2. *Cecil Medicine, 23rd Edition*, "Chronic Poisoning: Trace Metals," Saunders, an imprint of Elsevier Inc., 2008, Chap. 20.

3. Nagyova A, Galbavy S, Ginter E, "Histopathological evidence of vitamin C protection against Cd-nephrotoxicity in guinea pigs" *Experimental and Toxicologic Pathology* 1994 46(1):11-14.

4. Kubova J, et al, "The influence of ascorbic acid on selected parameters of cell immunity in guinea pigs exposed to cadmium" *Zeitschrift fur Ernahrungswissenschaft* 1993 32(2):113-120.

5. Hudecova A, Ginter E, "The influence of ascorbic acid on lipid peroxidation in guinea pigs intoxicated with cadmium" *Food and Chemical Toxicology* 1992 30(12):1011-1013.

6. Kadrabova J, Madaric A, Ginter, "The effect of ascorbic acid on cadmium accumulation in guinea pig tissues" *Experientia* 1992 48(10):989-991.

7. Shiraishi N, Uno H, Waalkes M, "Effect of L-ascorbic acid pretreatment on cadmium toxicity in the male Fischer (F344/NCr) rat" *Toxicology* 1993 85(2-3):85-100.

8. Fahmy M, Aly F, "*In vivo* and *in vitro* studies on the genotoxicity of cadmium chloride in mice" Journal of Applied *Toxicology* 2000 20(3):231-238.

9. Rambeck W, Guillot I, "Bioavailability of cadmium: effect of vitamin C and phytase in broiler chickens" [Article in German] *Tierarztliche Praxis* 1996 24(5):467-470.

10. Rothe S, et al, "The effect of vitamin C and zinc on the copper-induced increase of cadmium residues in swine" [Article in German] *Zeitschrift fur Ernahrungswissenshaft* 1994 33(1):61-67.

## Cancer

1. Online article at: http://en.wikipedia.org/wiki/Cancer

2. Definition," Saunders, an imprint of Elsevier Inc., 2008, Chap. 192

3. Riordan HD, et al, "Intravenous Vitamin C as a Chemotherapy Agent: A Report on Clinical Cases" *Puerto Rico Health Sci. J* 2004, 23-2:115.

4. Riordan HD, et al, "Intravenous Vitamin C as a Chemotherapy Agent: A Report on Clinical Cases" *Puerto Rico Health Sci. J* 2004, 23-2:117.

5. Riordan HD, et al, "Intravenous Vitamin C as a Chemotherapy Agent: A Report on Clinical Cases" *Puerto Rico Health Sci. J* 2004, 23-2:115.

6. Jackson JA, et al, "Sixteen-Year History with High Dose Intravenous Vitamin C Treatment for Various Types of Cancer and Other Diseases," *J Orthomol Med* 2002, 17-2:117-119.

7. Padayatty SJ, et al, "Intravenously administered vitamin C as cancer therapy: three cases" *Canadian Med. Assoc. Journal* Mar 28, 2006; 174(7).

8. Jackson JA, Riordan HD, Schultz M, "High-dose intravenous vitamin C in the treatment of a patient with adenocarcinoma of the kidneys – a case study" J *Orthomol Med* 1990; 5-1: 5-7.

10. Jackson JA, et al, "High-dose intravenous vitamin C and long time survival of a patient with Cancer of the head of the pancreas" *J Orthomol Med* 1995 10-2:87-88.

11. Riordan NH, Jackson JA, Riordan HD, "Intravenous vitamin C in a terminal cancer patient" *J Orthomol Med* 1996 11-2:80-82.

12. Riordan HD, et al., "High-dose intravenous vitamin C in the treatment of a patient with renal cell carcinoma of the kidney," *J Orthomol Med* 1998 13-2:72-73.

13. http://www.oasisofhope.com/irt_ch17_survival_statistics.php

14. Kurbacher C, et al, "Ascorbic acid (vitamin C) improves the antineoplastic activity of doxorubicin, cisplatin, and paclitaxel in human breast carcinoma cells *in vitro*" *Cancer Letters* 1996 103(2):183-189.

15. Shimpo K, et al, "Ascorbic acid and adriamycin toxicity" *The American Journal of Clinical Nutrition* 1991 54(6 Suppl):1298S-1301S.

16. Padayatty SJ, et al., "Intravenously administered vitamin C as cancer therapy: three cases" *Canadian Med. Assoc. Journal* Mar 28 2006 174(7).

17. Kurbacher C, et al, "Ascorbic acid (vitamin C) improves the antineoplastic activity of doxorubicin, cisplatin, and paclitaxel in human breast carcinoma cells *in vitro*" *Cancer Letters* 1996 103(2):183-189.

## Carbon Tetrachloride Poisoning

1. Online article at: http://en.wikipedia.org/wiki/Carbon_tetrachloride_poisoning

2. *Cecil Medicine, 23rd Edition*, "Acute Poisoning," Saunders, an imprint of Elsevier Inc., 2008, Chap. 111.

3. Sheweita S, El-Gabar M, Bastawy M, "Carbon tetrachloride changes the activity of cytochrome P450 system in the liver of male rats: role of antioxidants" *Toxicology* 2001 169(2):83-92.

4. Sheweita S, El-Gabar M, Bastawy M, "Carbon tetrachloride-induced changes in the activity of phase II drug-metabolizing enzyme in the liver of male rats: role of antioxidants" 2001 *Toxicology* 165(2-3):217-224.

5. Ademuyiwa O, Adesanya O, Ajuwon O, "Vitamin C in CCl4 hepatotoxicityča preliminary report" *Human & Experimental Toxicology* 1994 13(2):107-109.

6. Soliman M, et al, "Vitamin C as prophylactic drug against experimental hepatotoxicity" *The Journal of the Egyptian Medical Association* 1965 48(11):806-812.

7. Chatterjee A, "Role of ascorbic acid in the prevention of gonadal inhibition by carbon tetrachloride" Endokrinologie 1967 51(5-6):319-322.

## Cholesterol (High Levels of LDL)

1. *Cecil Medicine, 23rd Edition*, "Disorders of Lipid Metabolism," Saunders, an imprint of Elsevier Inc., 2008, Chap. 217.

2. Taylor F, et al, "Statins for the primary prevention of cardiovascular disease " Cochrane Database Syst Rev. 2011 Jan 19;(1):CD004816.

3. Willis G, "An experimental study of the intimal ground substance in atherosclerosis" *Canadian Medical Association Journal* 1953 69:17-22.

4. Duff G, "Experimental cholesterol arteriosclerosis and its relationship to human arteriosclerosis" *Archives of Pathology* 1935 20:81-123, 259-304.

5. Turley S, West C, Horton B, "The role of ascorbic acid in the regulation of cholesterol metabolism and in the pathogenesis of atherosclerosis" *Atherosclerosis* 1976 24(1-2):1-18.

6. Ginter E, "Ascorbic acid in cholesterol and bile acid metabolism" *Annals of the New York Academy of Sciences* 1975 258:410-421.

7. Ginter E, et al, "Lowered cholesterol catabolism in guinea pigs with chronic ascorbic acid deficiency" *American Journal of Clinical Nutrition* 1971 24(10):1238-1245.

8. Banerjee S, Singh H, "Cholesterol metabolism in scorbutic guinea pigs" *Journal of Biological Chemistry* 1958 233(1):336-339.

9. Maeda N, et al, "Aortic wall damage in mice unable to synthesize ascorbic acid" *Proceedings of the National Academy of Sciences of the United States of America* 2000 97(2):841-846.

10. Dent F, Hayes R, Booker W, "Further evidence of cholesterol-ascorbic acid antagonism in blood; role of adrenocortical hormones" *Federation Proceedings* 1951 18:291.

11. Booker W, et al, "Cholesterol-ascorbic acid relationship; changes in plasma and cell ascorbic acid and plasma cholesterol following administration of ascorbic acid and cholesterol" *American Journal of Physiology* 1957 189:75-77.

12. Sitaramayya C, Ali T, "Studies on experimental hypercholesterolemia and atherosclerosis" *Journal of Physiology and Pharmacology* 1962 6:192-204.

13. Sadava D, et al, "The effect of vitamin C on the rapid induction of aortic changes in rabbits" *Journal of Nutritional Science and Vitaminology* 1982 28(2):85-92.

14. Ginter E, Kajaba T, Nizner O, "The effect of ascorbic acid on cholesterolemia in healthy subjects with seasonal deficit of vitamin C" *Nutrition and Metabolism* 1970 2(2):76-86.

15. Ginter E, et al, "Effect of ascorbic acid on plasma cholesterol in humans in a long-term experiment" *International Journal for Vitamin and Nutrition Research* 1977 47(2):123-134.

16. Ginter E, "Marginal vitamin C deficiency, lipid metabolism, and atherogenesis" *Advances in Lipid Research* 1978 16:167-220.

17. Sokoloff B, et al, "Aging, atherosclerosis and ascorbic acid metabolism" *Journal of the American Geriatrics Society* 1966 14(12):1239-1260.

18. Turley S, West C, Horton B, "The role of ascorbic acid in the regulation of cholesterol metabolism and in the pathogenesis of atherosclerosis" *Atherosclerosis* 1976 24(1-2):1-18

19. Ginter E, et al, "Lowered cholesterol catabolism in guinea pigs with chronic ascorbic acid deficiency" *American Journal of Clinical Nutrition* 1971 24(10):1238-1245.

20. Willis G, "An experimental study of the intimal ground substance in atherosclerosis" *Canadian Medical Association Journal* 1953 69:17-22.

21. Datey K, et al, "Ascorbic acid and experimental atherosclerosis" *Journal of the Association of Physicians of India* 1968 16(9):567-570.

## Chromium Poisoning

1. Online article at: http://www.weitzlux.com/exposedchromiumpoisoning_712.html

2. *Cecil Medicine, 23rd Edition*, "Chronic Poisoning: Trace Metals," Saunders, an imprint of Elsevier Inc., 2008, Chap. 20.

3. Samitz M, Shrager J, Katz S, "Studies on the prevention of injurious effects of chromates in industry" *Industrial Medicine and Surgery* 1962 31:427-432.

4. Pirozzi D, Gross P, SamitzM, "The effect of ascorbic acid on chrome ulcers in guinea pigs" *Archives of Environmental Health* 1968 17(2):178-180.

328                                                     PRIMAL PANACEA

5. Samitz M, Katz S, "Protection against inhalation of chromic acid mist. Use of filters impregnated with ascorbic acid" *Archives of Environmental Health* 1965 11(6):770-772.

6. Korallus U, Harzdorf C, Lewalter J, "Experimental bases for ascorbic acid therapy of poisoning by hexavalent chromium compounds" *International Archives of Occupational and Environmental Health* 1984 53(3):247-256.

7. Na K, Jeong S, Lim C, "The role of glutathione in the acute nephrotoxicity of sodium dichromate" *Archives of Toxicology* 1992 66(9):646-651.

8. Ginter E, Chorvatovicova D, Kosinova A, "Vitamin C lowers mutagenic and toxic effect of hexavalent chromium in guinea pigs" *International Journal for Vitamin and Nutrition Research* 1989 59(2):161-166.

9. Tandon S, Gaur J, "Chelation in metal intoxication. IV. Removal of chromium from organs of experimentally poisoned animals" *Clinical Toxicology* 1977 11(2):257-264.

## Common Cold

1. *Cecil Medicine, 23rd Edition*, Chap. 384, Saunders, an imprint of Elsevier Inc., 2008.

2. Carr A, et al, "Vitamin C and the common cold: using identical twins as controls" *The Medical Journal of Australia* 1981 2(8):411-412.

3. Cathcart R, "Vitamin C, titrating to bowel tolerance, anascorbemia, and acute induced scurvy" *Medical Hypotheses* 1981 7(11):1359-1376.

4. Gorton H, Jarvis K, "The effectiveness of vitamin C in preventing and relieving the symptoms of virus-induced respiratory infections" *Journal of Manipulative and Physiological Therapeutics* 1999 22(8):530-533.

5. Hemila H, "Does vitamin C alleviate the symptoms of the common cold? — a review of current evidence" *Scandinavian Journal of Infectious Disease* 1994 26(1):1-6.

6. Hemila H, "Vitamin C, the placebo effect, and the common cold: a case study of how preconceptions influence the analysis of results" *Journal of Clinical Epidemiology* 1996 49(10):1079-1084.

7. Murphy B, et al, "Ascorbic acid (vitamin C) and its effects on parainfluenza type III virus infection in cotton-topped marmosets" *Laboratory Animal Science* 1974 24(1):229-232.

## Diphtheria

1. *Cecil Medicine, 23rd Edition*, Chap. 315, Saunders, an imprint of Elsevier Inc., 2008.

2. Harde E, Philippe M, "Observations sur le pouvoir antigene du melange toxine diphtherique et vitamin C" *Compt Rend Acad d Sc* 1934 199:738-739.

3. Greenwald C, Harde E, "Vitamin C and diphtheria toxin" *Proceedings of the Society for Experimental Biology and Medicine* 1935 32:1157-1160.

4. Jungeblut C, Zwemer R, "Inactivation of diphtheria toxin *in vivo* and *in vitro* by crystalline vitamin C (ascorbic acid)" *Proceedings of the Society for Experimental Biology and Medicine* 1935 32:1229-1234.

5. King C, Menten M, "Influence of vitamin level on resistance to diphtheria toxin" *Journal of Nutrition* 1935 10:129-155.

6. Hanzlik P, Terada B, "Protective measures in diphtheria intoxication" *Journal of Pharmacology and Experimental Therapeutics* 1936 56:269-277.

7. Klenner F, "The treatment of poliomyelitis and other virus diseases with vitamin C" *Southern Medicine & Surgery* 1949 Jul 111(7):209-214.

8. Klenner F, "Observations of the dose and administration of ascorbic acid when employed beyond the range of a vitamin in human pathology" *Journal of Applied Nutrition* 1971 23(3&4):61-88.

## Distemper (Cat & Dog)

1. http://en.wikipedia.org/wiki/Canine_distemper
2. Belfield W, "Vitamin C in treatment of canine and feline distemper complex" *Veterinary Medicine/Small Animal Clinician* 1967 62(4):345-348.
3. Klenner F, "Significance of high daily intake of ascorbic acid in preventive medicine" *Journal of the International Academy of Preventive Medicine* 1974 1(1):45-69.
4. Leveque J, "Ascorbic acid in treatment of the canine distemper complex" *Veterinary Medicine/Small Animal Clinician* 1969 64(11):997-999, 1001.

## Dysentery, Amebic

1. *Cecil Medicine, 23rd Edition*, Chap. 373, Saunders, an imprint of Elsevier Inc., 2008.
2. Sadun E, et al, "Effect of single inocula of *Endamoeba histolytica* trophozoites on guinea-pigs" *Proceedings of the Society for Experimental Biology and Medicine* 1950 73:362-366.
3. Sadun E, Bradin Jr J, Faust E, "The effect of ascorbic acid deficiency on the resistance of guinea-pigs to infection with *Endamoeba histolytica* of human origin" *American Journal of Tropical Medicine* 1951 31:426-437.
4. Veselovskaia T, "Effect of vitamin C on the clinical picture of dysentery" *Voenno-Meditsinskii Zhurnal* 1957 (Moskva) 3:32-37.
5. Sokolova V, "Application of vitamin C in treatment of dysentery" *Terapevticheskii Arkhiv* 1958 (Moskva) 30:59-64.

## Dysentery, Bacillary (Shigellosis)

1. *Cecil Medicine, 23rd Edition*, "Shigellosis," Saunders, an imprint of Elsevier Inc., 2008, Chap. 330
2. Online article at: http://en.wikipedia.org/wiki/Shigellosis
3. Klenner F, "The treatment of poliomyelitis and other virus diseases with vitamin C" *Southern Medicine & Surgery* 1949 Jul 111(7):209-214.
4. Honjo S, Imaizumi K, "Ascorbic acid content of adrenal and liver in cynomolgus monkeys suffering from bacillary dysentery" *Japanese Journal of Medical Science & Biology* 1967 20(1):97-102.
5. Honjo S, et al, "Shigellosis in cynomolgus monkeys (*Macaca irus*) VII. Experimental production of dysentery with a relatively small dose of *Shigella flexneri* 2a in ascorbic acid deficient monkeys" *Japanese Journal of Medical Science & Biology* 1969 22(3):149-162.

## Encephalitis

1. Online article at: http://www.ncbi.nlm.nih.gov/pubmedhealth/PMH0002388/
2. *Cecil Medicine, 23rd Edition*, "Acute Viral Encephalitis," Saunders, an imprint of Elsevier Inc., 2008, Chap. 439.
3. Klenner F, "The treatment of poliomyelitis and other virus diseases with vitamin C" *Southern Medicine & Surgery* 1949 Jul 111(7):209-214.
4. Klenner F, "Massive doses of vitamin C and the virus diseases" *Southern Medicine & Surgery* 1951 Apr 103(4):101-107.
5. Klenner F, "The use of vitamin C as an antibiotic" *Journal of Applied Nutrition* 1953 6:274-278.
6. Klenner F, "An 'insidious' virus" *Tri-State Medical Journal* 1957 Jul pp.10-12.
7. Klenner F, "The clinical evaluation and treatment of a deadly syndrome caused by an insidious virus" *Tri-State Medical Journal* 1958 Oct pp.11-15.
8. Klenner F, "Virus encephalitis as a sequela of the pneumonias" *Tri-State Medical Journal* 1960 Feb pp.7-11.
9. Klenner F, "Observations of the dose and administration of ascorbic acid when employed beyond the range of a vitamin in human pathology" *Journal of Applied Nutrition* 1971 23(3&4):61-88.

## Fluoride Poisoning

1. Online article at: http://www.fluoridation.com/skeletal.htm
2. Gupta S, Gupta R, Seth A, "Reversal of clinical and dental fluorosis" *Indian Pediatrics* 1994 31(4):439-443.
3. Gupta S, et al, "Reversal of fluorosis in children" *Acta Paediatrica Japonica* 1996 38(5):513-519.
4. Narayana M, Chinoy N, "Reversible effects of sodium fluoride ingestion on spermatozoa of the rat" *International Journal of Fertility and Menopausal Studies* 1994 39(6):337-346.

## Hepatitis, Acute Viral

1. *Cecil Medicine, 23rd Edition*, "Acute Vital Hepatitis," Saunders, an imprint of Elsevier Inc., 2008, Chap. 151.
2. Calleja H, Brooks R, "Acute hepatitis treated with high doses of vitamin C" *The Ohio State Medical Journal* 1960 56:821-823.
3. Cathcart R, "Vitamin C, titrating to bowel tolerance, anascorbemia, and acute induced scurvy" *Medical Hypotheses* 1981 7(11):1359-1376.
4. Komar V, Vasil'ev V, "The use of water-soluble vitamins in viral hepatitis A" [Article in Russian] *Klinicheskaia Meditsina* 1992 70(1):73-75.
5. Morishige F, Murata A, "Vitamin C for prophylaxis of viral hepatitis B in transfused patients" *Journal of the International Academy of Preventive Medicine* 1978 5(1):54-58.
6. Baur H, Staub H, "Therapy of hepatitis with ascorbic acid infusions" [Article in German] *Schweizerische Medizinische Wochenschrift* 1954 84:595-597.
7. Baetgen D, Results of the treatment of epidemic hepatitis in children with high doses of ascorbic acid in the years 1957-1958" [Article in German] *Medizinische Monatschrift* 1961 15:30-36.
8. Dalton W, "Massive doses of vitamin C in the treatment of viral diseases" *Journal of the Indiana State Medical Association* 1962 Aug pp.1151-1154.
9. Orens S, "Hepatitis B — a ten day cure: a personal history" Bulletin *Philadelphia Cty Dental Society* 1983 48(6):4-5.

## Herpes Infections

1. Online article at: http://www.medicinenet.com/acyclovir/article.htm
2. *Cecil Medicine, 23rd Edition*, "Herpes Simplex Virus Infections," Saunders, an imprint of Elsevier Inc., 2008, Chap. 307.
3. Terezhalmy G, Bottomley W, Pelleu G, "The use of water-soluble bioflavonoid-ascorbic acid complex in the treatment of recurrent herpes labialis" *Oral Surgery, Oral Medicine, Oral Pathology* 1978 45(1):56-62.
4. White L, et al, "*In vitro* effect of ascorbic acid on infectivity of herpesviruses and paramyxoviruses" *Journal of Clinical Microbiology* 1986 24(4):527-531.
5. Sagripanti J, et al, "Mechanism of copper-mediated inactivation of herpes simplex virus" *Antimicrobial Agents and Chemotherapy* 1997 41(4):812-817.
6. Hovi T, et al, "Topical treatment of recurrent mucocutaneous herpes with ascorbic acid-containing solution" *Antiviral Research* 1995 27(3):263-270.

## Hypertension (High Blood Pressure)

1. Online article at: www.ncbi.nlm.nih.gov/pubmedhealth/PMH0001502/
2. *Cecil Medicine, 23rd Edition*, "Arterial Hypertension," Saunders, an imprint of Elsevier Inc., 2008, Chap.66.
3. Bates C, et al, "Does vitamin C reduce blood pressure? Results of a large study of people aged 65 or older" *Journal of Hypertension* 1998 16(7):925-932.
4. Fotherby M, et al, "Effect of vitamin C on ambulatory blood pressure and plasma lipids in older persons" *Journal of Hypertension* 2000 18(4):411-415.

5. May J, "How does ascorbic acid prevent endothelial dysfunction?" *Free Radical Biology & Medicine* 2000 28(9):1421-1429.

6. Moran J, et al, "Plasma ascorbic acid concentrations relate inversely to blood pressure in human subjects" *The American Journal of Clinical Nutrition* 1993 57(2):213-217.

7. Ness A, et al, "Vitamin C status and blood pressure" *Journal of Hypertension* 1996 14(4):503-508.

8. Ness A, Chee D, Elliott P, "Vitamin C and blood pressure—an overview" *Journal of Human Hypertension* 1997 11(6):343-350.

9. Sakai N, et al, "An inverse relationship between serum vitamin C and blood pressure in a Japanese community" *Journal of Nutritional Science and Vitaminology* 1998 44(6):853-867.

10. Galley H, et al, "Combination oral antioxidant supplementation reduces blood pressure" *Clinical Science* 1997 92(4):361-365.

11. Duffy S, et al, "Treatment of hypertension with ascorbic acid" *Lancet* 1999 354(9195):2048-2049.

## Lead Poisoning

1. Online article at: http://www.mayoclinic.com/health/lead-poisoning/FL00068

2. *Cecil Medicine, 23rd Edition*, "Chronic Poisoning: Lead Poisoning," Saunders, an imprint of Elsevier Inc., 2008, Chap.20.

3. Holmes H, Campbell K, Amberg E, "Effect of vitamin C on lead poisoning" *Journal of Laboratory and Clinical Medicine* 1939 24:1119-1127.

4. Tandon S, et al, "Lead poisoning in Indian silver refiners" *The Science of the Total Environment* 2001 281(1-3):177-182.

5. Altmann P, et al, "Lead detoxication effect of a combined calcium phosphate and ascorbic acid therapy in pregnant women with increased lead burden" [Article in German] *Wiener Medizinische Wochenschrift* 1981 [131(12):311-314.

6. Flora S, Tandon S, "Preventive and therapeutic effects of thiamine, ascorbic acid and their combination in lead intoxication" *Acta Pharmacologica et Toxicologica* 1986 Copenh) 58(5):374-378.

7. Morton A, Partridge S, Blair J, "The intestinal uptake of lead" *Chemistry in Britain* 1985 15:923-927.

8. Niazi S, Lim J, Bederka J, "Effect of ascorbic acid on renal excretion of lead in the rat" *Journal of Pharmaceutical Sciences* 1982 71(10):1189-1190.

9. Goyer R, Cherian M, "Ascorbic acid and EDTA treatment of lead toxicity in rats" *Life Sciences* 1979 24(5):433-438.

10. Dhawan M, Kachru D, Tandon S, "Influence of thiamine and ascorbic acid supplementation on the antidotal efficacy of thiol chelators in experimental lead intoxication" *Archives of Toxicology* 1988 62(4):301-304.

11. Vij A, Satija N, Flora S, "Lead induced disorders in hematopoietic and drug metabolizing enzyme system and their protection by ascorbic acid supplementation" *Biomedical and Environmental Sciences* 1998 11(1):7-14.

12. Simon J, Hudes E, "Relationship of ascorbic acid to blood lead levels" *The Journal of the American Medical Association* 1999 281(24):2289-2293.

13. Houston D, Johnson M, "Does vitamin C intake protect against lead toxicity?" *Nutrition Reviews* 2000 58(3 Pt 1):73-75.

14. Cheng Y, et al, "Relation of nutrition to bone lead and blood lead levels in middle-aged to elderly men: The Normative Aging Study" *American Journal of Epidemiology* 1998 147(12):1162-1174.

15. Flanagan P, Chamberlain M, Valberg L, "The relationship between iron and lead absorption in humans" *The American Journal of Clinical Nutrition* 1982 36(5):823-829.

16. Dalley J, et al, "Interaction of L-ascorbic acid on the disposition of lead in rats" *Pharmacology & Toxicology* 1989 64(4):360-364.

17. Dawson E, et al, "The effect of ascorbic acid supplementation on the blood lead levels of smokers" *Journal of the American College of Nutrition* 1999 18(2):166-170.

## Leprosy

1. Online article at: http://www.ncbi.nlm.nih.gov/pubmedhealth/PMH0002323/

2. *Cecil Medicine, 23rd Edition*, "Leprosy," Saunders, an imprint of Elsevier Inc., 2008, Chap.347.

3. Sinha S, et al, "A study of blood ascorbic acid in leprosy" *International Journal of Leprosy and Other Mycobacterial Diseases* 1984 52(2):159-162.

4. Bechelli L, "Vitamin C therapy of the lepra reaction" *Revista Brasileira de Leprologia* (Sao Paulo) 1939 7:251-255.

5. Ferreira D, "Vitamin C in leprosy" *Publicacoes Medicas* 1950 20:25-28.

6. Gatti C, Gaona R, "Ascorbic acid in the treatment of leprosy" *Archiv Schiffe- und Tropenhygiene* 1939 43:32-33.

7. Hastings R, et al, "Activity of ascorbic acid in inhibiting the multiplication of *M. leprae* in the mouse foot pad" *International Journal of Leprosy and Other Mycobacterial Diseases* 1976 44(4):427-430.

## Malaria

1. Online article at: http://www.ncbi.nlm.nih.gov/pubmedhealth/PMH0001646/

2. Lotze H, "Clinical experimental investigations in benign tertian malaria" [Article in German] *Arch f Schiffs-u Trop-Hyg* 1938 42(7):287-305. Also cited in: *Tropical Diseases Bulletin* 1938 35:733.

3. Bourke G, Coleman R, Rencricca N, "Effect of ascorbic acid on host resistance in virulent rodent malaria" *Clinical Research* 1980 28(3):642A.

4. Marva E, et al, "Deleterious synergistic effects of ascorbate and copper on the development of *Plasmodium falciparum*: an *in vitro* study in normal and in G6PD-deficient erythrocytes" *International Journal of Parasitology* 1989 19(7):779-785.

5. Marva E, et al, "The effects of ascorbate-induced free radicals on *Plasmodium falciparum*" *Tropical Medicine and Parasitology* 1992 43(1):17-23.

6. Mohr W, "Vitamin C-stoffwechsel und malaria. Malaria and assimilation of vitamin C" [Article in German] *Deut Trop Zeitschrift* 1941 45(13):404-405. Also cited in: *Tropical Diseases Bulletin* 1943 40(1):13-14.

7. Naraqi S, et al, "Quinine blindness" *Papua and New Guinea Medical Journal* 1992 35(4):308-310.

8. Winter R, et al, "Potentiation of an antimalarial oxidant drug" *Antimicrobial Agents and Chemotherapy* 1997 41(7):1449-1454.

## Measles

1. Online article at: http://www.ncbi.nlm.nih.gov/pubmedhealth/PMH0000148/

2. *Cecil Medicine, 23rd Edition*, "Measles," Saunders, an imprint of Elsevier Inc., 2008, Chap.390.

3. Joffe M, Sukha N, Rabson A, "Lymphocyte subsets in measles. Depressed helper/inducer subpopulation reversed by *in vitro* treatment with levamisole and ascorbic acid" *The Journal of Clinical Investigation* 1983 72(3):971-980.

4. Klenner F, "Massive doses of vitamin C and the virus diseases" *Southern Medicine & Surgery* 1951 Apr 103(4):101-107.

5. Klenner F, "The treatment of poliomyelitis and other virus diseases with vitamin C" *Southern Medicine & Surgery* 1949 Jul 111(7):209-214.

6. Paez de la Torre J, "Ascorbic acid in measles" *Archives Argentinos de Pediatria* 1945 24:225-227.

## Mercury Poisoning

1. Online article at: http://en.wikipedia.org/wiki/Mercury_poisoning
2. *Cecil Medicine, 23rd Edition,* "Chronic Poisoning: Trace Metals," Saunders, an imprint of Elsevier Inc., 2008, Chap.20.
3. Ruskin A, Ruskin B, "Effect of mercurial diuretics upon the respiration of the rat heart and kidney. III. The protective action of ascorbic acid against Mercuhydrin *in vitro*" *Texas Reports on Biology and Medicine* 1952 10:429-438.
4. Huggins H, Levy T, *Uninformed Consent: The Hidden Dangers in Dental Care,* Charlottesville, VA: Hampton Roads Publishing Company, Inc. 1999.
5. Chapman D, Shaffer C, "Mercurial diuretics. A comparison of acute cardiac toxicity in animals and the effect of ascorbic acid on detoxification in their intravenous administration" *Archives of Internal Medicine* 1947 79:449-456.
6. Ruskin A, Johnson J, "Cardiodepressive effects of mercurial diuretics. Cardioprotective value of BAL, ascorbic acid and thiamin" *Proceedings of the Society for Experimental Biology and Medicine* 1949 72:577-583.
7. Blackstone S, Hurley R, Hughes R, "Some inter-relationships between vitamin C (L-ascorbic acid) and mercury in the guinea-pig" *Food and Cosmetics Toxicology* 1974 12(4):511-516.
8. Carroll R, Kovacs K, Tapp E, "Protection against mercuric chloride poisoning of the rat kidney" *Arzneimittelforschung* 1965 15(11):1361-1363.
9. Vauthey M, "Protective effect of vitamin C against poisons" *Praxis* (Bern) 1951 40:284-286.
10. Mokranjac M, Petrovic, "Vitamin C as an antidote in poisoning by fatal doses of mercury" *Comptes Rendus Hebdomadaires des Seances de l'Academie des Sciences* 1964 258:1341-1342.
11. Panda B, Subhadra A, Panda K "Prophylaxis of antioxidants against the genotoxicity of methyl mercuric chloride and maleic hydrazide in *Allium* micronucleus assay" *Mutation Research* 1995 343(2-3):75-84.
12. Gage J, "Mechanisms for the biodegradation of organic mercury compounds: the actions of ascorbate and of soluble proteins" *Toxicology and Applied Pharmacology* 1975 32(2):225-238.

## Mononucleosis

1. Online article at: http://www.ncbi.nlm.nih.gov/pubmedhealth/PMH0001617/
2. Cathcart R, "Vitamin C, titrating to bowel tolerance, anascorbemia, and acute induced scurvy" *Medical Hypotheses* 1981 7(11):1359-1376.
3. Dalton W, "Massive doses of vitamin C in the treatment of viral diseases" *Journal of the Indiana State Medical Association* 1962 Aug pp.1151-1154.
4. Klenner F, "Observations of the dose and administration of ascorbic acid when employed beyond the range of a vitamin in human pathology" *Journal of Applied Nutrition* 1971 23(3&4):61-88.

## Mumps

1. Online article at: http://www.ncbi.nlm.nih.gov/pubmedhealth/PMH0002524/
2. Klenner F, "The treatment of poliomyelitis and other virus diseases with vitamin C" *Southern Medicine & Surgery* 1949 Jul 111(7):209-214.

## Mushroom Poisoning

1. Online article at: http://emedicine.medscape.com/article/167398-overview
2. http://en.wikipedia.org/wiki/Mushroom_poisoning
3. .Online article at: http://emedicine.medscape.com/article/167398-treatment
4. Laing M, "A cure for mushroom poisoning" *South African Medical Journal* 1984 65(15):590.

## Nickel Poisoning

1. *Cecil Medicine, 23rd Edition*, "Chronic Poisoning: Trace Metals," Saunders, an imprint of Elsevier Inc., 2008, Chap.20.
2. Online article at: http://www.ehow.com/how_2085600_treat-nickel-poisoning.html
3. Chen C, Lin T, "Effects of nickel chloride on human platelets: enhancement of lipid peroxidation, inhibition of aggregation and interaction with ascorbic acid" *Journal of Toxicology and Environmental Health. Part A* 2001 62(6):431-438.
4. Chen C, Lin T, "Nickel toxicity to human term placenta: *in vitro* study on lipid peroxidation" *Journal of Toxicology and Environmental Health. Part A* 1998 54(1):37-47.
5. Wozniak K, Blasiak J, "Free radicals-mediated induction of oxidized DNA bases and DNA-protein cross-links by nickel chloride" *Mutation Research* 2002 514(1-2):233-243.
6. Osipova T, et al, "Repair processes in human cultured cells upon exposure to nickel salts and their modification" [Article in Russian] *Genetika* 1998 34(6):852-856.
7. Perminova I, et al, "Individual sensitivity to genotoxic effects of nickel and antimutagenic activity of ascorbic acid" *Bulletin of Experimental Biology and Medicine* 2001 131(4):367-370.
8. Chatterjee K, et al, "Biochemical studies on nickel toxicity in weanling rats — influence of vitamin C supplementation" *International Journal for Vitamin and Nutrition Research* 1979 49(3):264-275.
9. Das K, Das S, Das Gupta S "The influence of ascorbic acid on nickel-induced hepatic lipid peroxidation in rats" *Journal of Basic and Clinical Physiology and Pharmacology* 2001 12(3):187-195.
10. Chen C, Huang Y, Lin T, "Association between oxidative stress and cytokine production in nickel-treated rats" *Archives of Biochemistry and Biophysics* 1998 356(2):127-132.
11. Chen C, Huang Y, Lin T, "Lipid peroxidation in liver of mice administered with nickel chloride: with special reference to trace elements and antioxidants" *Biological Trace Element Research* 1998 61(2):193-205.
12. Memon A, Molokhia M, Friedmann P, "The inhibitory effects of topical chelating agents and antioxidants on nickel-induced hypersensitivity reactions" *Journal of the American Academy of Dermatology* 1994 30(4):560-565.

## Nitrate/Nitrite Toxicity

1. Whiteman M, Halliwell B, "Protection against peroxynitrite-dependent tyrosine nitration and alpha 1-antiproteinase inactivation by ascorbic acid. A comparison with other biological antioxidants" *Free Radical Research* 1996 25(3):275-283.
2. Sandoval M, et al, "Peroxynitrite-induced apoptosis in T84 and RAW 264.7 cells: attenuation by L-ascorbic acid" *Free Radical Biology & Medicine* 1997 22(3):489-495.
3. Bohm F, et al, "Beta-carotene with vitamins E and C offers synergistic cell protection against NOx" *FEBS Letters* 1998 436(3):387-389.
4. Shi X, et al, "Generation of thiyl and ascorbyl radicals in the reaction of peroxynitrite with thiols and ascorbate at physiological pH" *Journal of Inorganic Biochemistry* 1994 56(2):77-86.
5. Kirsch M, de Groot H, "Ascorbate is a potent antioxidant against peroxynitrite-induced oxidation reactions. Evidence that ascorbate acts by re-reducing substrate radicals produced by peroxynitrite" *The Journal of Biological Chemistry* 2000 275(22):16702-16708.
6. Carnes C, et al, "Ascorbate attenuates atrial pacing-induced peroxynitrite formation and electrical remodeling and decreases the incidence of postoperative atrial fibrillation" *Circulation Research* 2001 89(6):E32-E38.

7. Garcia-Roche M, et al, "Effect of ascorbic acid on the hepatoxicity due to the daily intake of nitrate, nitrite and dimethylamine" *Die Nahrung* 1987 31(2):99-104.

8. Fink B, et al, "Tolerance to nitrates with enhanced radical formation suppressed by carvedilol" *Journal of Cardiovascular Pharmacology* 1999 34(6):800-805.

9. Cummings J, "Dietary factors in the aetiology of gastrointestinal cancer" *Journal of Human Nutrition* 1978 32(6):455-465.

10. Schmahl D, Eisenbrand G, "Influence of ascorbic acid on the endogenous (intragastral) formation of N-nitroso compounds" *International Journal for Vitamin and Nutrition Research. Supplement* 1982 23:91-102.

11. Ohshima H, Bartsch H, "Monitoring endogenous nitrosamine formation in man" *IARC Scientific Publications* 1984 59:233-246.

12. Bartsch H, "N-nitroso compounds and human cancer: where do we stand?" *IARC Scientific Publications* 1991 105:1-10.

13. Sierra R, et al, "Exposure to N-nitrosamines and other risk factors for gastric cancer in Costa Rican children" *IARC Scientific Publications* 1991 105:162-167.

14. Srivatanakul P, et al, "Endogenous nitrosamines and liver fluke as risk factors for cholangiocarcinoma in Thailand" *IARC Scientific Publications* 1991 105:88-95.

15. Perez A, et al, "Mutagenicity of N-nitrosomorpholine biosynthesized from morpholine in the presence of nitrate and its inhibition by ascorbic acid" *Die Nahrung* 1990 34(7):661-664.

## Nitrogen Dioxide Poisoning

1. Online article at: http://emedicine.medscape.com/article/820431-overview

2. Online article at: http://emedicine.medscape.com/article/820431-treatment

3. Cooney R, Ross P, Bartolini G, "N-nitrosation and N-nitration of morpholine by nitrogen dioxide: inhibition by ascorbate, glutathione and alpha-tocopherol" *Cancer Letters* 1986 32(1):83-90.

4. Miyanishi K, et al, "*In vivo* formation of mutagens by intraperitoneal administration of polycyclic aromatic hydrocarbons in animals during exposure to nitrogen dioxide" *Carcinogenesis* 1996 17(7):1483-1490.

5. Bohm F, et al, "Beta-carotene with vitamins E and C offers synergistic cell protections against NOx" *FEBS Letters* 1998 436(3):387-389.

## Ochratoxin Toxicity

1. Online article at: http://en.wikipedia.org/wiki/Ochratoxin

2. Pfohl-Leszkowicz A, "Ochratoxin A, ubiquitous mycotoxin contaminating human food" [Article in French] *Comptes Rendus des Seances de la Societe de Biologie et de Ses Filiales* 1994 188(4):335-353.

3. Grosse Y, et al, "Retinol, ascorbic acid and alpha-tocopherol prevent DNA adduct formation in mice treated with the mycotoxins ochratoxin A and zearalenone" *Cancer Letters* 1997 114(1-2):225-229.

4. Marquardt R, Frohlich A, "A review of recent advances in understanding ochratoxicosis" *Journal of Animal Science* 1992 70(12):3968-3988.

5. Bose S, Sinha S, "Modulation of ochratoxin-produced genotoxicity in mice by vitamin C" *Food and Chemical Toxicology* 1994 32(6):533-537.

## Osteoporosis

1. Online article at: http://www.ncbi.nlm.nih.gov/pubmedhealth/PMH0001400/

2. *Cecil Medicine, 23rd Edition*, "Osteoporosis," Saunders, an imprint of Elsevier Inc., 2008, Chap.264.

3. Gabbay KH, et al, "Ascorbate synthesis pathway: dual role of ascorbate in bone homeostasis" *J Biol Chem.* 2010 Jun 18;285(25):19510-20.

4. Yalin S, et al. "Is there a role of free oxygen radicals in primary male osteoporosis?" *Clin Exp Rheumatol.* 2005 Sep-Oct;23(5):689-92.

5. Park JB, "The effects of dexamethasone, ascorbic acid, and β-glycerophosphate on osteoblastic differentiation by regulating estrogen receptor and osteopontin expression" *J Surg Res.* 2010 Oct 8.

6. Hie M, Tsukamoto I, "Vitamin C-deficiency stimulates osteoclastogenesis with an increase in RANK expression" *J Nutr Biochem.* 2011 Feb;22(2):164-71.

7. Sheweita SA, Khoshhal KI, "Calcium metabolism and oxidative stress in bone fractures: role of antioxidants" *Curr Drug Metab.* 2007 Jun;8(5):519-25.

8. Saito M, "Nutrition and bone health. Roles of vitamin C and vitamin B as regulators of bone mass and quality" [article in Japanese] *Clin Calcium.* 2009 Aug;19(8):1192-9.

9. Chuin A, et al, "Effect of antioxidants combined to resistance training on BMD in elderly women: a pilot study" *Osteoporos Int.* 2009 Jul;20(7):1253-8.

10. Sahni S, et al, "High vitamin C intake is associated with lower 4-year bone loss in elderly men"*J Nutr.* 2008 Oct;138(10):1931-8.

11. Pasco JA, et al, "Antioxidant vitamin supplements and markers of bone turnover in a community sample of nonsmoking women" *J Womens Health* (Larchmt). 2006 Apr;15(3):295-300.

12. Sugiura M, et al, "Dietary patterns of antioxidant vitamin and carotenoid intake associated with bone mineral density: findings from post-menopausal Japanese female subjects" *Osteoporos Int.* 2011 Jan;22(1):143-52.

13. Ruiz-Ramos M, et al, "Supplementation of ascorbic acid and alpha-tocopherol is useful to preventing bone loss linked to oxidative stress in elderly" *J Nutr Health Aging* 2010 Jun;14(6):467-72.

14. Zinnuroglu M, et al, "Prospective evaluation of free radicals and antioxidant activity following 6-month risedronate treatment in patients with postmenopausal osteoporosis" *Rheumatol Int.* 2011 Jan 8.

15. Sahni S, et al, "Protective effect of total and supplemental vitamin C intake on the risk of hip fracture — a 17-year follow-up from the Framingham Osteoporosis Study" *Osteoporos Int.* 2009 Nov;20(11):1853-61.

16. Falch JA, Mowé M, Bøhmer T, "Low levels of serum ascorbic acid in elderly patients with hip fracture" *Scand J Clin Lab Invest.* 1998 May;58(3):225-8.

17. Bourne, G. "Vitamin C and repair of injured tissues" *Lancet* 1942 2:661-664.

18. Morton D, Barrett-Connor E, Schneider D, "Vitamin C supplement use and bone mineral density in postmenopausal women" *Journal of Bone and Mineral Research* 2001 16(1):135-140.

19. Leveille S, et al, "Dietary vitamin C and bone mineral density in postmenopausal women in Washington State, USA" *Journal of Epidemiology and Community Health* 1997 51(5):479-485.

## Ozone Toxicity

1. Yeadon M, Payne A, "Ascorbic acid prevents ozone-induced bronchial hyperreactivity in guinea-pigs" *British Journal of Pharmacology* 1989 98 Suppl:790P.

2. Cotovio J, et al, "Generation of oxidative stress in human cutaneous models following *in vitro* ozone exposure" *Toxicology In Vitro* 2001 15(4-5):357-362.

3. Menzel D, "The toxicity of air pollution in experimental animals and humans: the role of oxidative stress" *Toxicology Letters* 1994 72(1-3):269-277.

## Paraquat Poisoning

1. Online article at: http://www.ncbi.nlm.nih.gov/pubmedhealth/PMH0002076/

2. Matkovics B, et al, "*In vivo* study of the mechanism of protective effects of ascorbic acid and reduced glutathione in paraquat poisoning" *General Pharmacology* 1980 11(5):455-461.

3. Hong S, et al, "Effect of vitamin C on plasma total antioxidant status in patients with paraquat intoxication" *Toxicology Letters* 2002 126(1):51-59.

4. Cappelletti G, Maggioni M, Maci R, "Apoptosis in human lung epithelial cells: triggering by paraquat and modulation by antioxidants" *Cell Biology International* 1998 22(9-10):671-678.

5. Vismara C, Vailati G, Bacchetta R "Reduction in paraquat embryotoxicity by ascorbic acid in *Xenopus laevis*" *Aquatic Toxicology* 2001 51(3):293-303.

6. Fujimoto Y, et al, "Inhibition of paraquat accumulation in rabbit kidney cortex slices by ascorbic acid" *Research Communications in Clinical Pathology and Pharmacology* 1989 65(2):245-248.

## Pertussis (Whooping Cough)

1. Online article at: http://www.ncbi.nlm.nih.gov/pubmedhealth/PMH0002528/

2. Meier K, "Vitamin C treatment of pertussis" *Annales de Pediatrie* (Paris) 1945 164:50-53.

3. Ormerod M, Unkauf B, "Ascorbic acid (vitamin C) treatment of whooping cough" *Canadian Medical Association Journal* 1937 37(2):134-136.

4. Omerod M, et al, "A further report on the ascorbic acid treatment of whooping cough" *Canadian Medical Association Journal* 1937 37(3):268-272

5. Otani T, "On the vitamin C therapy of pertussis" *Klinische Wochenschrift* 1936 15(51):1884-1885.

6. Sessa T, "Vitamin C therapy of whooping cough" *Riforma Medica* 1940 56:38-43.

7. Vermillion E, Stafford G, "A preliminary report on the use of cevitaminic acid in the treatment of whooping cough" *Journal of the Kansas Medical Society* 1938 39(11):469, 479.

## Pesticide/Herbicide Poisoning

1. Online article at: http://en.wikipedia.org/wiki/Diquat

2. Online article at: http://en.wikipedia.org/wiki/Endosulfan

3. Online article at: http://en.wikipedia.org/wiki/Phosphamidon

4. Online article at: http://pmep.cce.cornell.edu/profiles/extoxnet/haloxyfop-methylparathion/mancozeb-ext.html

5. Online article at: http://pmep.cce.cornell.edu/profiles/extoxnet/dienochlor-glyphosate/dimethoate-ext.html

6. Online article at: http://en.wikipedia.org/wiki/Malathion

7. Online article at: http://en.wikipedia.org/wiki/Parathion

8. Online article at: http://en.wikipedia.org/wiki/Lindane.

9. Klenner F, "Observations on the dose and administration of ascorbic acid when employed beyond the range of a vitamin in human pathology" *Journal of Applied Nutrition* 1971 23(3&4):61-88.

10. Nakagawa Y, Cotgreave I, Moldeus P, "Relationships between ascorbic acid and alpha-tocopherol during diquat-induced redox cycling in isolated rat hepatocytes" *Biochemical Pharmacology* 1991 42(4):883-888.

11. Khan P, Sinha S, "Ameliorating effect of vitamin C on murine sperm toxicity induced by three pesticides (endosulfan, phosphamidon and mancozeb)" *Mutagenesis* 1996 11(1):33-36.

12. Khan P, Sinha S, "Impact of higher doses of vitamin C in modulating pesticide genotoxicity" *Teratogenesis, Carcinogenesis, and Mutagenesis* 1994 14(4):175-181.

13. Geetanjali D, Rita P, Reddy P, "Effect of ascorbic acid in the detoxification of the insecticide dimethoate in the bone marrow erythrocytes of mice" *Food and Chemical Toxicology* 1993 31(6):435-437.

14. Hoda Q, Sinha S, "Minimization of cytogenetic toxicity of malathion by vitamin C" *Journal of Nutritional Science and Vitaminology* 1991 37(4):329-339.

15. Hoda Q, Sinha S, "Vitamin C-mediated minimisation of Rogor-induced genotoxicity" *Mutation Research* 1993 299(1):29-36.

16. Chakraborty D, et al, "Studies on L-ascorbic acid metabolism in rats under chronic toxicity due to organophosphorus insecticides: effects of supplementation of L-ascorbic acid in high doses" *The Journal of Nutrition* 1978 108(6):973-980.

17. Hoda Q, Azfer M, Sinha S, "Modificatory effect of vitamin C and vitamin B-complex on meiotic inhibition induced by organophosphorus pesticide in mice *Mus musculus*" *International Journal for Vitamin and Nutrition Research* 1993 63(1):48-51.

18. Tiwari R, Bandyopadhyayn S, Chatterjee G, "Protective effect of L-ascorbic acid in lindane intoxicated rats" *Acta Vitaminologica et Enzymologica* 1982 4(3):215-220.

19. Koner B, Banerjee B, Ray A, "Organochlorine pesticide-induced oxidative stress and immune suppression in rats" *Indian Journal of Experimental Biology* 1998 36(4):395-398.

## Phencyclidine (Angel Dust) Poisoning

1. Online article at: http://en.wikipedia.org/wiki/Phencyclidine

2. Aronow R, Miceli J, Done A "A therapeutic approach to the acutely overdosed PCP patient" *Journal of Psychedelic Drugs* 1980 12(3-4):259-267.

3. Rappolt R, Gay G, Farris R, "Emergency management of acute phencyclidine intoxication" *JACEP* 1979 8(2):68-76.

4. Giannini A, et al, "Augmentation of haloperidol by ascorbic acid in phencyclidine intoxication" *The American Journal of Psychiatry* 1987 144(9):1207-1209.

5. Welch M, Correa G, "PCP intoxication in young children and infants" *Clinical Pediatrics* 1980 19(8):510-514.

## Phenol Poisoning

1. Online article at: http://medical-dictionary.thefreedictionary.com/phenol+poisoning

2. Todorović V, "Acute phenol poisoning" [article in Serbian] Med Pregl. 2003;56 Suppl 1:37-41.

3. Skvortsova R, Pozniakovskii V, Agarkova I, "Role of the vitamin factor in preventing phenol poisoning" [Article in Russian] *Voprosy Pitaniia* 1981 2:32-35.

4. Valentovic M, et al, "2-Amino-5-chlorophenol toxicity in renal cortical slices from Fisher 344 rats: effect of antioxidants and sulfhydryl agents" *Toxicology and Applied Pharmacology* 1999 161(1):1-9.

5. Hong S, et al, "4-Amino-2,6-dichlorophenol nephrotoxicity in the Fisher 344 rat: protection by ascorbic acid, AT-125, and aminooxyacetic acid" *Toxicology and Applied Pharmacology* 1997 147(1):115-125.

6. Nagyova A, Ginter E, "The influence of ascorbic acid on the hepatic cytochrome P-450, and glutathione in guinea-pigs exposed to 2,4-dichlorophenol" *Physiological Research* 1995 44(5):301-305.

7. Satoh K, et al, "Effect of antioxidants on radical intensity and cytotoxic activity of eugenol" *Anticancer Research* 1998 18(3A):1549-1552.

8. Song H, Lang C, Chen T, "The role of glutathione in p-aminophenol-induced nephrotoxicity in the mouse" *Drug and Chemical Toxicology* 1999 22(3):529-544.

9. Lock E, Cross T, Schnellmann R, "Studies on the mechanism of 4-aminophenol-induced toxicity to renal proximal tubules" *Human & Experimental Toxicology* 1993 12(5):383-388.

## Pneumonia

1. Online article at: http://www.ncbi.nlm.nih.gov/pubmedhealth/PMH0001200/
2. Locke A, et al, "Fitness, sulfanilamide and pneumococcus infection in the rabbit" *Science* 1937 86(2227):228-229.
3. Kaiser A, Slavin B, "The incidence of hemolytic streptococci in the tonsils of children as related to the vitamin C content of tonsils and blood" *Journal of Pediatrics* 1938 13:322-333.
4. Sabin A, "Vitamin C in relation to experimental poliomyelitis with incidental observations on certain manifestations in *Macacus rhesus* monkeys on a scorbutic diet" *Journal of Experimental Medicine* 1939 69:507-515.
5. Gander J, Niederberger W, *Munchener Medizinische Wochenschrift* 1936 83:1386.
6. Vogl A, *Munchener Medizinische Wochenschrift* 1937 84:1569.
7. Bonnholtzer E, *Deutsches Med Wochenschrift* 1937 26:1001.
8. Hochwald A, *Deutsches Med Wochenschrift* 1937 63:182.
9. Gunzel W, Kroehnert G, "Experiences in the treatment of pneumonia with vitamin C" *Fortschrifte der Therapie* 1937 13:460-463.
10. Sennewald K, *Fortschrifte der Therapie* 1938 14:139.
11. Szirmai F, "Value of vitamin C in treatment of acute infectious diseases" *Deutsches Archive fur Klinische Medizin* 1940 85:434-443.
12. Kimbarowski J, Mokrow N, "Colored precipitation reaction of the urine according to Kimbarowski (FARK) as an index of the effect of ascorbic acid during treatment of viral influenza" [Article in German] *Das Deutsche Gesundheitswesen* 1967 22(51):2413-2418.
13. Slotkin G, Fletcher R, "Ascorbic acid in pulmonary complications following prostatic surgery: a preliminary report" *Journal of Urology* 1944 52:566-569.
14. Hamdy A, et al, "Effect of vitamin C on lamb pneumonia and mortality" *The Cornell Veterinarian* 1967 57(1):12-20.
15. Esposito A, "Ascorbate modulates antibacterial mechanisms in experimental pneumococcal pneumonia" *The American Review of Respiratory Disease* 1986 133(4):643-647.
16. Pitt H, Costrini A, "Vitamin C prophylaxis in marine recruits" *Journal of the American Medical Association* 1979 241(9):908-911.
17. Dalton W, "Massive doses of vitamin C in the treatment of viral diseases" *Journal of the Indiana State Medical Association* (1962) Aug pp.1151-1154.
18. Klenner F, "Virus pneumonia and its treatment with vitamin C" *Southern Medicine & Surgery* 1948 Feb 110(2):36-38,46.
19. Klenner F, "The use of vitamin C as an antibiotic" *Journal of Applied Nutrition* 1953 6:274-278.

## Polio

1. Online article at: http://www.ncbi.nlm.nih.gov/pubmedhealth/PMH0002375/
2. Jungeblut C, "Inactivation of poliomyelitis virus *in vitro* by crystalline vitamin C (ascorbic acid)" *Journal of Experimental Medicine* 1935 62:517-521.
3. Jungeblut C, "Vitamin C therapy and prophylaxis in experimental poliomyelitis" *Journal of Experimental Medicine* 1937 65:127-146.
4. Jungeblut C, "A further contribution to vitamin C therapy in experimental poliomyelitis" *Journal of Experimental Medicine* 1939 70:315-332.
5. Klenner F, "The treatment of poliomyelitis and other virus diseases with vitamin C" *Southern Medicine & Surgery* 1949 Jul 111(7):209-214.
6. Baur H, "Poliomyelitis therapy with ascorbic acid" [German] *Helvetia Medica Acta* 1952 19:470-474.
7. Greer E, "Vitamin C in acute poliomyelitis" *Medical Times* 1955 83(11):1160-1161.

8. Peloux Y, et al, "Inactivation du virus polio-myelitique par des systemes chimique generateurs du radical libre hydroxide Mechanism de l'activite virulicide du peroxide d'hydrogene et de l'acide ascorbique" *Annls Inst Pasteur, Paris* 1962 102:6.

9. Klenner F, "Massive doses of vitamin C and the virus diseases" *Southern Medicine & Surgery* 1951 Apr 103(4):101-107.

## PCB Toxicity

1. Online article al: http://en.wikipedia.org/wiki/Polychlorinated_biphenyl

2. Online article at: http://www.atsdr.cdc.gov/csem/pcb/

3. Kawai-Kobayashi K, Yoshidan A, "Effect of dietary ascorbic acid and vitamin E on metabolic changes in rats and guinea pigs exposed to PCB" *The Journal of Nutrition* 1986 116(1):98-106.

4. Saito M, "Polychlorinated biphenyls-induced lipid peroxidation as measured by thiobarbituric acid-reactive substances in liver subcellular fractions of rats" *Biochimica et Biophysica Acta* 1990 1046(3):301-308.

5. Horio F, et al, "Ascorbic acid requirement for the induction of microsomal drug-metabolizing enzymes in a rat mutant unable to synthesize ascorbic acid" *The Journal of Nutrition* 1986 116(11):2278-2289.

6. Suzuki H, et al, "Ascorbate-dependent elevation of mRNA levels for cytochrome P450s induced by polychlorinated biphenyls" *Biochemical Pharmacology* 1993 46(1):186-189.

7. Matsushita N, et al, "Ascorbic acid deficiency reduces the level of mRNA for cytochrome P-450 on the induction of polychlorinated biphenyls" *Journal of Nutritional Science and Vitaminology* 1993 39(4):289-302.

8. Chakraborty D, et al, "Biochemical studies on polychlorinated biphenyl toxicity in rats: manipulation by vitamin C" *International Journal for Vitamin and Nutrition Research* 1978 48(1):22-31.

## Pseudomonas Infections

1. Online article at: http://emedicine.medscape.com/article/970904-overview

2. Online article at: http://emedicine.medscape.com/article/970904-treatment

3. Carlsson S, et al, "Effects of pH, nitrite, and ascorbic acid on nonenzymatic nitric oxide generation and bacterial growth in urine" *Nitric Oxide: Biology and Chemistry* 2001 5(6):580-586.

4. Klenner F, "Observations of the dose and administration of ascorbic acid when employed beyond the range of a vitamin in human pathology" *Journal of Applied Nutrition* 1971 23(3&4):61-88.

5. Nakanishi T, "A report on a clinical experience of which has successfully made several antibiotics-resistant bacteria (MRSA etc.) negative on a bedsore" [Article in Japanese] *Igaku Kenkyu. Acta Medica* 1992 62(1):31-37.

6. Nakanishi T, "A report on the therapeutical experiences of which have successfully made several antibiotics-resistant bacteria (MRSA etc.) negative on bedsores and respiratory organs" [Article in Japanese] *Igaku Kenkyu. Acta Medica* 1993 63(3):95-100.

7. Rawal B, "Bactericidal action of ascorbic acid on *Pseudomonas aeruginosa*: alteration of cell surface as a possible mechanism" *Chemotherapy* 1978 24(3):166-171.

8. Rawal B, Charles B, "Inhibition of *Pseudomonas aeruginosa* by ascorbic acid-sulphamethoxazole-trimethoprim combination" *The Southeast Asian Journal of Tropical Medicine and Public Health* 1972 3(2):225-228.

9. Rawal B, McKay G, Blackhall M, "Inhibition of *Pseudomonas aeruginosa* by ascorbic acid acting singly and in combination with antimicrobials: *in-vitro* and *in-vivo* studies" *Medical Journal of Australia* 1974 1(6):169-174.

## Rabies

1. Online article at: http://www.ncbi.nlm.nih.gov/pubmedhealth/PMH0002310/
2. Amato, G. "Azione dell'acido ascorbico sul virus fisso della rabbia e sulla tossina tetanica" *Giornale di Batteriologia, Virologia et Immunologia* (Torino) 1937 19:843-847.
3. Banic S, "Prevention of rabies by vitamin C" *Nature* 1975 258(5531):153-154.

## Radiation Toxicity

1. Online article at: http://www.nlm.nih.gov/medlineplus/radiationexposure.html
2. Online article at: http://en.wikipedia.org/wiki/Acute_radiation_syndrome
3. Ala-Ketola L, Varis R, Kiviniitty K, "Effect of ascorbic acid on the survival of rats after whole body irradiation" *Strahlentherapie* 1974 148(6):643-644.
4. Blumenthal R, et al, "Anti-oxidant vitamins reduce normal tissue Poisoning induced by radio-immunotherapy" *International Journal of Cancer* 2000 86(2):276-280.
5. Okunieff P, "Interactions between ascorbic acid and the radiation of bone marrow, skin, and tumor" *The American Journal of Clinical Nutrition* 1991 54(6 Suppl):1281S-1283S.
6. Kennedy M, et al, "Successful and sustained treatment of chronic radiation proctitis with antioxidant vitamins E and C" *The American Journal of Gastroenterology* 2001 96(4):1080-1084.
7. Kretzschmar C, Ellis F, "The effect of x rays on ascorbic acid concentration in plasma and in tissues" *The British Journal of Radiology* 1974 20(231):94-99.
8. Koyama S, et al, "Radiation-induced long-lived radicals which cause mutation and transformation" *Mutation Research* 1998 421(1):45-54.
9. Sarma L, Kesavan P, "Protective effects of vitamins C and E against gamma-ray-induced chromosomal damage in mice" *International Journal of Radiation Biology* 1993 63(6):759-764.
10. Konopacka M, Widel M, Rzeszowska-Wolny J. "Modifying effect of vitamins C, E and beta-carotene against gamma-ray-induced DNA damage in mouse cells" *Mutation Research* 1998 417(2-3):85-94.
11. Fomenko L, et al, "A vitamin-antioxidant diet decreases the level of chromosomal damages and the frequency of gene mutations in irradiated mice" [Article in Russian] *Izvestiia Akademii Nauk. Seriia Biologicheskaia* 1997 4:419-424.
12. Narra V, et al, "Vitamin C as a radioprotector against iodine-131 *in vivo*" *Journal of Nuclear Medicine* 1993 34(4):637-640.
13. Konopacka M, Rzeszowska-Wolny J, "Antioxidant vitamins C, E and beta-carotene reduce DNA damage before as well as after gamma-ray irradiation of human lymphocytes *in vitro*" *Mutation Research* 2001 491(1-2):1-7.
14. Riabchenko N, et al, "The molecular, cellular and systemic mechanisms of the radioprotective action of multivitamin antioxidant complexes" [Article in Russian] *Radiatsionnaia Biologiia, Radioecologiia* 1996 36(6):895-899.
15. Yasukawa M, Terasima T, Seki M, "Radiation-induced neoplastic transformation of C3H10T1/2 cells is suppressed by ascorbic acid" *Radiation Research* 1989 120(3):456-467.
16. Mireles-Rocha H, et al, "UVB photoprotection with antioxidants: effects of oral therapy with d-alpha-tocopherol and ascorbic acid on the minimal erythema dose" *Acta Dermato-Venereologica* 2002 82(1):21-24.
17. Eberlein-Konig B, Placzek M, Przybilla R, "Protective effect against sunburn of combined systemic ascorbic acid (vitamin C) and d-alpha-tocopherol (vitamin E)" *Journal of the American Academy of Dermatology* 1998 38(1):45-48.
18. Moison R, Beijersbergen van Henegouwen G, "Topical antioxidant vitamins C and E prevent UVB-radiation-induced peroxidation of eicosapentaenoic acid in pig skin" *Radiation Research* 2002 157(4):402-409.

19. Kobayashi S, et al, "Protective effect of magnesium-L-ascorbyl-2 phosphate against skin damage induced by UVB irradiation" *Photochemistry and Photobiology* 1996 64(1):224-228.

20. Neumann N, et al, "The photoprotective effect of ascorbic acid, acetylsalicylic acid, and indomethacin evaluated by the photo hen's egg test" *Photodermatology, Photoimmunology & Photomedicine* 1999 15(5):166-170.

21. Miyai E, et al, "Ascorbic acid 2-O-alpha-glucoside, a stable form of ascorbic acid, rescues human keratinocyte cell line, SCC, from cytotoxicity of ultraviolet light B" *Biological & Pharmaceutical Bulletin* 1996 19(7):984-987.

22. He Y, Hader D, "UV-B-induced formation of reactive oxygen species and oxidative damage of the cyanobacterium *Anabaena* sp.: protective effects of ascorbic acid and N-acetyl-L-cysteine" *Journal of Photochemistry and Photobiology. B, Biology* 2002 66(2):115-124.

23. Dreosti I, McGown M, "Antioxidants and UV-induced genotoxicity" *Research Communications in Chemical Pathology and Pharmacology* 1992 75(2):251-254.

24. Dunham W, et al, "Effects of intake of L-ascorbic acid on the incidence of dermal neoplasms induced in mice by ultraviolet light" *Proceedings of the National Academy of Sciences of the United States of America* 1982 79(23):7532-7536.

25. Mothersill C, Malone J, O'Connor M, "Vitamin C and radioprotection" *British Journal of Radiology* 1978 51(606):474.

## Selenium Poisoning

1. *Cecil Medicine, 23rd Edition*, "Chronic Poisoning: Trace Metals," Saunders, an imprint of Elsevier Inc., 2008, Chap.20.

2. Civil I, McDonald M, "Acute selenium poisoning: case report" *New Zealand Medical Journal* 1978 87(612):354-356.

3. Svirbely J, "Vitamin C studies in the rat. The effect of selenium dioxide, sodium selenate and tellurate" *The Biochemical Journal* 1938 32:467-473.

4. Terada A, et al, "Influence of combined use of selenious acid and SH compounds in parenteral preparations" *Journal of Trace Elements in Medicine and Biology* 1997 11(2):105-109.

5. Hill C, "Studies on the ameliorating effect of ascorbic acid on mineral toxicities in the chick" *The Journal of Nutrition* 1979 109(1):84-90.

6. Jacques-Silva M, et al, "Diphenyl diselenide and ascorbic acid changes deposition of selenium and ascorbic acid in liver and brain of mice" *Pharmacology & Toxicology* 2001 88(3):119-125.

## Shingles

1. Online article at: http://www.ncbi.nlm.nih.gov/pubmedhealth/PMH0001861/

2. *Cecil Medicine, 23rd Edition*, "Macular, Papular, Vesiculobullos, and Pustular Disease," Saunders, an imprint of Elsevier Inc., 2008, Chap.465.

3. Dainow I, "Treatment of herpes zoster with vitamin C" *Dermatologia* 1943 68:197-201.

4. Klenner F, "The treatment of poliomyelitis and other virus diseases with vitamin C" *Southern Medicine & Surgery* 1949 Jul 111(7):209-214.

5. Klenner F, "The use of vitamin C as an antibiotic" *Journal of Applied Nutrition* 1953 6:274-278.

6. Klenner F, "Significance of high daily intake of ascorbic acid in preventive medicine" *Journal of the International Academy of Preventive Medicine* 1974 1(1):45-69.

7. Zureick M, "Treatment of shingles and herpes with vitamin C intravenously" *Journal des Praticiens* 1950 64:586.

## Staph Infections

1. Online article at: http://www.emedicinehealth.com/staphylococcus/article_em.htm

2. *Cecil Medicine, 23rd Edition*, "Staphylococcal Infections," Saunders, an imprint of Elsevier Inc., 2008, Chap.310.

3. Andreasen C, Frank D, "The effects of ascorbic acid on *in vitro* heterophil function" *Avian Diseases* 1999 43(4):656-663.

4. Gupta G, Guha B, "The effect of vitamin C and certain other substances on the growth of microorganisms" *Annals of Biochemistry and Experimental Medicine* 1941 1(1):14-26.

5. Klenner F, "Significance of high daily intake of ascorbic acid in preventive medicine" *Journal of the International Academy of Preventive Medicine* 1974 1(1):45-69.

6. Kodama T, Kojima T, "Studies of the staphylococcal toxin, toxoid and antitoxin; effect of ascorbic acid on staphylococcal lysins and organisms" *Kitasato Archives of Experimental Medicine* 1939 16:36-55.

7. Ledermann E, "Vitamin-C deficiency and ulceration of the face" *The Lancet* 1962 2:1382.

8. Nakanishi T, "A report on a clinical experience of which has successfully made several antibiotics-resistant bacteria (MRSA etc.) negative on a bedsore" [Article in Japanese] *Igaku Kenkyu. Acta Medica* 1992 62(1):31-37.

9. Nakanishi T, "A report on the therapeutical experiences of which have successfully made several antibiotics-resistant bacteria (MRSA etc.) negative on bedsores and respiratory organs" [Article in Japanese] *Igaku Kenkyu. Acta Medica* 1993 63(3):95-100.

10. Nelson J, et al, "Metabolic and immune effects of enteral ascorbic acid after burn trauma" *Burns: Journal of the International Society for Burn Injuries* 1992 18(2):92-97.

## Strep Infections

1. Article online at: http://www.nlm.nih.gov/medlineplus/streptococcalinfections.html

2. *Cecil Medicine, 23rd Edition*, "Streptococcal Infections," Saunders, an imprint of Elsevier Inc., 2008, Chap.312.

3. Gnarpe H, Michaelsson M, Dreborg S, "The *in vitro* effect of ascorbic acid on the bacterial growth in urine" *Acta Pathologica et Microbiologica Scandinavica* 1968 74(1):41-50.

4. Klenner F, "Significance of high daily intake of ascorbic acid in preventive medicine" *Journal of the International Academy of Preventive Medicine* 1974 1(1):45-69.

5. Witt W, Hubbard G, Fanton J, "*Streptococcus pneumoniae* arthritis and osteomyelitis with vitamin C deficiency in guinea pigs" *Laboratory Animal Science* 1988 38(2):192-194.

6. Devasena T, Lalitha S, Padma K, "Lipid peroxidation, osmotic fragility and antioxidant status in children with acute post-streptococcal glomerulonephritis" *Clinica Chimica Acta* 2001 308(1-2):155-161.

7. Ruskin S, "Contribution to the study of grippe otitis, myringitis bullosa hemorrhagica, and its relationship to latent scurvy" *Laryngoscope* 1938 48:327-334.

8. Massell B, et al, "Antirheumatic activity of ascorbic acid in large doses. Preliminary observations on seven patients with rheumatic fever" *The New England Journal of Medicine* 1950 242(16):614-615.

9. Glazebrook A, Thomson S, "The administration of vitamin C in a large institution and its effect on general health and resistance to infection" *Journal of Hygiene* 1942 42(1):1-19.

10. McCormick W, "Vitamin C in the prophylaxis and therapy of infectious diseases" *Archives of Pediatrics* 1951 68(1):1-9.

11. Cathcart R, "Vitamin C, titrating to bowel tolerance, anascorbemia, and acute induced scurvy" *Medical Hypotheses* 1981 7(11):1359-1376.

12. Coulehan J, et al, "Vitamin C and acute illness in Navajo school children" *The New England Journal of Medicine* 1976 295(18):973-977.

## Strychnine Poisoning

1. Online article at: http://en.wikipedia.org/wiki/Strychnine_poisoning

2. Dey P, "Protective action of lemon juice and ascorbic acid against lethality and convulsive property of strychnine" *Die Naturwissenschaften* 1965 52:164.

3. Dey P, "Protective action of ascorbic acid & its precursors on the convulsive & lethal actions of strychnine" *Indian Journal of Experimental Biology* 1967 5(2):110-112.

4. Jahan K, Ahmad K, Ali M, "Effect of ascorbic acid in the treatment of tetanus" *Bangladesh Medical Research Council Bulletin* 1984 10(1):24-28.

## Tetanus

1. Online article at: http://www.ncbi.nlm.nih.gov/pubmedhealth/PMH0001640/

2. *Cecil Medicine, 23rd Edition*, "Clostridial Infections," Saunders, an imprint of Elsevier Inc., 2008, Chap.319.

3. Jungeblut C, "Inactivation of tetanus toxin by crystalline vitamin C (L-ascorbic acid)" *Journal of Immunology* 1937 33:203-214.

4. Kligler I, Guggenheim K, Warburg F, "Influence of ascorbic acid on the growth and toxin production of *Cl. tetani* and on the detoxication of tetanus toxin" *Journal of Pathology* 1938 46:619-629.

5. Klenner F, "Case history: cure of a 4-year-old child bitten by a mature highland moccasin with vitamin C" *Tri-State Medical Journal* 1954 Jul.

6. Dey P, "Efficacy of vitamin C in counteracting tetanus toxicity" *Die Naturwissenschaften* 1966 53(12):310.

7. Dey P, "Protective action of ascorbic acid & its precursors on the convulsive & lethal actions of strychnine" *Indian Journal of Experimental Biology* 1967 5(2):110-112.

8. Klenner F, "Case history: cure of a 4-year-old child bitten by a mature highland moccasin with vitamin C" *Tri-State Medical Journal* 1954 Jul.

9. Jahan K, Ahmad K, Ali M, "Effect of ascorbic acid in the treatment of tetanus" *Bangladesh Medical Research Council Bulletin* 1984 10(1):24-28.

## Toxic Drugs

1. Online article at: http://www.ncbi.nlm.nih.gov/pubmedhealth/PMH0000521/

2. Online article at: http://en.wikipedia.org/wiki/Acetaminophen

3. Peterson F, Knodell R, "Ascorbic acid protects against acetaminophen- and cocaine-induced hepatic damage in mice" *Drug-Nutrient Interactions* 1984 3(1):33-41.

4. Ilkiw J, Ratcliffe R, "Paracetamol toxicity in a cat" *Australian Veterinary Journal* 1987 64(8):245-247.

5. Axelrod J, Udenfriend S, Brodie B, "Ascorbic acid in aromatic hydroxylation. III. Effect of ascorbic acid on hydroxylation of acetanilide, aniline and antipyrine *in vivo*" *The Journal of Pharmacology and Experimental Therapeutics* 1954 111:176-181.

6. Online article at: http://en.wikipedia.org/wiki/Arsphenamine

7. Sulzberger M, Oser B, "The influence of ascorbic acid in diet on sensitization of guinea pigs to neoarsphenamine" *Proceedings of the Society for Experimental Biology and Medicine* 1935 32:716.

8. Dainow I, "Desensitizing action of L-ascorbic acid" *Ann Dermat et Syph.* 1935 6:830.

9. Online article at: http://en.wikipedia.org/wiki/Chloroform

10. Tamura T, et al, "Studies on the antidotal action of drugs. Part 2. Vitamin C and its antidotal effect against chloroform and carbon tetrachloridum" *The Journal of Nihon University School of Dentistry* 1970 12(1):25-28.

11. Online article at: http://www.nlm.nih.gov/medlineplus/druginfo/meds/a684036. html

12. Nefic H, "Anticlastogenic effect of vitamin C on cisplatin induced chromosome aberrations in human lymphocyte cultures" *Mutation Research* 2001 498(1-2):89-98.

13. Giri A, Khynriam D, Prasad S, "Vitamin C mediated protection on cisplatin induced mutagenicity in mice" *Mutation Research* 1998 421(2):139-148.

14. Greggi Antunes L, Darin J, Bianchi M, "Protective effects of vitamin C against cisplatin-induced nephrotoxicity and lipid peroxidation in adult rats: a dose-dependent study" 2000 *Pharmacological Research* 41(4):405-411.

15. Appenroth D, et al, "Protective effects of vitamin E and C on cisplatin nephrotoxicity in developing rats" *Archives of Toxicology* 1997 71(11):677-683.

16. Lopez-Gonzalez M, et al, "Ototoxicity caused by cisplatin is ameliorated by melatonin and other antioxidants" *Journal of Pineal Research* 2000 28(2):73-80.

17. Rybak L, Whitworth C, Somani S, "Application of antioxidants and other agents to prevent cisplatin ototoxicity" *The Laryngoscope* 1999 109(11):1740-1744.

18. Olas B, Wachowicz B, Buczynski A, "Vitamin C suppresses the cisplatin toxicity on blood platelets" *Anti-cancer Drugs* 2000 11(6):487-493.

19. Online article at: http://www.nlm.nih.gov/medlineplus/druginfo/meds/a682080. html

20. Lee C, et al, "Fatal cyclophosphamide cardiomyopathy: its clinical course and treatment" *Bone Marrow Transplantation* 1996 18(3):573-577.

21. Ghosh S, et al, "Effect of ascorbic acid supplementation on liver and kidney toxicity in cyclophosphamide-treated female albino rats" *The Journal of Toxicological Sciences* 1999 24(3):141-144.

22. Vasavi H, et al, "The salubrious effects of ascorbic acid on cyclophosphamide instigated lipid abnormalities in fibrosarcoma bearing rats" *Cancer Biochemistry Biophysics* 1998 16(1-2):71-83.

23. Vijayalaxmi K, Venu R, "*In vivo* anticlastogenic effects of L-ascorbic acid in mice" *Mutation Research* 1999 438(1):47-51.

24. Ghaskadbi S, et al, "Modulation of cyclophosphamide mutagenicity by vitamin C in the *in vivo* rodent micronucleus assay" *Teratogenesis, Carcinogenesis, and Mutagenesis* 1992 12(1):11-17.

25. Kola I, Vogel R, Spielmann H, "Co-administration of ascorbic acid with cyclophosphamide (CPA) to pregnant mice inhibits the clastogenic activity of CPA in preimplantation murine blastocysts" *Mutagenesis* 1989 4(4):297-301.

26. Vogel R, Spielmann H, "Beneficial effects of ascorbic acid on preimplantation mouse embryos after exposure to cyclophosphamide *in vivo*" *Teratogenesis, Carcinogenesis, and Mutagenesis* 1989 9(1):51-59.

27. Pillans P, Ponzi S, Parker M, "Effects of ascorbic acid on the mouse embryo and on cyclophosphamide-induced cephalic DNA strand breaks *in vivo*" *Archives of Toxicology* 1990 64(5):423-425.

28. Online article at: http://www.nlm.nih.gov/medlineplus/druginfo/meds/a601207. html

29. Durak I, et al, (1998) Impaired antioxidant defense system in the kidney tissues from rabbits treated with cyclosporine. Protective effects of vitamins E and C. *Nephron* 1990 78(2):207-211.

30. Rojas M, et al, "Differential modulation of apoptosis and necrosis by antioxidants in immunosuppressed human lymphocytes" *Toxicology and Applied Pharmacology* 2002 180(2):67-73.

31. Slakey D, et al, "Delayed cardiac allograft rejection due to combined cyclosporine and antioxidant therapy" *Transplantation* 1993 56(6):1305-1309.

32. Slakey D, et al, "Ascorbic acid and alpha-tocopherol prolong rat cardiac allograft survival" *Transplantation Proceedings* 1993 25(1):610-611.

33. Online article at: http://www.nlm.nih.gov/medlineplus/druginfo/meds/a682301.html

34. De K, et al, "Evaluation of alpha-tocopherol, probucol and ascorbic acid as suppressors of digoxin induced lipid peroxidation" *Acta Poloniae Pharmaceutica* 2001 58(5):391-400.

35. Online article at: http://www.nlm.nih.gov/medlineplus/druginfo/meds/a682221.html

36. Geetha A, Catherine J, Shyamala Devi C, "Effect of alpha-tocopherol on the microsomal lipid peroxidation induced by doxorubicin: influence of ascorbic acid" *Indian Journal of Physiology and Pharmacology* 1989 33(1):53-58.

37. Fujita K, et al, "Reduction of adriamycin toxicity by ascorbate in mice and guinea pigs" *Cancer Research* 1982 42(1):309-316.

38. Kurbacher C, et al, "Ascorbic acid (vitamin C) improves the antineoplastic activity of doxorubicin, cisplatin, and paclitaxel in human breast carcinoma cells *in vitro*" *Cancer Letters* 1996 103(2):183-189.

39. Kojima S, et al, "Antioxidative activity of benzylideneascorbate and its effect on adriamycin-induced cardiotoxicity" *Anticancer Research* 1994 14(5A):1875-1880.

40. Shimpo K, et al, "Ascorbic acid and adriamycin toxicity" *The American Journal of Clinical Nutrition* 1991 54(6 Suppl):1298S-1301S.

41. Hajarizadeh H, et al, "Protective effect of doxorubicin in vitamin C or dimethyl sulfoxide against skin ulceration in the pig" *Annals of Surgical Oncology* 1994 1(5):411-414.

42. Tavares D, et al, "Protective effects of the amino acid glutamine and of ascorbic acid against chromosomal damage induced by doxorubicin in mammalian cells" *Teratogenesis, Carcinogenesis, and Mutagenesis* 1998 18(4):153-161.

43. Antunes L, Takahashi C, "Effects of high doses of vitamins C and E against doxorubicin-induced chromosomal damage in Wistar rat bone marrow cells" *Mutation Research* 1998 419(1-3):137-143.

44. Online Article at: http://www.britannica.com/EBchecked/topic/293288/iproniazid

45. Matsuki Y, et al, "Effects of ascorbic acid on the metabolic fate and the free radical formation of iproniazid" [Article in Japanese] *Yakugaku Zasshi. Journal of the Pharmaceutical Society of Japan* 1992 112(12):926-933.

46. Matsuki Y, et al, "Effects of ascorbic acid on iproniazid-induced hepatitis in phenobarbital-treated rats" *Biological & Pharmaceutical Bulletin* 1994 17(8):1078-1082.

47. Online article at: http://en.wikipedia.org/wiki/Isoprenaline

48. Ramos K, Acosta D, "Prevention by L(-)ascorbic acid of isoproterenol-induced cardiotoxicity in primary cultures of rat myocytes" *Toxicology* 1983 26(1):81-90.

49. Acosta D, Combs A, Ramos K, "Attenuation by antioxidants of Na+/K+ ATPase inhibition by toxic concentrations of isoproterenol in cultured rat myocardial cells" *Journal of Molecular and Cellular Cardiology* 1984 16(3):281-284.

50. Persoon-Rothert M, et al, "Isoproterenol-induced cytotoxicity in neonatal rat heart cell cultures is mediated by free radical formation" *Journal of Molecular and Cellular Cardiology* 1989 21(12):1285-1291.

51. Mohan P, Bloom S, "Lipolysis is an important determinant of isoproterenol-induced myocardial necrosis" *Cardiovascular Pathology* 1999 8(5):255-261.

52. Ramos K, Combs A, Acosta D, "Role of calcium in isoproterenol cytotoxicity to cultured myocardial cells" *Biochemical Pharmacology* 1984 33(12):1989-1992.

53. Laky D, et al, "Morphophysiological studies in experimental myocardial stress induced by isoproterenol. Note II. The myocardioprotector effect of magnesium ascorbate" *Morphologie et Embryologie* 1984 30(1):55-59.

54. Online article at: http://en.wikipedia.org/wiki/Neosalvarsan

55. Cormia F, "Experimental arsphenamine dermatitis: the influence of vitamin C in the production of arsphenamine sensitiveness" *Canadian Medical Association Journal* 1937 36:392.

56. McChesney E, Barlow O, Klinck Jr G, "The detoxication of neoarsphenamine by means of various organic acids" *The Journal of Pharmacology and Experimental Therapeutics* 1942 80:81-92.

57. McChesney E, "Further studies on the detoxication of the arsphenamines by ascorbic acid" *The Journal of Pharmacology and Experimental Therapeutics* 1945 84:222-235.

58. Bundesen H, et al, "The detoxifying action of vitamin C (ascorbic acid) in arsenical therapy. I. Ascorbic acid as a preventive of reactions of human skin to neoarsphenamine" *The Journal of the American Medical Association* 1941 117(20):1692-1695.

59. Ruskin S, Silberstein R, "Practical therapeutics. The influence of vitamin C on the therapeutic activity of bismuth, antimony and the arsenic group of metals" *Medical Record* 1938 153:327-330.

60. Online article at: http://en.wikipedia.org/wiki/Sulfonamide_%28medicine%29

61. Schropp J, "Case reports: sulfapyridine sensitivity checked by ascorbic acid" *Canadian Medical Association Journal* 1943 49:515.

62. McCormick W, "Sulfonamide sensitivity and C-avitaminosis" *Canadian Medical Association Journal* 1945 52:68-70.

63. Landauer W, Sopher D, "Succinate, glycerophosphate and ascorbate as sources of cellular energy and as antiteratogens" *Journal of Embryology and Experimental Morphology* 1970 24(1):187-202.

64. Online article at: http://www.nlm.nih.gov/medlineplus/druginfo/meds/a682098.html

65. Polec R, Yeh S, Shils M, "Protective effect of ascorbic acid, isoascorbic acid and mannitol against tetracycline-induced nephrotoxicity" *The Journal of Pharmacology and Experimental Therapeutics* 1971 178(1):152-158.

66. Online article at: http://www.nlm.nih.gov/medlineplus/druginfo/meds/a682412.html

67. Jurima-Romet M, et al, "Cytotoxicity of unsaturated metabolites of valproic acid and protection by vitamins C and E in glutathione-depleted rat hepatocytes" *Toxicology* 1996 112(1):69-85.

## Trichinosis

1. Online article at: http://www.ncbi.nlm.nih.gov/pubmedhealth/PMH0001655/

2. Daoud A, et al, "The effect of antioxidant preparation (antox) on the course and efficacy of treatment of trichinosis" *Journal of the Egyptian Society of Parasitology* 2000 30(1):305-314.

3. Senutaite J, Biziulevicius S, "Influence of vitamin C on the resistance of rats to *Trichinella spiralis* infection" *Wiadomosci Parazytologiczne* 1986 32(3):261-262.

## Trypanosomal Infections

1. *Cecil Medicine, 23rd Edition*, "African Trypanosomaisis," Saunders, an imprint of Elsevier Inc., 2008, Chap. 367.

2. Perla D, "The effect of an excess of vitamin C on the natural resistance of mice and guinea pigs to trypanosome infections" *American Journal of Hygiene* 1937 26:374-381.

3. Ramirez L, et al, "Prevention of transfusion-associated Chagas' disease by sterilization of *Trypanosoma cruzi*-infected blood with gentian violet, ascorbic acid, and light" *Transfusion* 1995 35(3):226-230.

4. Strangeways W, "Observations on the trypanocidal action *in vitro* of solutions of glutathione and ascorbic acid" *Annals of Tropical Medicine and Parasitology* 1937 31:405-416.

5. Umar I, et al, "Effects of combined parenteral vitamins C and E administration on the severity of anaemia, hepatic and renal damage in *Trypanosoma brucei brucei* infected rabbits" *Veterinary Parasitology* 1999 85(1):43-47.

## Tuberculosis

1. Online article at: http://www.ncbi.nlm.nih.gov/pubmedhealth/PMH0001141/

2. Steinbach M, Klein S, "Vitamin C in experimental tuberculosis" *American Review of Tuberculosis* 1941 43:403-414.

3. Albrecht E, "Vitamin C as an adjuvant in the therapy of lung tuberculosis" *Medizinische Klinic* (Munchen) 1938 34:972-973.

4. Babbar I, "Observations of ascorbic acid. Part XI. Therapeutic effect of ascorbic acid in tuberculosis" *The Indian Medical Gazette* 1948 83:409-410.

5. Birkhaug K, "The role of vitamin C in the pathogenesis of tuberculosis in the guinea pig. I. Daily excretion of vitamin C in urine of L-ascorbic acid treated and control tuberculous animals. II. Vitamin C content of suprarenals of L-ascorbic acid treated and control tuberculous animals" *Acta Tuberculosea Scandinavica* 1938 12:89-104 & III. "Quantitative variations in the haemogram of L-ascorbic acid treated and control tuberculous animals" *Acta Tuberculosea Scandinavica* 1938 12:359-372.

6. Birkhaug K, "IV. Effect of L-ascorbic acid on the tuberculin reaction in tuberculous animals" *Acta Tuberculosea Scandinavica* 13:45-51. & "V. Degree of tuberculosis in L-ascorbic acid treated and control tuberculosis animals" *Acta Tuberculosea Scandinavica* 1939 13:52-66.

7. Bogen E, Hawkins L, Bennett E, "Vitamin C treatment of mucous membrane tuberculosis" *American Review of Tuberculosis* (1941) 44:596-603.

8. Bossevain C, Spillane J, "A note on the effect of synthetic ascorbic acid (vitamin C) on the growth of the tubercle bacillus" *American Review of Tuberculosis* 1937 35:661-662.

9. Borsalino G, "La fragilita capillare nella tubercolosi polmonare e le sue modificazioni per azione della vitamin C" *Giornale di Clinica Medica* (Bologna) 1937 18:273-294.

10. Charpy J, "Ascorbic acid in very large doses alone or with vitamin D2 in tuberculosis" *Bulletin de l'academie Nationale de Medecine* (Paris) 1948 132:421-423.

11. Downes J, "An experiment in the control of tuberculosis among Negroes" *The Milbank Memorial Fund Quarterly* 1950 28:127-159.

12. Faulkner J, Taylor F, "Vitamin C and infection" *Annals of Internal Medicine* 1937 10:1867-1873.

13. Getz H, Long E, Henderson H, "A study of the relation of nutrition to the development of tuberculosis. Influence of ascorbic acid and vitamin A" *American Review of Tuberculosis* 1951 64:381-393.

14. Grant A, *American Review of Tuberculosis* 1930 21:115.

15. Heise F, Martin G, "Ascorbic acid metabolism in tuberculosis" *Proceedings of the Society for Experimental Biology and Medicine* 1936 34:642-644.

16. Heise F, Martin G, "Supervitaminosis C in tuberculosis" *Proceedings of the Society for Experimental Biology and Medicine* 1936 35:337-338.

17. Hemila H, et al, "Vitamin C and other compounds in vitamin C rich food in relation to risk of tuberculosis in male smokers" *American Journal of Epidemiology* 1999 150(6):632-641.

18. Klenner F, "Significance of high daily intake of ascorbic acid in preventive medicine" *Journal of the International Academy of Preventive Medicine* 1974 1(1):45-69.

19. Leichtentritt B, *Deutsche Medizinische Wochenschrift* 1924 40:672.

20. McConkey M, Smith D, "The relation of vitamin C deficiency to intestinal tuberculosis in the guinea pig" *Journal of Experimental Medicine* 1933 58:503-512.

21. McCormick W, "Vitamin C in the prophylaxis and therapy of infectious diseases" *Archives of Pediatrics* 1951 68(1):1-9.

22. Myrvik Q, et al, "Studies on the tuberculoinhibitory properties of ascorbic acid derivatives and their possible role in inhibition of tubercle bacilli by urine" *American Review of Tuberculosis* (1954) 69:406-418.

23. Petter C, "Vitamin C and tuberculosis" *The Journal-Lancet* (Minneapolis) 1937 57:221-224.

24. Pijoan M, Sedlacek B, "Ascorbic acid in tuberculous Navajo Indians" *American Review of Tuberculosis* 1943 48:342-346.

25. Rudra M, Roy S, "Haematological study in pulmonary tuberculosis and the effect upon it of large doses of vitamin C" *Tubercle* 1946 27:93-94.

26. Steinbach M, Klein S, "Effect of crystalline vitamin C (ascorbic acid) on tolerance to tuberculin" *Proceedings of the Society for Experimental Biology and Medicine* 1936 35:151-154.

## Typhoid Fever

1. Online article at: http://www.ncbi.nlm.nih.gov/pubmedhealth/PMH0002308/

2. Drummond J, "Recent advances in the treatment of enteric fever" *Clinical Proceedings* (South Africa) 1943 2:65-93.

3. Farah N, "Enteric fever treated with suprarenal cortex extract and vitamin C intravenously" *Lancet* 1938 1:777-779.

4. Foster D, Obineche E, Traub N, "The effect of pyridoxine, folic acid and ascorbic acid therapy on the incidence of sideroblastic anaemia in Zambians with chloramphenicol treated typhoid. A preliminary report" *East African Medical Journal* 1974 51(1):20-25.

5. Hill C, Garren H, "The effect of high levels of vitamins on the resistance of chicks to fowl typhoid" *Annals of the New York Academy of Sciences* 1955 63:186-194.

## Vanadium Poisoning

1. Online article at: http://en.wikipedia.org/wiki/Vanadium#Safety

2. Online article at: http://www.atsdr.cdc.gov/substances/toxsubstance. asp?toxid=50

3. Chandra AK, et al, "Vanadium-induced testicular toxicity and its prevention by oral supplementation of zinc sulphate" *Toxicol Mech Methods* 2007 17(4):175-87.

4. Venkataraman B, Sudha S "Vanadium toxicity" *Asian J Exp Sci* 2005 19(2):127-134

5. Domingo J, Llobet J, Corbella J, "Protection of mice against the lethal effects of sodium metavanadate: a quantitative comparison of a number of chelating agents" *Toxicology Letters* 1985 26(2-3):95-99.

6. Jones M, Basinger M, "Chelate antidotes for sodium vanadate and vanadyl sulfate intoxication in mice" *Journal of Toxicology and Environmental Health* 1983 12(4-6):749-756.

7. Domingo J, et al, "Influence of chelating agents on the toxicity, distribution and excretion of vanadium in mice" *Journal of Applied Toxicology* 1986 6(5):337-341.

8. Donaldson J, Hemming R, LaBella F, "Vanadium exposure enhances lipid peroxidation in the kidney of rats and mice" *Canadian Journal of Physiology and Pharmacology* 1985 63(3):196-199.

9. Hill C, "Studies on the ameliorating effect of ascorbic acid on mineral toxicities in the chick" *The Journal of Nutrition* 1979 109(1):84-90.

10. Ousterhout L, Berg L, "Effects of diet composition on vanadium toxicity in laying hens" *Poultry Science* 1981 60(6):1152-1159.

11. Benabdeljelil K, Jensen L, "Effectiveness of ascorbic acid and chromium in counteracting the negative effects of dietary vanadium on interior egg quality" *Poultry Science* 1990 69(5):781-786.

12. Domingo J, et al, "Chelating agents in the treatment of acute vanadyl sulphate intoxication in mice" *Toxicology* 1990 62(2):203-211.

13. Ferrer E, Baran E, "Reduction of vanadium(V) with ascorbic acid and isolation of the generated oxovanadium(IV) species" *Biological Trace Element Research* 2001 83(2):111-119.

14. Song B, Aebischer N, Orvig C, "Reduction of [VO2(ma)2]- and [VO2(ema)2]- by ascorbic acid and glutathione: kinetic studies of pro-drugs for the enhancement of insulin action" *Inorganic Chemistry* 2002 41(6):1357-1364.

15. Adam-Vizi V, Varadi G, Simon P, "Reduction of vanadate by ascorbic acid and noradrenaline in synaptosomes" *Journal of Neurochemistry* 1981 36(5):1616-1620.

## Venoms

1. *Cecil Medicine, 23rd Edition*, "Arthropods and Leeches," Saunders, an imprint of Elsevier Inc., 2008, Chap.380.

2. *Cecil Medicine, 23rd Edition*, "Venoms and Poisons from Marine Organisms," Saunders, an imprint of Elsevier Inc., 2008, Chap 382.

3. Cilento P, et al, "Venomous bites and vitamin C status" *The Australasian Nurses Journal* 1980 9(6):19.

4. Klenner F, "Significance of high daily intake of ascorbic acid in preventive medicine" *Journal of the International Academy of Preventive Medicine* 1974 1(1):45-69.

5. Klenner F, "The black widow spider: case history" *Tri-State Medical Journal* 1957 Dec pp.15-18.

6. Klenner F, "Observations of the dose and administration of ascorbic acid when employed beyond the range of a vitamin in human pathology" *Journal of Applied Nutrition* 1971 23(3&4):61-88.

7. Klenner F, "Case history: cure of a 4-year-old child bitten by a mature highland moccasin with vitamin C" *Tri-State Medical Journal* 1954 Jul.

8. Smith L, "The Clinical Experiences of Frederick R. Klenner, M.D.: Clinical Guide to the Use of Vitamin C" Portland, OR: Life Sciences Press 1988.

For a Special Offer

from the Publisher

See Next Page

# A Special Offer from the Publisher

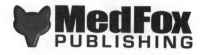

Get this essential information into the hands
of your family, friends, and doctors.

Order additional copies of this book for
$19.95 plus $3.57 shipping each
(regularly $29.95 plus $6.95 shipping each)
and receive two (2) powerful DVDs with each book:

1) The *60 Minutes* "Living Proof"
   documentary and sequel

2) Dr. Levy's recorded lecture at the
   *Vitamin-C-Can-Cure Convention*
   in New Zealand

*To order call*

## 1-866-359-5589

*— or go to —*

## www.primalpanacea.com

*Promotion Code:* **PRP19**

*This offer may be discontinued at the publisher's discretion.*